KATHERINE F. JETER, EdD, ET
Staff Affiliate in Enterostomal Therapy
Spartanburg Regional Medical Center
Director, HIP, Inc. (Help for Incontinent People)
Clinical Assistant Professor of Urology
Medical University of South Carolina
Adjunct Professor of Nursing
Mary Black School of Nursing
University of South Carolina, Spartanburg

NANCY FALLER, RN, BSN, CETN
Consultant at the Vermont Achievement Center,
Vermont Department of Health,
Pleasant Manor Nursing Home, and the
Rutland Area Visiting Nurse Association
ET Nurse at the Rutland Regional Center
Rutland, Vermont

CHRISTINE NORTON, MA, SRN
Formerly Senior Nurse/Continence Advisor
Bloomsbury Health Authority
London, United Kingdom

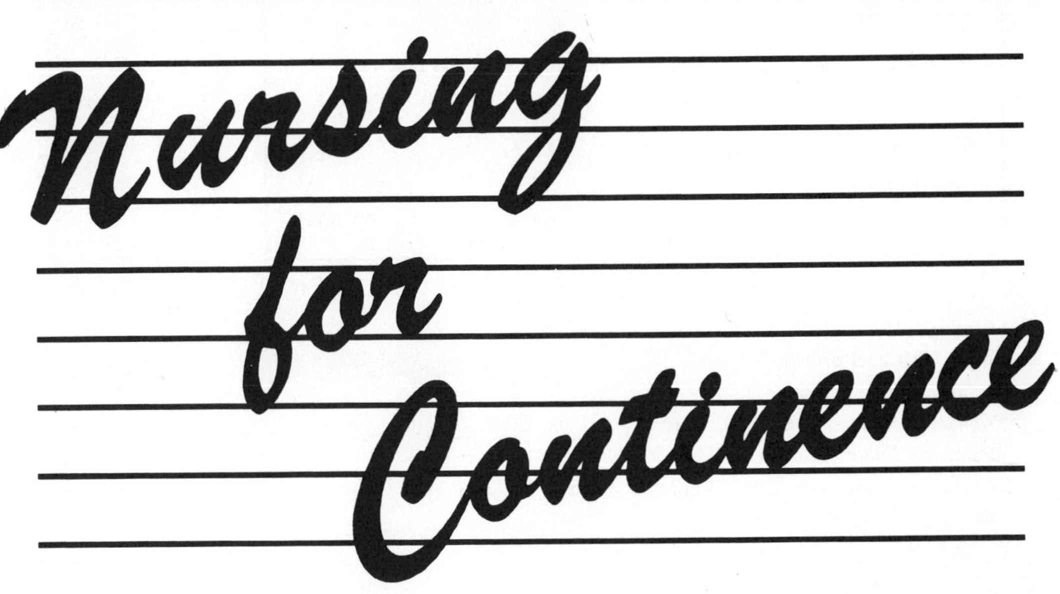

1990
W.B. SAUNDERS COMPANY
Harcourt Brace Jovanovich, Inc.
Philadelphia
London Toronto Montreal Sydney Tokyo

W. B. SAUNDERS COMPANY
Harcourt Brace Jovanovich, Inc.

The Curtis Center
Independence Square West
Philadelphia, PA 19106

Library of Congress Cataloging-in-Publication Data

Nursing for continence/[edited by] Katherine F. Jeter, Nancy Faller, Christine Norton.—1st ed.

p. cm.

ISBN 0-7216-2892-3

1. Urinary incontinence—Nursing. 2. Fecal incontinence—Nursing. I. Jeter, Katherine F. II. Faller, Nancy. III. Norton, Christine.

[DNLM: 1. Urinary Incontinence—nursing. WY 164 N9745]

RC921.I5N87 1990

616.6′2—dc20

DNLM/DLC

90-8081

Editor: Michael Brown
Designer: Joan Wendt
Production Manager: Linda R. Turner
Manuscript Editor: Louise Robinson
Illustration Coordinator: Walt Verbitski
Indexer: Diana Witt
Cover Designer: Ellen Bodner

Nursing for Continence ISBN 0-7216-2892-3

Printed in the United States of America

Last digit is the print number: 9 8 7 6 5 4 3 2 1

Contributors

Georgeann L. Constantino, RN, MS, ANP-C
Nurse Practitioner, Department of Urology, Erie County Medical Center, Buffalo, New York
Chapter 15: Catheterization

Brenda J. Donovan, RN, BSN, CURN
Chapter 6: Female Incontinence

Linda M. Duffy, RN, C, MS
Adjunct Assistant Professor, School of Nursing, University of Minnesota; Geriatric Consultation Team, Geriatric Research, Education, and Clinical Center, Minneapolis Veterans Administration Medical Center, Minneapolis, Minnesota
Chapter 7: Male Incontinence

Nancy Faller, RN, BSN, CETN
Consultant at the Vermont Achievement Center, Vermont Department of Health, Pleasant Manor Nursing Home, and the Rutland Area Visiting Nurse Association; ET Nurse at the Rutland Regional Center, Rutland, Vermont
Chapter 5: Incontinence in Childhood, and *Chapter 12: Toilet-Training People with Mental Retardation*

Mikel L. Gray, CURN, MSN
Clinical Associate, Nell Hodgson Woodruff School of Nursing, Emory University, Atlanta, Georgia
Chapter 3: Assessment and Investigation of Urinary Incontinence

Ted P. Hammon, RN, CRT
Clinical Director, Urology Associates and Willis-Knighton Urology Institute, Shreveport, Louisiana
Chapter 2: The Development of Continence and Causes of Incontinence

Linda L. Jensen, RN
Clinical Research Director, Colon and Rectal Surgery Associates, Minneapolis, Minnesota
Chapter 14: Fecal Incontinence

Katherine F. Jeter, EdD, ET
Staff Affiliate in Enterostomal Therapy, Spartanburg Regional Medical Center; Director, HIP, Inc. (Help for Incontinent People); Clinical Assistant Professor of Urology, Medical University of South Carolina; Adjunct Professor of Nursing, Mary Black School of Nursing, University of South Carolina, Spartanburg, South Carolina
Chapter 4: Treating and Managing Incontinence, and *Chapter 13: The Use of Incontinence Products*

Karen A. Karlowicz, RN, MSN
Educational Development Coordinator, American Urological Association Allied, Inc., Riderwood, Maryland
Chapter 1: The Problem of Incontinence

Diane L. Krasner, RN, MS, ET
ET Nurse Consultant and Part-time Staff, Harbor Hospital Center, Baltimore, Maryland
Chapter 11: Incontinence in Varied Settings

Diane K. Newman, RN, MSN, CRNP
Vice President, Golden Horizons, Inc., Newtown Square, Pennsylvania; Director of Clinical Services, Continence Management Specialists, Inc., Trenton, New Jersey
Chapter 16: The Role of Continence Nurse Specialists

Leslie Oliver, RN, BS
Supervisor, Urodynamic Laboratory, Columbia-Presbyterian Medical Center, New York, New York
Chapter 10: The Neurogenic Bladder

Mary H. Palmer, RN, C, MS
Doctoral Student, Johns Hopkins University, Baltimore, Maryland
Chapter 8: Incontinence in the Elderly

Marilyn Pires, RN, MS
Clinical Nurse Specialist and Spinal Injury Specialist, Rancho Los Amigos Medical Center, Downey, California
Chapter 9: Promoting Continence for the Physically Impaired

Nancy J. Reilly, RN, MSN, CURN
Gastrointestinal/Genitourinary Nurse Specialist, Hospital of the University of Pennsylvania, Philadelphia, Pennsylvania
Chapter 1: The Problem of Incontinence

Diane A. Smith, RN, MSN, CRNP
President, Golden Horizons, Inc., Newtown Square, Pennsylvania; Director of Research, Continence Management Specialists, Inc., Trenton, New Jersey
Chapter 16: The Role of Continence Nurse Specialists

Preface

In 1988 the National Institutes of Health noted that incontinence affects an estimated 10 million Americans; it is epidemic in nursing homes (NIH, 1988). Nurses interact intimately with their patients and have a unique opportunity to discover secretive behavior regarding voiding dysfunction, to design or reinforce treatment regimens, and to ease the management of intractable incontinence.

A nursing text on the subject of incontinence across the life span has been lacking. Many nurse researchers and clinicians have intended to write or edit one. In 1986 an English nurse, Christine Norton, first published *Nursing for Continence,* which addressed the diagnosis, treatment, and management of incontinence in all age groups and in special populations and circumstances in a practical, thorough, and sensitive manner. To begin again in the United States would have been redundant and presumptuous.

Since the concept and content had been organized, it seemed most logical to "Americanize" Norton's text. The idea evolved into an urgent project as American nurses began requesting more information about voiding dysfunction. The task was catalyzed by Diane Krasner, RN, MSN, CETN; Karen Karlowicz, RN, MSN; Michael Brown of the W. B. Saunders Company; and Katherine Jeter, EdD, ET.

Invitations were issued to a stellar panel of nurses who have distinguished themselves in the field to help update and Americanize Norton's work. For most this required sublimating their own rich experience and clinical biases. If we had set out to write an original work, we might have organized and written it differently. But we did not—we endeavored to improve on a good product. We applaud our contributors.

We welcome the interest of our readers. We advise you to consult this book purposefully. If you are working with older people, begin by reading Chapter 8, Incontinence in the Elderly. If time permits and interest motivates you, continue with Chapter 4, Treating and Managing

Incontinence. If your patient is female, proceed to Chapter 6, Female Incontinence. Each chapter can be read alone; together, chapters reiterate, clarify, and amplify the material in the other chapters.

You have decided to learn more about a complex subject. Your nursing practice will be enhanced. Your patients will benefit.

KATHERINE F. JETER, EdD, ET
NANCY FALLER, BSN, CETN

Contents

Nancy J. Reilly, RN, MSN, CURN
Karen A. Karlowicz, RN, MSN

1 The Problem of Incontinence

What Is Incontinence? Who Is Incontinent?

Attitudes and Incontinence

Incontinence is one of the most unpleasant and distressing symptoms an individual can suffer. Those affected usually feel embarrassed, ashamed, and alone. Such feelings are often validated by the reactions of society, family, and friends. Incontinent people frequently choose to hide or disguise their problem; some deny it exists, even to themselves. Nurses and other health professionals may see only a small part of the misery and distress that accompany incontinence.

Most health professionals are profoundly ignorant of the causes and management of incontinence. Incontinence is often regarded as a condition over which there is no control, rather than as a symptom of an underlying physiologic disorder. The unfortunate result of such limited understanding is a passive acceptance by caregivers of the symptom of incontinence, which is tolerated or circumvented. This book hopes to show that, in most cases, incontinence is treatable.

There has been more open discussion of incontinence in recent years. As public recognition of the implications of incontinence increases, the stigma associated with it will slowly decrease. Radio and television commercials now promote products for those with "bladder control problems." Finally, it has become common knowledge that millions of Americans suffer from incontinence. Most pharmacies and supermarkets have a section for incontinence products. Larger chain stores sell incontinence products under their own name. The availability of these products denotes acceptability.

At one time incontinence was primarily regarded as a "nursing" problem, with nurses providing custodial care—keeping the patient as clean and comfortable as possible and preventing pressure ulcers from developing. Currently, nursing interventions encompass various assessment and management skills. Nurses have advanced to the point of viewing incontinence as a nursing challenge, rather than as a problem to be tolerated. As nurses, we understand that "regular toileting" or "frequent offering of the bedpan" will manage, but not solve, the problem.

Nurses are not alone in acknowledging that incontinence is a symptom requiring investigation and intervention; those in other health professions are also realizing this need. Research dollars are being allocated for the study of incontinence. Federal health care agencies have convened work sessions to develop strategies for diagnosing and treating incontinence. This book highlights the role of the nurse within the context of a multidisciplinary approach to incontinence.

WHAT IS INCONTINENCE?

Imagine asking a nurse this question! All nurses deal with incontinence at some point in their career. We have become attuned to the wet bed, the puddle on the floor, the odor. Nurses in some settings deal with incontinence many times a day. They may have various definitions for it.

We generally label patients as incontinent when they urinate or have a bowel movement somewhere other than the toilet. This is not a clear-cut definition, though. For example, people who pull their car off to the side of the road at night to relieve themselves are not considered to be incontinent. If they relieved themselves in the middle of a crowded street in broad daylight, they might find themselves in the local jail, but they would not be called incontinent. Continence is culturally and socially dictated.

The International Continence Society has defined urinary incontinence as "a condition in which involuntary loss of urine is a social or hygienic problem and is objectively demonstrable" (Bates et al., 1979). This definition was agreed on by the ICS Committee for Standardization of Terminology (1977). Uniform use of one definition lessens confusion among researchers and clinicians, while providing a common basis for all involved in the care of incontinent persons.

The use of "involuntary" in the definition is important. In some situations we might consider a patient who voluntarily passes urine (or stool) in the "wrong" place to be incontinent. Actually, this behavior is a social problem. Most incontinent patients we care for fall into the involuntary category. Involuntary loss of urine is considered to be incontinence regardless of how often it occurs or how much wetness the patient reports.

As incontinence becomes recognized by the public as a health problem rather than as an inevitable part of aging, it is expected that more people will admit to having the symptom of incontinence, and more people will seek medical attention. This will have a greater impact on health care financing and public health policy in the United States. The Surgeon General has estimated that eight billion dollars is spent by the federal government on incontinence in the United States annually (Abdellah, 1988). As this amount has risen, so has the recognition and sensitivity of the government to this problem. The federal government finances well over one-third of all medical expenditures in this country (Abdellah, 1988). Given the enormous expense of nursing home care, and the fact that the cost of incontinence alone can tip the balance between living independently and assisted living, it would certainly behoove government officials to allocate research grants and to collect information about epidemiologic, medical, and nursing aspects on incontinence.

WHO IS INCONTINENT?

Most nurses, if asked to associate the term "incontinent" with a particular group of people, would immediately think of the elderly. The usual image is of a confused and dependent elderly person in a nursing home. Occasionally, the child with enuresis or the mentally or physically disabled come to mind. Usually, though, it is the elderly. Few people realize that incontinence affects people of both sexes across their life span. The prevalence of incontinence does increase with age and illness, but most incontinent people live at home and lead otherwise normal lives.

Data on the prevalence of incontinence in the United States are difficult to obtain and hard to interpret. Prevalence means all cases that are present during a specific time frame established by the investigator(s) in any particular study. Most information is collected in the community, in nursing homes, or in acute care facilities. Some investigators have used two of these three settings. Large-scale studies designed to report the overall prevalence in the community in this country are lacking. Information about the prevalence in each of the three settings will be presented in this book, but it must be remembered that these figures do not represent the overall prevalence.

There are other problems inherent in published prevalence reports. A few of these are mentioned here to provide some basis for understanding the limitations on such data. Common terminology and the consistent use of one definition of incontinence have not been used in prevalence reports until recently. Each investigator has defined incontinence somewhat differently. Many factors affect prevalence reports, including under-reporting, erroneous reporting, and the availability of medical care (Abdellah, 1988). Current emphasis on early discharge might increase under-reporting. When incontinence is not severe enough to require changing the bed linens or clothing by the nursing staff, it will often go undetected (Sullivan and Lindsay, 1984). The use of indwelling catheters also complicates data collection. In many settings routine indwelling catheterization is still used to manage incontinence—a most unfortunate scenario for the patient. Finally, reports of prevalence rates are affected by the duration of an individual's incontinence. Many patients have transient or temporary incontinence, which affects data collection differently than does chronic incontinence.

Only a few studies have attempted to describe the prevalence of incontinence in the general population. None of these are from the United States. Thomas and associates (1980) conducted one of the largest prevalence studies ever reported. Based on over 18,000 replies to a postal survey in Great Britain, prevalence was reported for two age groups, those over and those under the age of 65. The results showed that 8.5% of women and 1.6% of men under the age of 65 were incontinent, as were 11.6% of women and 6.9% of men over the age of 65. The overall prevalence of incontinence in this study was reported to be 17%. Yarnell and colleagues (1981) found that 54 of 388 women (14%) in South Wales were incontinent. Mohide (1986) reported an incontinence rate of 22% in 2850 people over 16 years of age in Ontario, Canada. The range for these community-based studies is 14 to 22%, which certainly indicates how common is some degree of incontinence.

In long-term care facilities in the United States, the incidence of incontinence ranges from 40 to 60% (Ouslander and Uman, 1985). A further breakdown of the frequency of incontinence indicates that 70% of nursing home residents have some degree of urinary incontinence, whereas 50% are incontinent daily (Cella, 1988). Urinary incontinence in nursing homes is often associated with fecal incontinence (Palmer, 1988). These rates are high because the prevalence of incontinence increases with age, and most nursing home residents in this country are elderly (Abdellah, 1988; Palmer, 1988). The health care needs of the elderly in the United States are currently of major concern, considering the enormous costs of nursing home care and the uncertain financial future of the Social Security and Medicare programs. The expense associated with incontinence care in nursing homes ranges from $1.20 to $5.50 per day for labor alone, not including laundry and supply costs (Cella, 1988). On the average, nursing homes devote the equivalent of two full-time staff members per day to the care and treatment of those with urinary incontinence (Cella, 1988).

In acute care settings, the incidence of incontinence varies from 5.5 to 48% (Palmer, 1988), with most figures reflecting a large proportion of elderly patients. The lowest figure, 5.5%, was obtained in a study of over 400 patients under the age of 70 who were admitted to general medical units at Boston City Hospital (Gillick, 1982).

Is all this incontinence unavoidable or inevitable? Probably not. Many types of incontinence are curable. More than one-third of those with incontinence can be cured, another third dramatically improved, and most of the remainder significantly improved (Resnick, 1986). Probably many more could benefit than are presently receiving treatment. The potential of preventive measures is still largely unexplored.

ATTITUDES AND INCONTINENCE

Attitudes toward incontinence present a major problem. As nurses we can begin by examining our own attitudes. Passive acceptance of the symptom of incontinence, as an inevitable part of working in certain situations or with certain patient populations, is common. With increased knowledge and awareness this is gradually changing toward a more positive problem-solving approach for each individual. As we have moved toward primary nursing, incontinence can be identified as a symptom of a patient with a unique combination of problems, needs, and potentials, rather than as an inevitable part of working with the elderly.

Incontinence may arouse as much revulsion in a nurse as in anyone else. Few people enjoy dealing with other people's excreta, or even with their own, but nurses are expected, from the beginning of their education, to ignore their own automatic reactions. Emptying bed pans and cleaning patients who are incontinent must be one of the most unpleasant aspects of nursing, and is usually what members of the public mean when they say that they "could never be a nurse," or that "nurses are wonderful for putting up with the things they have to do for people." Nurses are not encouraged to discuss or express their emotions about this aspect of their work. Feelings of distaste are frowned on, and best ignored: "you will soon get used to it." It is this "getting used to it" that causes nurses to deal with incontinence as quickly as possible, usually in a manner that detaches the nurse from the personal reality of the situation. Incontinence is cleared away and forgotten to make way for the more pleasant aspects of care—until the next time. This, combined with the patient's embarrassment, can lead to a situation of "mutual pretense" between the nurse and the patient, as if nothing out of the ordinary had occurred (Schwartz, 1977). The nurse wishes to spare the patient's feelings, and the patient is ashamed and assumes it cannot be helped. The problem is seldom openly and frankly discussed. Alternatively, the nurse might take a patronizing attitude, reassuring the patient that it does not matter and that "it happens all the time." Neither pretense nor bland platitudes help to get at the cause of the incontinence.

Nurses need a forum to discuss their own feelings more openly, without fear of censure. They may feel embarrassed, both for themselves and for the patient. The nurse might feel guilty, because incontinence could be interpreted by some as a sign of poor nursing care. Anger with a patient is common, and difficult for the nurse to admit. Anger can result from the extra and unpleasant work created by incontinence or because the nurse thinks that the patient is being lazy or voluntarily incontinent to gain attention or to annoy the staff. Many of these feelings—revulsion, guilt, embarrassment, and anger—are understandable. They should be examined openly, instead of being repressed as unworthy of a professional nurse, if the nurse is to view the patient's incontinence objectively and help to formulate a rational plan of care. Constructive assessment begins with nurses' awareness of their own attitudes toward the problem.

Nurses have a tradition of coping, whatever the situation, of putting up with problems, however great or unpleasant, and of making the best of problems. For the sake of incontinent patients, as well as for nurses themselves, it is time to look at how the situation can be altered. The nursing profession has a responsibility to patients and their families to use the best expertise available in providing care, both for the promotion of continence and the management of incontinence, and to foster a more positive approach among caregivers.

References

Abdellah, F.G.: Incontinence: Implications for health care policy. Nurs. Clin. North Am., *23:*291, 1988.

Bates, P., et al.: The standardization of terminology of lower urinary tract function. J. Urol., *121:*551, 1979.

Cella, M.: The nursing costs of urinary incontinence in a nursing home population. Nurs. Clin. North Am., *23:*159, 1988.

Gillick, M., Serrell, N., and Gillick, L.: Adverse consequences of hospitalization in the elderly. Social Sci. Med., *16:*1033, 1982.

International Continence Society Standardization Committee: First report of the standardization of terminology related to lower urinary tract function. Scand. J. Urol. Nephrol., *2:*193, 1977.

Mohide, E.: The prevalence and scope of urinary incontinence. Clin. Geriatr. Med., *2:*639, 1986.

Ouslander, J., and Uman, G.: Urinary incontinence: Opportunities for research, education and improvements in medical care in the nursing home setting. *In* Schreider, E., et al. (eds.): The Teaching Nursing Home. New York, Raven Press, 1985, pp. 73–196.

Palmer, N.H.: Incontinence: The magnitude of the problem. Nurs. Clin. North Am., *23:*139, 1988.

Resnick, N.: Urinary incontinence in the elderly. Hosp. Pract., *21:*80C, 1986.
Schwartz, D.R.: Personal point of view—a report of 17 elderly patients with a persistent problem of urinary incontinence. Health Bull. (Edinb.), *35:*197, 1977.
Staskin, D.R., Nehra, A. and Ouslander, J.: Urinary incontinence in the elderly. Hosp. Pract., 133, 1988.
Sullivan, D., and Lindsay, R.: Urinary incontinence in the geriatric population of an acute care hospital. J. Am. Geriatr. Soc., *32:*646, 1984.
Thomas, T., et al.: Prevalence of urinary incontinence. Br. J. Med., *281:*1243, 1980.
Yarnell, J., et al.: The prevalence and severity of urinary incontinence in women. J. Epidemiol. Community Health, *35:*71, 1981.

Ted Hammon, RN

2 The Development of Continence and Causes of Incontinence

No one is born continent. Continence is a skill acquired, at a variable age, and retained often only with difficulty. This chapter aims to provide a framework for understanding, in a simplified form, the mechanism of continence and the common causes of incontinence. Subsequent chapters explain in greater depth many of the types of incontinence introduced here.

Any health professional who wishes to help incontinent patients needs a thorough understanding of normal voiding function and the ways in which it can become dysfunctional. This will make it possible to assess the causes of an individual's incontinence (Chap. 3) and to set appropriate and realistic goals during the planning of care.

THE BABY'S BLADDER AND THE ACQUISITION OF CONTINENCE

The bladder of the newborn baby is controlled by a complex reflex arc (Fig. 2–1). As the bladder fills with urine (which drains down from the kidneys by way of the ureters), stretch and pain receptors in the bladder wall send sensory impulses to the pontine micturition center by way of the sacral bladder center in the spinal cord (located in sacral segments S2, S3, S4). When these impulses become strong and persistent enough a reflex arc is completed and motor impulses cause a bladder contraction, coordinated with relaxation of the urethral sphincter. The bladder empties completely; the filling and emptying cycle is then repeated. Babies are therefore not continuously wet, but "incontinent" in episodes throughout the 24-hour period. At this stage the immature central nervous system cannot consciously appreciate or voluntarily control this cycle.

Continence is acquired by the interaction of two processes: (1) socialization of the infant; and (2) maturation of the central nervous system. Potty training is dealt with in Chapter 5. Without society's expectation of continence, and without broadly accepted definitions of

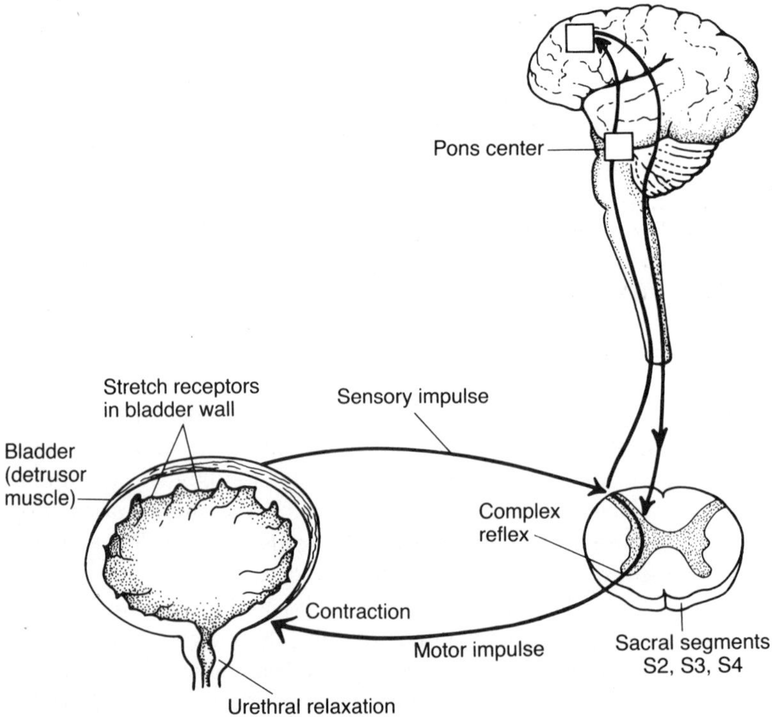

Figure 2–1. *Complex reflex arc.*

correct behavior, the whole concept of "incontinence" would be meaningless.

As the central nervous system matures with age, the baby is increasingly aware of the various bodily functions, including bladder emptying. With practice voluntary control becomes possible, just as control of limb movements becomes more purposeful. Figure 2–2 shows that the sensory messages from the bladder are relayed through several intermediate centers to the cerebral cortex, where a micturition control center is situated in the frontal lobe. As maturation progresses infants become able to interpret these signals as indicating a full bladder. With practice, children learn to inhibit motor impulses that block the completion of the micturition reflex arc, thus preventing urination. Continence involves an active inhibition of nerve impulses, not merely the passive absence of micturition. Eventually children learn to delay voiding reliably until the appropriate time and place have been reached. The cerebral inhibition is then removed, the reflex arc is completed, and the bladder contracts and empties (Fig. 2–3). Micturition is coordinated by a complex feedback loop between the bladder and pons. This feedback loop ensures that bladder contraction is

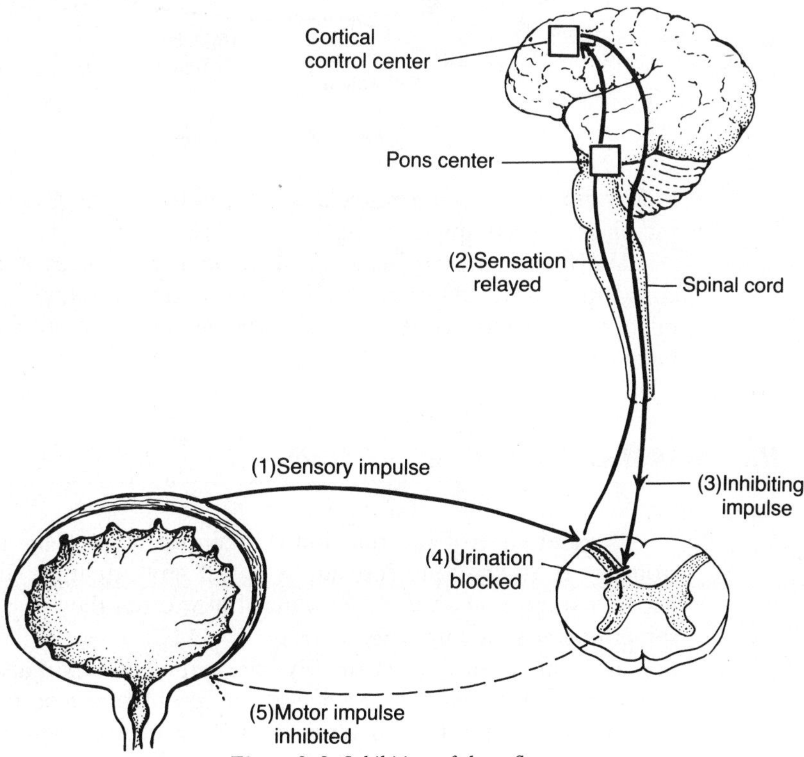

Figure 2–2. *Inhibition of the reflex arc.*

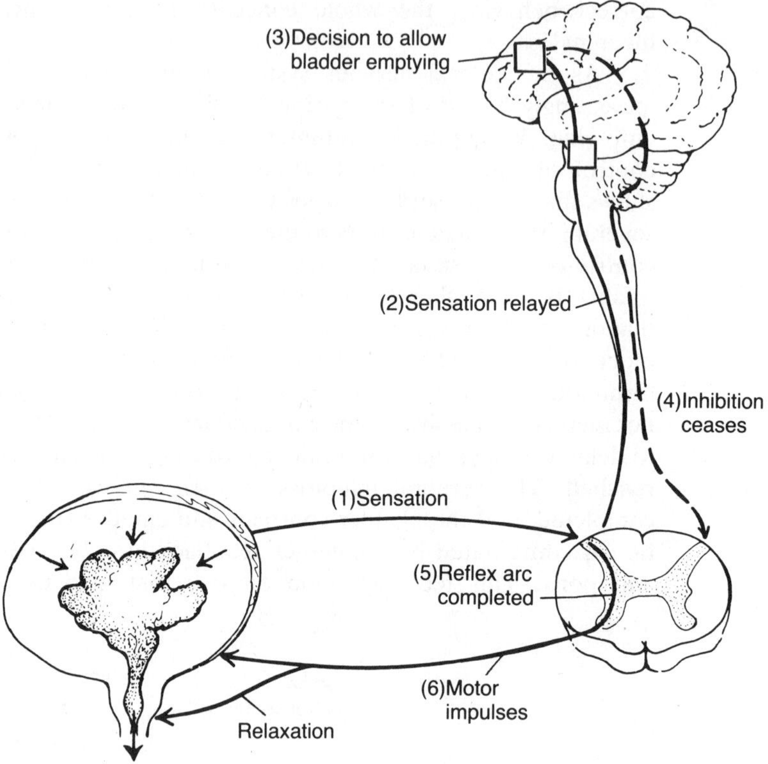

Figure 2–3. *Micturition.*

synchronous with sphincter relaxation and that voiding continues until the bladder is completely empty.

With time, this reflex control no longer involves a continuous, conscious effort between the first sensation of bladder filling and micturition. Continence becomes subconscious and automatic under most circumstances.

THE "NORMAL" ADULT BLADDER

Bladder control and function is taken for granted by most people from an early age, and few adults pay it any attention. Indeed, few people can give an accurate account of how often they pass urine until something goes wrong with control.

The boundaries of "normality" are quite wide; perhaps "normal" should be defined as the absence of any problem for each individual. Most people empty their bladder between four and eight times within a 24-hour period. Some people do so more or less often than this, and would still describe themselves as normal. Most individuals seldom have to get up at night, but a few always have to get up once. Urgency (having to rush to the toilet) should be rare, and only experienced if bladder sensations have been ignored for too long or if fluid intake has been excessive. Generally, the bladder has an effective early warning system—most people have a margin of 1 to 2 hours between the first conscious appreciation of bladder sensation and reaching the limit of bladder capacity. During this interval it should be possible to find the time and the appropriate place to empty the bladder. Sensation is usually felt at about one-half of total bladder capacity. It is usually registered consciously as the need to take advantage of the next convenient opportunity to pass urine. The sensation should then fade from consciousness; it is not constantly present until urination. It returns with increasing intensity, at decreasing intervals, until the bladder is finally emptied. Between these periodic reminders it can usually be forgotten until the bladder is almost full.

A useful skill is the ability to empty the bladder at will, even in the absence of any sensation of the need to do so. Most people can empty the bladder at any time, even with little volume. This enables anticipatory voiding (e.g., before a long journey, meeting, or during a meal break), thereby avoiding the need to interrupt future activities because of a full bladder. Ordinary civilized life would be more difficult if we all waited until the bladder was absolutely full and then rushed off to empty it. Movies, lectures, meetings, and other such structured activities would be constantly interrupted. The remarkable ability of most people to inhibit and activate urination enables organized modern life to proceed uninterrupted by the "call of nature."

Most adult bladders hold between 300 and 600 ml (10 to 20 ounces) at capacity, although many people urinate before this volume is reached. Leakage should not occur at any time, even if voiding has been delayed and urgency is severe.

CAUSES OF URINARY INCONTINENCE

There are many reasons why some people never acquire the control described above, or why it may break down at some point in life, so any classification of the causes is arbitrary. Some scheme for considering the causes is needed, however, and in this book they are divided into three broad categories: (1) physiologic voiding dysfunction; (2) factors directly influencing voiding function; and (3) factors affecting the individual's ability to manage voiding. Table 2–1 summarizes the major types of incontinence and common associated symptoms. It should be remembered that these categories are intimately interrelated, and often overlap.

Table 2–1. COMMON CAUSES OF URINARY INCONTINENCE

Cause	Usual Symptoms
Physiologic voiding dysfunction	
Bladder instability	Urgency, frequency, urge incontinence, nocturia
Genuine stress incontinence	Leakage upon physical exertion, increased intra-abdominal pressure (e.g., cough)
Outflow obstruction with overflow incontinence	Dribbling continually, frequency, urgency, nocturia
Atonic bladder (insufficient bladder strength)	Feelings of incomplete emptying, frequency, high postvoid residual volume
Factors influencing bladder function	
Urinary tract infection	Frequency, urgency, painful urination, potential urge incontinence
Fecal impaction	Voiding difficulty with incomplete emptying
Drug therapy	Various symptoms
Endocrine disorder	Various symptoms
Miscellaneous voiding dysfunction	Various symptoms
Factors affecting ability to manage voiding	
Immobility	Functional incontinence or voluntary wetting
Environment	Various symptoms
Mental function	Behavioral, functional incontinence
Emotions	Urge incontinence, apathetic incontinence
Inadequate patient care	Functional incontinence

Physiologic Voiding Dysfunction

The causes of incontinence that are included in this category involve an abnormality in bladder or sphincter function, or in both. The bladder and sphincter have only two functions: to store urine until the correct time for urination, and then to empty it completely. Voiding dysfunction involves the failure of one or both of these mechanisms.

Most, but not all, of those who are incontinent have some underlying degree of voiding dysfunction. For some it is the only cause of incontinence. For others it is a necessary, but not sufficient, predisposing reason. Alone, it does not explain entirely why they are wet—and many are actually precipitated into frank incontinence by the coincidence of another problem from one of the other categories described below. A few incontinent people do not have any physiologic abnormality, and are wet solely for reasons to be discussed.

Four basic types of voiding dysfunction can be distinguished: detrusor instability, genuine stress incontinence, outflow obstruction, and atonic bladder.

Detrusor Instability

Detrusor instability (which can also be referred to as bladder instability, uninhibited bladder, detrusor hyperreflexia, or the unstable bladder) is a condition characterized by involuntary bladder (detrusor muscle) contractions during filling. All the causes of bladder instability are not fully understood, but it can be associated with the following: neurologic disease (brain and spinal cord abnormalities), inflammation of the bladder wall, bladder outlet obstruction, stress urinary incontinence, and idiopathic dysfunction (Fig. 2–4). Detrusor instability will usually cause symptoms of frequency, urgency, urge incontinence, and possibly nocturia or even nocturnal enuresis.

The unstable bladder, contracting outside voluntary control, can result from an abnormality of the brain, such as a cerebrovascular accident or brain tumor affecting the micturition centers. Sensation is left intact; the person appreciates the need to pass urine, but cannot delay this until the toilet is reached. Sometimes urgency is total—voiding occurs simultaneously with sensation. At other times urgency is less severe, with a diminished warning between sensation and capacity. Incontinence can occur if the toilet is not reached in time. Aging also causes some degree of bladder instability (Chap. 8).

Many people with an unstable bladder have no obvious neurologic lesion to explain their inability to inhibit bladder contractions. This

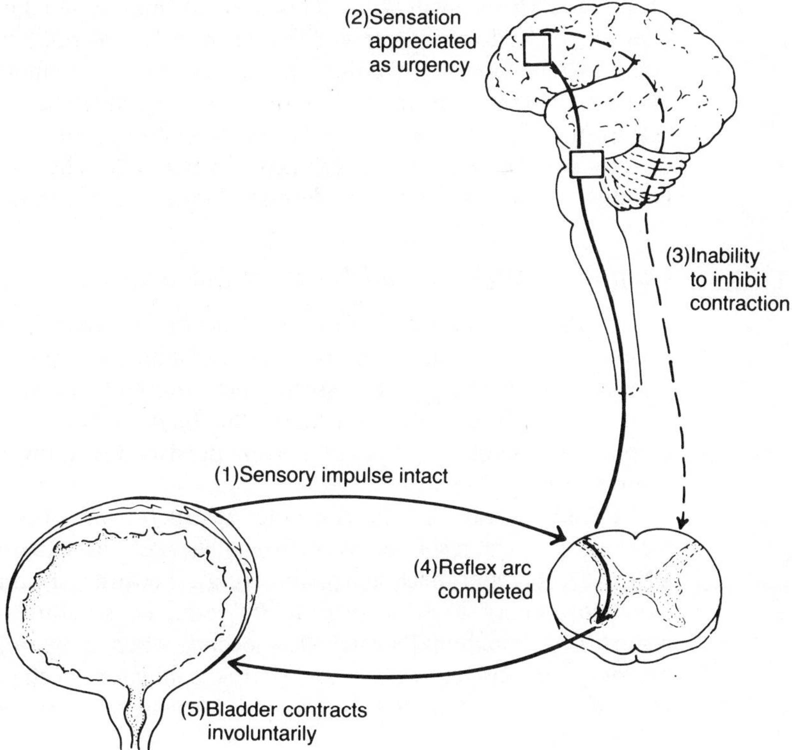

Figure 2–4. *Detrusor instability.*

category can include life-long nocturnal enuretics (bed wetters) and others without overt neuropathy. The condition often presents in the second, third, or fourth decade of life with no obvious preceding cause. It is then called idiopathic detrusor instability, causing exactly the same symptoms as the unstable bladder occurring secondarily to a neurologic lesion. In children, detrusor instability predominantly affects boys; in young adults, it is more common in women. Some investigators have theorized a psychosomatic causation, whereas others have suggested that the bladder control center in the brain is congenitally malformed. Other investigators have hypothesized that it might be caused by a failure to learn effective subconscious bladder control. Undetected neurologic or neurochemical imbalances have also been suggested. None of these explanations has been conclusively proven so the condition, for the present, remains idiopathic.

Genuine Stress Incontinence

Genuine stress incontinence is caused by a failure to hold urine during bladder filling as a result of an incompetent urethral sphincter mechanism. If the closure mechanism of the bladder outlet fails to hold urine, incontinence will occur. This is usually manifested during physical exertion or abdominal stress. (The term does not refer to emotional stress.) It can occur in either sex, but is more common in women because of their shorter urethra and the physical trauma of childbirth (Chap. 6). Men can experience stress incontinence following traumatic or surgical damage to the sphincter (Chap. 7). The mechanism of genuine stress incontinence is described in detail in Chapters 6 and 7.

Outflow Obstruction and Overflow Incontinence

Obstruction of the outflow of urine during voiding can produce various symptoms, including frequency, straining to void, poor urinary stream, preurination and posturination dribbling, and urgency with urge incontinence. In severe cases the bladder is never completely emptied and a volume of residual urine persists. Overflow incontinence can result (Fig. 2–5).

Common causes of bladder outlet obstruction are prostatic enlargement (e.g., as a result of hypertrophy, cancer, or inflammation; see Chap. 7), bladder neck narrowing (e.g., because of contracture or hypertrophy), or urethral obstruction (e.g., by stricture or anatomic distortion). Functional obstruction occurs when a neurologic lesion prevents coordinated relaxation of the sphincter mechanism during voiding. This phenomenon is termed "detrusor-sphincter dyssynergia" (Chap. 10).

The detrusor muscle of an obstructed bladder can become powerful

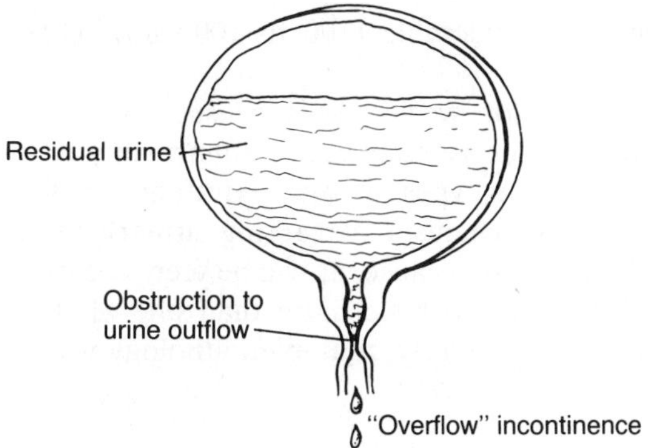

Figure 2–5. *Outflow obstruction.*

and hypertrophied in an attempt to overcome the high outflow resistance. In some instances secondary detrusor instability might develop. If the obstruction is of long standing the bladder can eventually "decompensate"—give up the unequal struggle to empty and become atonic.

Atonic Bladder

The atonic bladder does not produce a sufficient contraction to empty completely. Emptying can be enhanced by abdominal straining or manual expression, but a large residual volume persists. Sensation might or might not be present. Frequency is common if sensation is present, because only a small portion of the bladder volume is emptied (Fig. 2–6). Sensation is often diminished and the residual urine volume

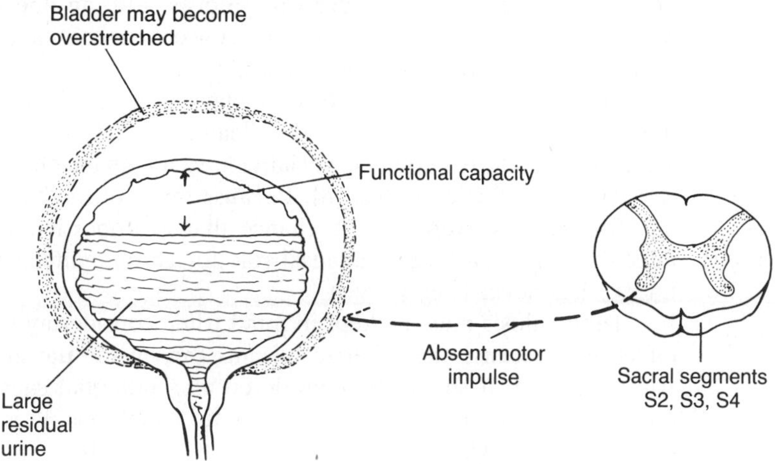

Figure 2–6. *Atonic bladder.*

can be considerable (100 to 1000 ml). Overflow incontinence often occurs.

Detrusor weakness is caused by smooth muscle insufficiency, peripheral nerve damage, or abnormality of the sacral spinal cord.

The four types of voiding dysfunction differ considerably in regard to their mechanism of causing urinary incontinence. They must be differentiated because, as will be seen, the treatments are also different. It is possible to have more than one of these problems at the same time. In the elderly, multiple pathology is common.

Factors Directly Influencing Voiding Function

Some problems directly affect and upset normal voiding function. Any of these factors, if severe enough, can cause incontinence, even in someone with otherwise normal function. More often they combine with one of the above problems and lead to incontinence.

Urinary Tract Infection

An acute urinary tract infection (UTI) can cause transient incontinence, even in a fit, healthy young person who normally has no voiding dysfunction. Acute frequency and urgency with disturbed sensation and pain can result in the inability to get to the toilet in time, or to tell when incontinence is occurring. If an underlying voiding dysfunction is also present, an acute UTI is likely to cause incontinence. Infection especially aggravates an unstable bladder and can increase the number and frequency of uninhibited contractions. The presence of residual urine in the bladder will predispose to an infection, which will be difficult to eradicate. The presence of incontinence might in turn increase the risks of acquiring a UTI.

The role that chronic infection plays in causing incontinence is more doubtful (Brocklehurst and colleagues, 1968; Milne and associates, 1972). Elderly people, especially, have a high incidence of chronic urinary tract infection (Chap. 8). Because many of the elderly are also incontinent it is likely just by chance that a proportion will be both infected and incontinent. A causal role for chronic infection in incontinence has never been proven.

Tuberculosis must be kept in mind when considering urinary tract infections, because the tubercle bacillus can invade the urinary tract. Although rare, it should be considered as a potential cause of symptoms, especially among those living in poor conditions, those who have lived abroad or who are recent immigrants, and/or those with a history of tuberculosis.

Fecal Impaction

Severe constipation with fecal impaction can disturb normal function, making voiding difficult—bladder contractions can be affected, and emptying might be incomplete. Fecal impaction might also cause the individual to feel lethargic, and generally disinclined to activity. Many causes of fecal impaction also disturb continence—for example, immobility, inadequate diet, low fluid intake, and poor living conditions (Chap. 14).

Drug Therapy

Many drugs can disturb the delicate balance of normal functioning. The most obvious category is diuretics; a large, swift diuresis will give most people frequency and urgency. If the bladder is unstable it might not be able to handle a sudden influx of urine, and urge incontinence can result. Sedation can affect voiding function directly (e.g., diazepam can lower urethral resistance), or can make the individual less responsive to signals from the bladder and thus fail to maintain continence. (For example, people with an unstable bladder might find that night sedation means a good night's sleep and a wet bed, whereas without medication they wake up several times to pass urine.)

Other drugs have secondary actions on voiding function. Table 2–2 summarizes the possible effects of some commonly prescribed drugs on continence. Not all patients, however, will experience urinary side effects from these drugs. In some people the side effects might actually be therapeutic (e.g., a drug that makes voiding more difficult for someone with a "normal" bladder might decrease frequency and urgency for the patient with an unstable bladder).

Every drug that has the potential to affect voiding function cannot be listed here. The main point to remember is that many medications can do so, and that it is always important to ascertain which drugs are being taken by an incontinent patient. Nurses often have more contact with the patient than the prescribing physician. Therefore, nurses might be more aware of unwanted side effects, and could suggest a medication review to the physician.

Endocrine Disorders

Various endocrine disorders can upset normal voiding function. Diabetes can cause polydypsia, with a consequent large volume of urine to be contained. Glycosuria might encourage urinary tract infection. Thyroid imbalances might aggravate an overactive or underactive bladder. Pituitary gland disorders can result in the production of excessive urine volumes because of an antidiuretic hormone deficiency.

Table 2–2. *POSSIBLE SIDE EFFECTS OF COMMONLY PRESCRIBED DRUGS ON CONTINENCE*

Drug	Main Uses	Action On Urinary Tract*	Possible Effect on Continence
Phenothiazines (e.g., promethazine)	Neuroleptic, sedative, antiemetic, antipsychotic	Relaxes smooth muscle (e.g., detrusor muscle); possibly affects the CNS micturition centers	Voiding difficulties and retention
Butyrophenone (e.g., haloperidol)	Neuroleptic, antipsychotic	Relaxes smooth muscle; possibly affects CNS	Voiding difficulties and retention
Imipramine, amitriptyline	Antidepressant	Anticholinergic	Voiding difficulties and retention
Propantheline	Peptic ulcer, pancreatitis	Anticholinergic	Voiding difficulties and retention
Diazepam	Muscle relaxant, sedative	Decreases muscle tone in outflow tract; decreases responsiveness to bladder signals	Outlet failure incontinence
Phenylpropanolamine	Nasal decongestant	Increases smooth muscle tone in outflow tract	Voiding difficulties and retention (might help with incompetent sphincters)
Reserpine, methyldopa, prazosin	Antihypertensive	Decreases outlet resistance	Possible stress incontinence
Hydralazine	Antihypertensive	Relaxes smooth muscle	Voiding difficulties and retention
Propranolol	Antihypertensive	Increases smooth muscle tone in outflow tract	Voiding difficulties and retention
Hydrochlorothiazide, furosemide, bumetanide, methyclothiazide	Diuretic	Large and swift increase in volume of urine	Frequency, urgency, urge incontinence precipitated by diuresis
Digoxin	Cardiac arrhythmia	Increases detrusor muscle tone	Increased bladder pressure and decreased capacity
Levodopa	Antiparkinsonian	Relaxes smooth muscle	Voiding difficulties and retention
Ergotamine	Migraine	Increases smooth muscle tone in outflow tract	Voiding difficulties and retention

*Not all patients taking these drugs will experience urinary tract symptoms.

Estrogen deficiency in postmenopausal women causes atrophic changes in the vaginal and urethral tissues, and will worsen stress incontinence and an unstable bladder (Chap. 8).

Miscellaneous Pathology

Several different bladder pathologies can cause incontinence by disrupting normal functioning. A patient with a neoplasm, whether benign or malignant, or a stone in the bladder occasionally presents with incontinence as a symptom. These are infrequent causes of incontinence.

Factors Affecting Ability to Manage Voiding

Many people can have one or more of the conditions discussed above without actually wetting themselves. Those with an unstable bladder or urinary tract infection, or who are taking diuretics, often learn to prevent incontinence. They achieve this by visiting the toilet at every available opportunity, never moving too far from a rest room, or keeping a receptacle nearby, such as a commode by the bed or a bucket under the sink, in case of being "caught short." They will only go shopping in a mall where they know the location of all the rest rooms; the first thing they do on any outing (if they will go on one) is to ascertain the quickest route to the nearest toilet. Some isolate themselves completely and refuse to go out or mix socially. Younger people with an unstable bladder are often not incontinent, because they can respond quickly to urgency. Many people with a tendency to stress incontinence avoid leakage by avoiding physical exertion—for example, they stop playing sports, they do not go shopping if heavy objects have to be carried, they refuse to dance, and they try not to laugh when they go out. When they have a cough they are more likely to stay at home to avoid potential embarrassment. People with difficulties in bladder emptying might spend excessive time on the toilet trying to strain until the bladder is empty. Many incontinent people restrict fluid intake, often completely, in an attempt to prevent incontinence.

Often it takes something else in addition to the underlying problem to tip the balance and produce incontinence. This is especially true for elderly and disabled persons who are delicately balanced between continence and incontinence. Any one of the following factors is sometimes a sufficient reason alone for incontinence. More often they combine with an actual dysfunction to produce incontinence.

Immobility

To pass urine in the "correct" place you must be able to get there. Thus, anything that impedes access is likely to induce incontinence. Immobility can be the result of the gradual worsening of a chronic condition, such as arthritis, multiple sclerosis, or Parkinson's disease, until eventually the individual simply cannot get to the toilet in time. Or the condition can be acute—an accident or illness that suddenly renders a person immobile might be the start of failure to control the bladder.

The importance of immobility is closely related to the degree of urgency experienced. If it takes longer to get to the toilet or to obtain an alternative receptacle (e.g., a bed pan), than it takes for the person to hold on, incontinence is the inevitable result. Disabled people can become incontinent simply because they cannot get to or onto a toilet, or because no one is available to help them.

Closely associated with mobility are factors such as manual dexterity, eyesight, condition of the feet (and shoes), and suitability of clothing. (Chap. 9 discusses incontinence and its relationship to the physically disabled.)

Environment

The physical design and layout of surroundings might not be ideal for easy continence. The situation of the bathroom, ease of access, and number of other people who share it (and might be using it) are important. In public places, including hospitals, many rest rooms are a considerable distance from main areas, and might be poorly marked and difficult to use if someone is disabled. At home, there could be stairs to negotiate or the toilet might be outside.

The social environment is also important. In some situations incontinence becomes the norm (especially in extended care facilities), and the social pressure to be continent disappears. In a socially impoverished atmosphere people might lose their grip on reality and exhibit disordered behaviors, including incontinence. At home the isolated and incontinent person might lose all motivation to try to maintain continence. The well-supported person with a good social network, who is seen as a valid and useful member of the community, is most likely to make every effort to avoid incontinence and to seek help early if it does occur.

Mental Function

People with lowered mental abilities, whether because of mental retardation, confusion, or dementia, might not recognize the social need for continence or what is considered acceptable behavior. This is seldom a sufficient reason on its own to explain incontinence. Many of these people also have an underlying voiding dysfunction (see above). Most people with disordered mental function can maintain continence with appropriate management (Chaps. 8 and 9), except possibly those with profound retardation or advanced dementia. The confused elderly, however, are easily disoriented, and many who can cope well in their own surroundings cannot manage in a strange environment.

Emotions

The bladder has been said to be a sensitive emotional barometer, and many people find their bladder function upset when they are—witness the lines for the rest rooms outside an examination or interview room. The causal relationship of emotional problems to incontinence is unclear. There can be little doubt that many incontinent people appear depressed or anxious, but whether this is a cause or an outcome of incontinence is not yet known.

Incontinence can also be associated with emotional regression under stress, and in rare situations might be a symptom of protest or despair at an unacceptable situation. The onset of incontinence might follow the reaction to a traumatic event, such as bereavement. It might also be used as manipulative or "attention-seeking" behavior by a few patients. As mentioned above, some clinicians believe that idiopathic detrusor instability is psychosomatic in origin (although the evidence for this is inconclusive).

Inadequate Patient Care

Those who depend to some degree on other people for their continence are at risk of becoming incontinent unless their caregivers—whether relatives, nurses, or others—are sensitive to their needs and oriented toward the promotion of continence. If the attitude of the caregiver is to expect and accept incontinence in the dependent, incontinence becomes much more likely.

In some instances, caregivers can actually promote incontinence by making it easier to be wet than dry. An individual might find that it is much less bother for someone to come and help change a pad at intervals than to struggle to get to the toilet. If incontinence seems to be the expected norm, and if it is rewarded by attention and physical and social contact, it can soon become established behavior.

These and other possible causes of incontinence are described in more detail in subsequent chapters. Any combination of problems is possible. Young, otherwise fit, incontinent people tend to have only a single dysfunction underlying their symptom. Older and disabled people tend to have complex problems, with many different factors combining to render them incontinent. The multiplicity of possible causes emphasizes the importance of regarding incontinence as a symptom, the causes of which must be investigated and diagnosed accurately if treatment is to be successful. Incontinence should never simply be accepted as an inevitable consequence of aging, disease, or disability. Often the assumed cause is only part of the story. Today it is possible to modify most of the underlying causes of incontinence and in many cases to remedy them completely.

It is never pointless to ask why someone is incontinent. There must always be a cause—incontinence does not just happen. If nurses and other health providers can keep that in the forefront of their thinking when caring for incontinent people, many who are currently suffering will stand a good chance of regaining continence.

References and Further Reading

Brocklehurst, J.C., et al.: The prevalence and symptomatology of urinary tract infection in an aged population. Gerontol. Clin., *10:*242, 1968.

Gartley, C.B.: Managing Incontinence. Ottawa, Jameson Books, 1985.

Gray, M.L., and Dougherty, M.C.: Urinary incontinence—pathophysiology and treatment. J. Enterost. Ther., *14:*152, 1987.

Krane, R.J., and Sirosky, M.B.: Clinical Neuro-Urology. Boston, Little, Brown, & Co., 1979.

Milne, J.S., et al.: Urinary symptoms in older people. Mod. Geriatr., *5:*198, 1972.

Mundy, A.R., Stephenson, T.P., and Wein, A.J.: Urodynamics: Principles, Practice and Application. London, Churchill-Livingstone, 1984.

Mikel Gray, CURN, MSN

3 Assessment and Investigation of Urinary Incontinence

Several health care professionals are involved in assessing and managing urinary incontinence. The multidisciplinary team approach offers optimum help for any patient. This chapter focuses on the nursing and medical aspects of assessment. It should be remembered, however, that other health care professionals often contribute to a complete assessment.

The individual presenting for help with incontinence is generally assessed by a nurse or physician. Ideally, a joint nursing and medical assessment should be made to determine the causes of incontinence and how the condition affects the patient. Unfortunately, nursing and medical assessments are often made independently, and in many cases one or more aspects of the assessment are omitted completely. This chapter describes a comprehensive assessment, without specifying which health professional should do what; the issue is affected by time, interest, and expertise in a local setting. Nurses can do much of the assessment alone, but the best diagnosis is made in the context of medical support and interest.

PRESENTATION: WHO IS THE INCONTINENT PERSON?

The first task in assessing incontinence is determining who has the problem. Sometimes the answer is obvious such as in the assessment of patients in an extended care facility. In contrast, others who suffer from incontinence live in a community setting and rarely seek professional health care. Many hide their incontinence because of embarrassment or guilt, or accept it as an inevitable concomitant of age or disability. Many persons do not wish to admit to a friend, neighbor, or relative that they are incontinent. Others feel that incontinence is not a serious condition (i.e., life-threatening), and does not warrant consulting their physician. Some patients are too shy to discuss their symptom with a health care professional of the opposite sex.

Once incontinence is admitted, the patient is often advised by a nurse or physician that it is a chronic, untreatable condition. Remarks like "What do you expect at your age?" or "You'll have to learn to live with it" are often heard by the patient. In certain cases the physician or nurse might not know alternative treatments for incontinence, or the clinician might feel inadequate or helpless to find a "complete" cure. Health care professionals can unknowingly compound the stigma of incontinence by expressing embarrassment when confronting patients with the condition or by avoiding discussion of such problems. Patients are particularly sensitive to this. Often incontinence is mentioned during the course of a consultation or hospitalization for another health problem, but discussion is rapidly abandoned in preference to "safer" topics.

HISTORY AND INTERVIEW

An accurate and full history comprises the first step in assessing the nature and extent of incontinence. A history of incontinence is obtained through the use of a loosely structured interview, with a checklist for pertinent information. The person taking the history must have a basic knowledge of incontinence to know what questions to ask and why, must understand the significance of the patient's responses to questions, and should recognize important "leads" elicited in the interview. The history is not gathered for its own sake, but is used as a tool to help in the accurate diagnosis and management of incontinence. A history also provides a baseline from which to monitor progress and a point of reference for other health care professionals who participate in the patient's care.

The interview should take place in an informal, relaxed setting, preferably one that is familiar to the patient. Adequate time is provided to allow the patient to discuss problems with incontinence fully and to express feelings related to the condition. This interview is often the first time that the patient has discussed the problem with anyone; a hurried consultation could result in the omission of important information or in misdiagnosis of the condition.

The patient is usually a reasonably reliable historian. When a patient cannot answer questions adequately, because of poor memory, impaired communication skills, or altered mental status, other sources of information are used. Medical records, reports from family members or health care providers, and observation of the person's environment (including clothing) provide helpful information. Much of this information may have been obtained in a routine assessment, which is included in the evaluation of urinary incontinence (Norton, 1980).

An example of an assessment checklist is provided in Figure 3–1. It is used as a guide for the interview rather than as a formal, rigid questionnaire. Some items require only "yes" or "no" responses, whereas others allow the patient to elaborate. The goal of the checklist is to ensure that all relevant issues affecting incontinence are addressed, and that records are kept in a cogent, systematic fashion. The interviewer must be aware of the relevance and implications of each question.

Main Complaint

It is important to differentiate whether the presenting problem arises from the patient's, family's, or health care provider's perspective. People can experience various symptoms that are of greater or less importance, depending on their perspective. Treatment is directed at relieving symptoms that are causing the patient the greatest physical and emotional distress. Because patients often rate the severity of symptoms differently from health care providers, it is essential to ask their opinion. "What, to you, is the *main* problem with your bladder (waterworks)?" is a useful question. The answer might be a common symptom, such as urinary leakage or frequency, or it might be a reflection of altered lifestyle secondary to urinary incontinence, such as an inability to engage in sports or have sexual intercourse without leakage.

Urinary Symptoms

Urinary symptoms are nonspecific indicators of underlying voiding dysfunction; it is not possible to make a reliable diagnosis of voiding

Name: Date of birth:

Address:

Family physician:

Assessed by: Date: Referred by:

1. Main complaint

2. Urinary symptoms

   Frequency: Nocturia (woken?):

   Urgency: Average warning time: Urge incontinence:

   Stress incontinence: Constant incontinence:

   Nocturnal enuresis: Number of nights per week:

   Symptoms of voiding difficulty:

   Hesitancy: Poor stream: Straining:

   Manual expression: Postmicturition dribble:

   Dysuria: Hematuria:

   Incontinence

   Onset—when? Circumstances:

   Is incontinence improving/static/worsening?

   How often does incontinence occur? How much is lost?

   Are containment devices used? Type:

   Number per day: Source of supply:

   Are devices effective? Problems:

   Type and amount of fluid intake: Fluid restriction?

   Other urinary symptoms:

3. Past medical history

   Previous illnesses and operations:

   Parity: Difficult deliveries?

   Current medication:

   Any previous treatment for incontinence?

4. Bowels

   Usual bowel habit: Constipation?

   Laxatives or diet regulation used?

   Fecal incontinence?

5. Mobility

   Problems with mobility: Aids used?

   Needs assistance? Who is available?

   Difficulties in transfer to/onto toilet? Comments:

   Foot problems: Manual dexterity:

Figure 3–1. *Incontinence assessment checklist. These headings will elicit the basic information needed for an assessment. You should construct a checklist using these headings (and any others found necessary and relevant for specific circumstances), leaving adequate space for filling in answers and comments.*

Clothing suitability: Eyesight:

Observe self-toileting and comment on problems:

Problems with personal hygiene:

6. Psychological state

Attitude to incontinence:

Anxiety? Depression?

Impaired mental abilities?

7. Social network

Usual activities: Are these restricted by incontinence?

Who does patient live with? Who visits regularly?

Relationship problems because of incontinence?

Official services received:

8. Environment

Toilet facilities: Are urinals or commode used?

Obstacles to using lavatory: Washing and laundry facilities:

Comments on general physical and social environment:

9. Results of physical examination

Skin problems: Prolapse (women): Atrophic changes (women):

Rectal examination: Postmicturition residual urine volume:

Urine test result: Other findings:

10. Results from chart

Summary of problems:

Aims and goals:

Planned action: Review date:

Follow-up notes:

Figure 3–1 Continued

dysfunction based solely on patient history. Symptoms do provide clues to a possible diagnosis, however, and, when combined with a comprehensive history and thorough examination, allow a provisional diagnosis of voiding dysfunction. Conservative treatment is often begun immediately after a history and initial physical assessment to alleviate problematic symptoms of voiding dysfunction. Further investigation (e.g., complex urodynamic testing) is instituted when the initial treatment strategy fails to correct the problem or when surgical management is contemplated. Patients with a complex mixture of symptoms often require urodynamic testing as part of their initial assessment.

Frequency of passing urine during the daytime is assessed by recording the number of times urine is passed between rising and retiring and the length of the intervals between visits to the rest room. Most people pass urine three to six times each day. Frequency exists when people urinate more than seven times a day, or when the interval between urination is 2 hours or less.

Nocturia occurs when the urge to urinate interrupts sleep. It is important to distinguish whether the patient is awakened by the desire to void or whether sleep is interrupted because of other factors. One episode of nocturia each night is considered normal. Awaking two or more times at night is abnormal although it is more common among the elderly, perhaps because of increased urinary excretion from the kidneys when the patient is recumbent at night.

When abnormal daytime frequency or nocturia is reported it is important to explore possible reasons with the patient. Usually a patient voids frequently because of sensory urgency or an attempt to avoid urinary leakage. Rarely, a patient might void frequently because of lifelong habits (e.g., following childhood advice not to hold urine for too long). Or, a patient might feel a compulsion to use every available opportunity to empty the bladder because of an anxious or obsessional personality trait. Urinary frequency accompanied by discomfort can indicate inflammation of the urinary tract. Urinary frequency and nocturia without discomfort can indicate excessive fluid intake or use of diuretics.

Dysfunctional voiding states also cause diurnal urinary frequency and nocturia. Detrusor instability, the occurrence of uncontrolled bladder contractions, causes frequent sensations of the desire to void and compromises functional bladder capacity. Genuine stress urinary incontinence causes diurnal urinary frequency, because urine in an open bladder neck can intensify the desire to empty the bladder. A patient with urinary retention caused by bladder outlet obstruction or insufficient muscle function experiences nocturia and diurnal frequency because the *functional* bladder capacity is paradoxically reduced as residual volumes increase.

Infrequent voiding might be reported. Patients may learn to void infrequently because of perceived inability to interrupt work or because of a lifelong habit of refraining from voiding in a public rest room. Retention of urine resulting from deficient bladder muscle function, loss of sensations of bladder filling, low fluid intake, or dehydration can also lead to urinary infrequency.

Urgency is the symptom of having to hurry to pass urine. The warning time between the first sensation of bladder filling and an urgent need to urinate is reduced. In the normal individual the time between these sensations is typically 1 hour or longer; in the person with urgency this time interval can be as short as 10 minutes. The result is an interruption of normal activities so that a rest room can be found quickly. Sometimes urgency is precipitant and the bladder contracts without prior warning.

Urge incontinence is the inability to reach the rest room or move onto the toilet before urination begins. This can occur if urgency is not responded to or if the environment is unsuitable. Precipitant bladder emptying can be partial or complete, depending on the patient's mobility and dexterity and on the distance to the nearest available rest room. Urgency and urge incontinence are characteristic symptoms of bladder instability, but they are also observed in association with other dysfunctional voiding states.

Stress incontinence is the symptom of leaking urine in conjunction with physical exertion (in contrast to emotional stress), such as coughing, laughing, or exercising. Stress urinary incontinence can range from mild to severe; the affected individual might leak only minimal volumes of urine with strenuous exercise or might leak large volumes of urine even with mild exertion, such as standing or walking. Stress urinary incontinence is caused by pelvic descent and by incompetence of the urethral sphincter mechanism (Gray and Dougherty, 1987).

Constant incontinence is the leakage of urine without noticeable exertion or sensation. The patient typically complains of "just finding myself wet." Extraurethral leakage can cause constant incontinence; urinary fistula or ureteral ectopia are common findings. Severe sphincter incompetence also can result in continuous incontinence.

Nocturnal enuresis is bed-wetting while asleep. This condition is distinct from nocturia with urge incontinence, in which people awaken with the desire to void and then leak before they can act on this desire. The cause of nocturnal enuresis remains unclear (Gray and Broadwell, 1986).

Symptoms of voiding difficulty should be explored. They are caused by deficient bladder muscle function or bladder outlet obstruction. *Hesitancy* is the symptom of having to wait for a urinary stream to begin, even after the person is in position and ready to urinate. Often hesitancy is associated with a decrease in the force of the urinary stream. Men readily notice this phenomenon; women are rarely aware of a decreased force in urinary stream until the condition becomes severe and the stream is reduced to a dribble. A patient might report straining or the need for manual expression (Credé's maneuver) to empty the bladder, although many patients, particularly children, remain unaware of this behavior.

Postvoid dribbling is a small passive leakage after the patient has completed voiding. It can indicate incomplete bladder emptying, trappage of urine in the bulbar urethra in men, or periurethral diverticulum in women. Some persons complain of a feeling of incomplete bladder emptying.

Dysuria is the symptom of pain or burning while passing urine. It is usually caused by inflammation of the bladder or urethra.

Hematuria, or blood in the urine, is a sign of potentially serious urinary tract abnormality. Visible blood in the urine (gross hematuria) should be investigated immediately and can indicate bladder tumor or severe infection.

Other Important Assessment Questions

The subjective report of incontinence only implies uncontrolled urinary leakage. This report is followed up by questions concerning the onset of the incontinence, circumstances that precipitate incontinence, and conditions that alleviate or worsen the condition. The frequency of urinary leakage and the volume of urine lost offer important clues to proper management. Estimating the volume of incontinence is difficult because the patient's clothing, use of collection devices, and subjective perceptions of the severity of leakage confound attempts to quantify the amount of urine lost. A simple indication of the volume (i.e., a few drops, a moderate amount, or completely wet pants) is generally sufficient. Weighing pads before and after urinary leakage offers a quantitative assessment of the volume of urinary leakage, but is seldom necessary except for research purposes.

Individual tolerance and perceptions of incontinence vary greatly. Occasional urinary leakage might be interpreted as severe by one person and tolerated as "normal" by another. The volume and frequency of urinary loss correlate poorly with the amount of distress experienced by the affected individual. Reactions to incontinence are interpreted within each individual's context of meaning. Exploring expectations of voiding behaviors and premorbid bladder habits assist in understanding the patient's perceptions of current symptoms.

Incontinence containment devices, such as pads or dribble pouches, might be in use when a patient presents for evaluation of incontinence. If this is the case, how many and what type of pads are used should be noted. Pad usage offers only an approximate indicator of frequency and volume of incontinence; many people change pads routinely rather than waiting until they are soaked to capacity. Incontinence containment devices are also assessed for suitability, availability, economy, and appropriate application.

Manipulation of fluid intake is often done in an attempt to control urinary leakage. Some patients will associate certain types of beverages with increased symptoms of bladder dysfunction. Tea, coffee, and alcohol are common offenders.

Past Medical History

Multiple aspects of a patient's medical history affect urinary incontinence and should be noted. Any genitourinary abnormality or urologic surgical procedure can affect urinary incontinence. An obstetric history should be obtained from a female patient, including the number of babies, how delivered, difficult or prolonged deliveries, and the use of forceps assistance in childbirth. Neurologic disease is particularly significant, as is a history of any neurologic or neuro-orthopedic surgical procedures. Psychiatric or mental deficiency states should be noted, as well as the general state of physical and emotional health. Any drugs a patient is taking are recorded because many have a subtle or direct influence on bladder function.

Bowel Function

Careful inquiry is essential to elicit information about usual bowel habits and to uncover any changes that might have occurred. Bowel function varies among individuals (Chap. 14), and care must be taken not to impose arbitrary criteria for abnormal states. "Constipation" refers to difficulty in passing stool and the consistency of the stool rather than to frequency of defecation. The history must include direct questions related to fecal incontinence, because it is even more embarrassing than urinary incontinence and patients are even more reticent to volunteer information concerning this problem.

Mobility and Manual Dexterity

Information about mobility is gathered both by interview and observation. Mobility might be impaired directly because of abnormality of bones, muscles, joints, or nervous control, or indirectly by pain or fear. Any mobility aids (e.g., walking canes, crutches, or wheelchairs) are inspected for suitability and ease of use in the context of a patient's usual surroundings. For the physically disabled, speed of mobility is assessed and correlated to the degree of urgency, amount of assistance needed to urinate, and availability of urinary receptacles. The patient's ability to transfer is affected by physical ability and equipment and by the physical design of bathrooms. Mobility can be restricted by common environmental factors such as inappropriate footwear (e.g., loose-fitting house slippers that make ambulation difficult), loose floor mats, slippery floors, or poor lighting.

Manual dexterity is closely linked to mobility. The ability to walk or move to the bathroom is useless if the patient cannot transfer to the toilet or remove clothing. Manual dexterity is assessed by watching the patient use the toilet. The observer must resist the temptation to assist the person during this assessment period, even when attempts to toilet appear awkward or inadequate.

Assess the style of clothing and incontinence devices used to determine how they influence a patient's dexterity when urinating. Multiple layers of tight clothing, buttons, or stiff zippers require significant time to remove when attempting to urinate, and might promote urinary leakage for the person who experiences urgency and urge incontinence. Pads might be incorrectly applied and interfere with the passage of urine into the toilet. Persons who have praxis disorders will have particular difficulty with performing the manual tasks necessary to empty their bladder into a toilet successfully.

Vision also affects the mobility and dexterity needed to empty the bladder into an appropriate receptacle successfully. Impaired vision can limit the ability to move onto the toilet or impair complete removal of clothing. This is a particular problem for men attempting to use a hand-held urinal.

Personal hygiene can indicate a loss of mobility and manual dexterity that contribute to urinary incontinence. Effective bathing relies on dexterity of the hands and arms. Even the use of toilet paper is impossible for a person with limited mobility of the arms and shoulders. Adequate personal hygiene is essential for preventing odor and skin problems. Occasionally, the incontinent person is unconcerned about hygiene and the odor produced by urinary leakage. More commonly, the incontinent person is greatly concerned about odor, and poor hygiene is the result of limited dexterity rather than apathy.

Psychologic State

Psychologic factors alone do not provide a complete picture of an individual's incontinence, but are essential to the comprehensive assessment of incontinence. For example, the patient's attitude toward incontinence profoundly affects the feasibility of treatment options. Most people are distressed by their leakage and are anxious to try any strategy that might help. Others are less amenable to treatment. They might be apathetic toward the problem and consider it to be untreatable, or they might deny incontinence because of shame. Some individuals deny a problem with incontinence even to themselves. This reflects a significant psychologic conflict between self-image and reality. Successful treatment is unlikely until the affected person admits the problem and agrees to participate in care.

Anxiety and depression are two common psychologic reactions to incontinence. All incontinent patients are likely to experience these feelings to some degree; for some, these symptoms are severe enough to constitute a psychiatric illness. Anxiety and depression are typically a secondary reaction to incontinence and can worsen existing urinary leakage, which further intensifies the depression and anxiety. Once the two problems coexist the patient becomes trapped in a vicious cycle, so that each problem only exacerbates the other.

Those with impaired mental function caused by mental handicap, delusional state, or organic brain condition are less able to cope with the complex social skills needed to manage incontinence. A formal assessment of cognitive and social function (Chap. 12) might be useful. Often a psychiatrist or psychologist is needed for the assessment of incontinence in the mentally handicapped.

Social Network

An individual's social network influences the ability to cope with a problem. A supportive network of friends and family can provide needed assistance and encouragement when a person faces a crisis or chronic stressor such as incontinence. Unfortunately, because of the social stigma associated with incontinence, many people deliberately isolate themselves and refuse to participate in former social activities.

The presence of incontinence disrupts the entire family or intimate social network. Stress factors, such as having to do extra laundry, fear of managing incontinence in public, and the unpleasantness of urinary leakage, can place significant strain on relationships within the family or social network. Families can feel trapped within their home because of fear of managing their relative's urinary leakage in unfamiliar surroundings. Many are afraid to invite friends into their homes because of embarrassment related to the odor created by incontinence. These problems can lead to acute crises such as child abuse, marital difficulties, altered sexual relationships, or refusal to participate in the care of an incontinent person.

Whether the victim of incontinence is a resident in an extended care facility or is living at home, the social environment will support continence or encourage incontinence. Assessment of the social network should include an impression of the social factors in which the individual is functioning that could affect continence.

Environment

The importance of the physical environment to the individual's ability to cope with bladder function has been previously emphasized. An assessment of the incontinent person's environment should focus on bathroom facilities in the home or health care facility and on any obstacles to reaching them (e.g., poor lighting, stairs, long distance from bed or chair to toilet, chairs or beds that obstruct walkways). In institutions, clearly visible signs and adequate lighting can help those who are disoriented or visually handicapped. The toilet is assessed for proper height, cleanliness, and accessibility. The privacy of the bathroom also is evaluated.

Assessment of the environment should also focus on access to laundry facilities and waste disposal services. Incontinence can contaminate the environment unless properly contained. Soiled linen and clothing must be washed and dried and incontinent aids must be disposed of properly. Inadequate laundry or garbage facilities often result in significant squalor and health risks as individuals try unsuccessfully to rid themselves of the evidence of their condition.

PHYSICAL EXAMINATION

Every incontinent person should have a full medical examination, with emphasis on genitourinary and neurologic systems. Because this evaluation is not always done, nursing assessment of the incontinent patient should include a basic physical examination. Careful inspection of the patient will reveal much about the general state of health, mobility, and mental state. The female genital area is inspected for altered skin integrity or signs of estrogen deficiency. The male genitalia are examined for signs of altered skin integrity and a digital rectal examination is performed if fecal impaction or prostatic enlargement is suspected.

A midstream or catheterized urine specimen is collected for routine urinalysis, including microscopic examination, culture, and sensitivity determination. Urinalysis allows detection of glucose, ketones (proteinuria), pH, specific gravity, and hemoglobin (gross or microscopic hematuria). Microscopic examination will detect the presence of bacteria, white blood cells, and other signs of infection.

URODYNAMIC STUDIES

Simple Urodynamic Strategies

Urodynamics involves a set of strategies for assessing incontinence. In the United States, the concept of urodynamics is typically limited to complex, technologic tests used to measure lower urinary tract function. In contrast, European health care professionals often advocate a broader definition of the concept, which includes simple (nontechnologic) urodynamic strategies, such as observation of voiding stream, continence charts, and postvoid residual measurement, as well as complex testing (Turner-Warwick, 1984). This definition of urodynamics is most useful for the nurse who assesses and manages patients with urinary incontinence.

Observation of Urinary Stream and Measurement of Residual Urine

Urodynamic assessment of the incontinent patient often begins with observation of the voided urinary stream and measurement of residual urine. In the male, the urinary stream is directly observed by asking the male to urinate to completion into a toilet. The nurse stands behind the patient at an oblique angle to observe the urinary stream. The length of time between assuming the position to void and onset of the stream is measured to distinguish urinary urgency versus hesitancy. The voided stream is assessed for its force, caliber, and trimness. The patient should void with an uninterrupted stream until the last several spurts; the stream should not spray to the side of the penis. At the termination of voiding several drops of urine are expressed within 10 to 30 seconds. The voiding time can be assessed by using a stopwatch; micturition time will vary according to the volume expelled. Even a relatively large bladder volume should be emptied within 30 to 60 seconds.

Observation of urination is more difficult in a female. The stream can be assessed by measuring voiding time and listening for the noise created when the patient empties her bladder. The stream should begin from 5 to 60 seconds after the woman has removed appropriate clothing and is ready to void. The stream should be uninterrupted, but the woman should be able to stop her stream volitionally on command.

The volume of residual urine is measured after observation of voiding is completed. The patient is catheterized and residual volume is measured. This volume is added to the amount voided and a total bladder volume is calculated. The residual volume is then divided into the total bladder volume and the percentage of residual versus amount voided is obtained. Among children and young adults the postvoid residual might approach 0 ml, although a residual of less than 20% of total bladder volume is considered to be within normal limits. Among older adults the residual volume is often greater and can approach 100 ml, or 25% of total bladder volume. Residual volumes greater than these amounts represent significant urinary retention.

Continence Chart Results

The continence chart is probably the single most useful nursing tool for assessing incontinence. Used properly, the chart is not an end in itself; but is a record that is interpreted in conjunction with other findings in an incontinence assessment.

The chart has two main uses, as part of the baseline assessment and later as a record of progress to monitor the effectiveness of therapy. It forms the cornerstone of bladder training programs. To be useful the chart must be accurate. The patient, family, or caregivers must be educated in regard to its proper use and importance in a bladder training program. This includes the evening and night staff in a hospital or extended care facility and several members of the patient's family. The patient should be allowed to take maximum responsibility for this task whenever feasible.

The patient or caregiver should be encouraged to fill out the record as soon as possible after the event occurs, rather than allowing reliance on memory at the end of the day. The place where the chart is kept will influence the likelihood of charting occurring promptly after significant events occur. The chart should be kept in a sufficiently private place to avoid embarrassment, but should be prominently displayed and easily accessible. Charts can be kept in the bathroom, near the door of the toilet, or in a purse or briefcase for active persons.

Many different charts are available. Some are interchangeable, whereas some have different functions. Before choosing a chart it is important to decide what information is needed. A simple chart shows continent voiding and episodes of incontinence. The chart shown in Figure 3–2*A* was designed for ease of use and suitability for inpatient and community use. The less information requested, the greater the likelihood that the information gathered will be accurate. Bold coloring and simple instructions make the chart easier to fill in for both patients and nurses. This type of chart, kept for approximately 1 week, provides a good baseline assessment of patterns of incontinence.

In some cases more information than that provided by a simple chart is needed. A frequency-volume chart provides an estimate of functional bladder capacity that can be combined with an estimate of fluid intake to obtain a fluid balance chart. Measuring input will detect polydipsia or excessively low fluid intake. When interpreting results it is important to note whether input was actually measured or simply estimated.

Some charts do not specify times, but are left blank to be filled in as necessary. This allows times to be filled in more accurately than to the nearest hour. The continence chart shown in Figure 3–2*B* also incorporates information about the patient's behavior. It is filled in by a nurse or caregiver for patients who cannot complete the record themselves. It demonstrates the patient's patterns of continence and incontinence, ability to indicate needs, and the success of any program being used. It is also used to distinguish between patient-initiated and caregiver-initiated toileting. Repeated caregiver-initiated toileting at-

Continence Chart

Week beginning ______________ Name ______________________________

Please put a check in LEFT column each time urine is passed

Please put a check in RIGHT column each time you are wet

	Monday	Tuesday	Wednesday	Thursday	Friday	Saturday	Sunday
6 am							
7 am							
8 am							
11 pm							
12 am							
1 am							
2 am							
3 am							
4 am							
5 am							
Totals							

A Special Instructions:

Continence Chart

Name..

TOILETING REGIME
- No
✓ Yes

Date	Time	Is patient incontinent of urine?	Did patient ask for toilet? or Routine toileting?	Did patient pass urine?	Signatures

B

Figure 3–2. *Various types of continence charts.* A, *Simple chart.* B, *Continence assessment chart.* (B, *Courtesy of Longmore Hospital, Edinburgh, Scotland.)*

Illustration continued on following page

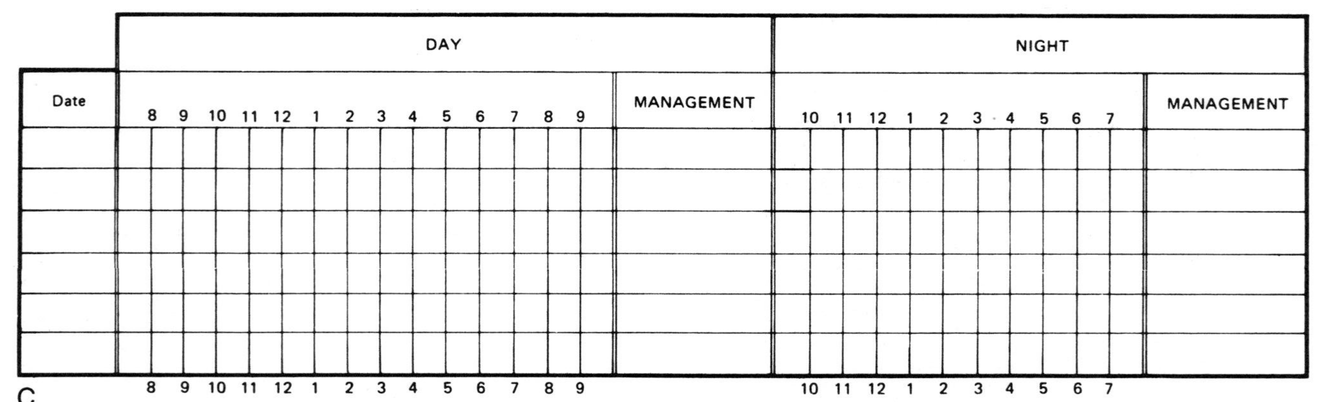

Date	DAY															NIGHT										
	8	9	10	11	12	1	2	3	4	5	6	7	8	9	MANAGEMENT	10	11	12	1	2	3	4	5	6	7	MANAGEMENT
	8	9	10	11	12	1	2	3	4	5	6	7	8	9		10	11	12	1	2	3	4	5	6	7	

C

Figure 3–2 Continued C, *Habit retraining chart (state of patient: dry, green dot; incontinent of urine, red dot; result of toileting: urine passed in toilet, blue dot; urine not passed in toilet, yellow dot; refused or absent: X in blue). (C, Courtesy of Geriatric Department, Dudley Road Hospital, Birmingham, England.)*

tempts that do not result in micturition might indicate an inappropriate schedule, inaccurate report of sensation to void, or inadequate mentation to associate toileting and passage of urine. Toileting a patient without results, followed by incontinence shortly afterwards, can indicate inhibition caused by lack of privacy during assisted toileting or feelings of being rushed by caregivers. Unsuccessful patient-initiated toileting usually indicates altered mentation or confusion concerning voiding behaviors or inaccurate sensations to void.

Figure 3–2*C* shows a continence chart designed for baseline assessment of urinary incontinence (Clay, 1978). It presupposes regular assessment (every 2 hours) of the patient (recorded to the left of the hour column) and nurse-initiated toileting, followed by recording of results in the column to the right of the hour line. Some caregivers will find recording on the chart complicated at first, but soon master the format. The chart requires four colored pens and provides a clear visual impression of voiding patterns.

Some charts use letters rather than checks or dots as their symbols. This increases the amount of information obtained within a single entry, but can cause confusion if too many symbols are used.

Other charts allow patients to record events that occur simultaneously with incontinence, such as coughing, exercise, or sensation of urgency. Patients can also indicate the amount of incontinence. This can be done when a pad is changed or by estimating how far the leakage spreads. Such measures are subjective, however, and accurate interpretation of findings is difficult.

Recording behavioral assessments can assist in the assessment of incontinence of confused patients. This should include what activities the patient was doing prior to incontinence, any indications of impending micturition or leakage (e.g., verbal or motor activity), and what actions were taken in response to these cues. This record also includes the events that precede and succeed continent voiding.

A continence assessment is kept for 4 to 7 days to obtain an accurate picture of voiding patterns. The chart helps to put the incontinence into perspective and can reduce the problem by focusing attention on toileting schedules. It also can show patterns of predictability in patients in whom incontinence has been considered out of control and intractable.

Assessment and Plan of Action

A careful history, thoughtful physical examination, and simple urodynamic assessment offer a detailed picture of a patient's incontinence, as well as the physical, social, and psychologic context within which incontinence occurs. Table 3–1 summarizes common relationships among urinary symptoms, dysfunctional states, and associated

*Table 3–1. RELATIONSHIP OF SYMPTOMS TO VOIDING DYSFUNCTION**

Presenting Symptoms	Most Likely Voiding Dysfunction	Common Associated or Causative Factors	Factors Likely to Exacerbate Symptoms
Urinary frequency; urgency, urge incontinence; nocturia	Detrusor instability	Neurologic disorders: brain (CVA, closed head injury, tumor), spinal cord (injury, spinovascular disease); irritative bladder disorder; bladder outlet obstruction; stress urinary incontinence; idiopathic factors	Immobility, impaired dexterity; visual deficit; poorly designed environment; anxiety; urinary tract infection
Stress incontinence (subjective report of leakage with physical exertion)	Genuine stress incontinence	Pelvic descent: multiple vaginal deliveries, estrogen deficiency; urethral sphincter incompetence: radical prostatectomy, transurethral prostatectomy, trauma denervation	Chronic cough; obesity
Poor force of stream; hesitancy; dribbling incontinence; urinary frequency, nocturia	Deficient detrusor function *or* bladder outlet obstruction	Deficient detrusor function: sacral spinal cord disorders, peripheral polyneuropathies, pelvic trauma, herpes zoster, chronic anemia; obstruction: prostatic enlargement (prostatic hyperplasia, cancer, inflammation), bladder neck hypertrophy, contracture or dyssynergia, detrusor-striated sphincter dyssynergia, urethral stricture or distortion	Fecal impaction; acute, debilitating illness; immobility
Continuous incontinence (absent warning or sensations of urgency)	Extraurethral leakage: vesicovaginal, urethrovaginal; urethrocutaneous fistula; urethral ectopia; epispadias, bladder exstrophy	Urinary ectopia, fistula; severe urethral sphincter incompetence; sphincteric incompetence: urethral trauma, iatrogenic trauma (multiple anti-incontinence procedures, etc.), denervation	
Unpredictable incontinence; no apparent reason	Functional incontinence	Alzheimer's disease	Disorientation, unfamiliar surroundings; immobility, deficient dexterity, vision; caregiver unaware of patient needs; depression, poor motivation; institutionalization or other crisis

*The relationships presented here are broad generalizations only.

medical conditions. Many patients, unfortunately, do not have a simple, readily identifiable, dysfunctional voiding state. A history, nursing assessment, and simple urodynamic assessment allow the clinician to establish a likely diagnosis of voiding dysfunction, probable causative medical conditions, and factors that affect the individual's ability to cope with incontinence. These findings are used to establish management goals and formulate a plan of action. A date is then set to review the outcome of this treatment plan.

Complex Urodynamic Studies

When symptoms are mixed or ambiguous, when surgery is contemplated, or when empiric treatment does not resolve urinary leakage, complex urodynamic testing is indicated. Complex urodynamic testing, performed as a portion of a more comprehensive assessment, provides invaluable information to help manage incontinence. In contrast, complex urodynamic test results obtained in the absence of an adequate nursing and medical assessment often do not completely determine why a person is incontinent, and do not identify the context and exacerbating factors that contribute to urinary leakage.

Complex urodynamics is a set of tests used to measure the transportation, storage, and expulsive function of the urinary tract (Webster, 1982). Common urodynamic tests include determination of the urinary flow rate, cystometry, electromyography, pressure-flow study, and urethral pressure study.

Flow Rate

The urinary flow rate can be measured simply by the use of a noninvasive uroflowmeter (Figs. 3–3*A* and *B*). The rate at which urine is expelled from the bladder is measured by a weight transducer, disruption of a spinning disk, light beam, or electromagnetic field. The patient is asked to refrain from voiding prior to testing and should void with a comfortably full bladder. The resulting uroflow chart plots flow rate (in milliliters per second) versus time (in seconds).

The urinary flow rate chart allows determination of several parameters. Maximum or peak flow is the highest flow rate achieved during micturition. In the normal adult this rate typically meets or exceeds 12 ml/second with a normal bladder volume (300 to 600 ml). The average or mean flow is determined by dividing volume voided by time. In normal adults the mean flow is 8 ml/second or more. Voided volume, postvoid residual, and voiding time are also obtained. A flow pattern is then diagnosed, which is used for screening or comparative purposes.

A normal flow pattern is characterized by adequate maximum and

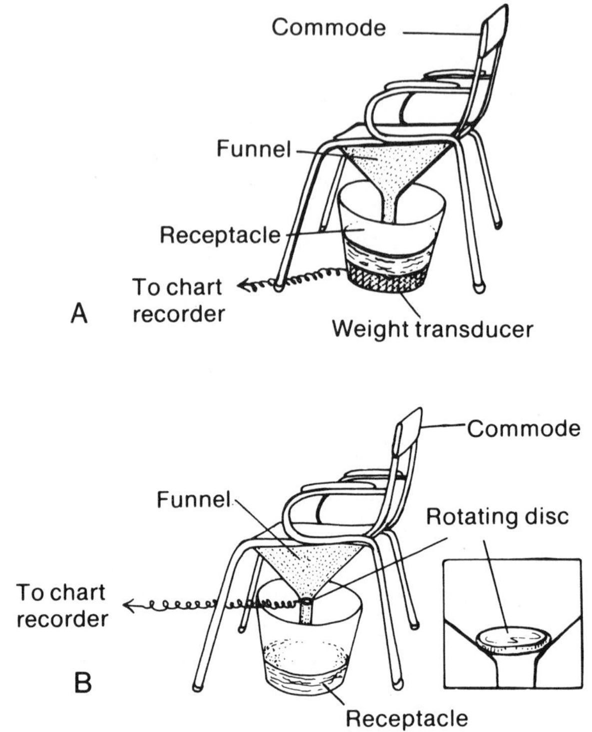

Figure 3–3. A, *Weight transducer flowmeter.* B, *Rotating disk flowmeter.*

mean flow, normal voided volume, and minimal residual. Women often have somewhat greater values than do men. Small voided volumes will result in lower values; use of a flow rate nomogram allows assessment of urine flow using volumes as low as 90 to 100 ml (Krane and Siroky, 1979). The normal flow pattern is shaped like a bell curve and can be slightly skewed to the left. It is uncommon in the presence of obstruction, but does not rule out the possibility of unstable bladder (Fig. 3–4).

An intermittent flow pattern is distinguished by a low mean flow and a characteristic saw-toothed configuration. The maximum flow can be normal or below normal; the residual is often elevated (Fig. 3–5*A*). An intermittent flow pattern occurs as a result of deficient detrusor function (weak bladder muscle tone) or bladder outlet obstruction. A poor flow pattern is characterized by a low maximum and mean flow and by a prolonged voiding time (Fig. 3–5*B*). It is characteristic of bladder outlet obstruction, but deficient detrusor function cannot be excluded. An explosive flow pattern is distinguished by a high peak and mean flow and by its characteristically brief voiding time (Fig. 3–

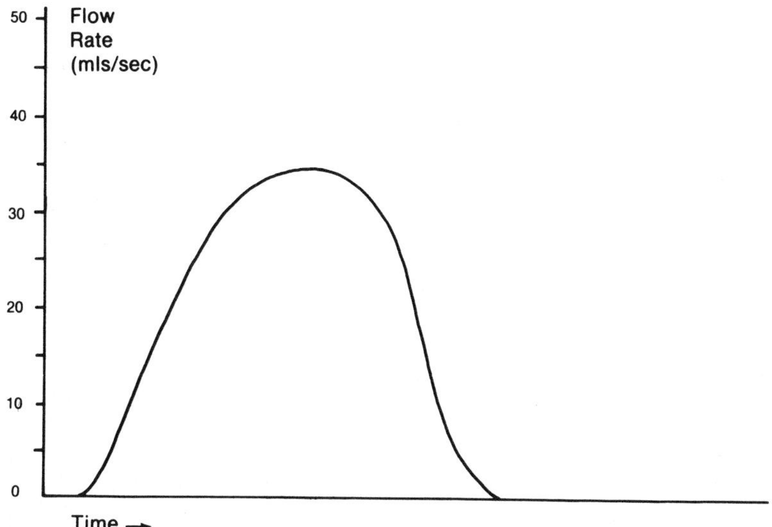

Figure 3–4. Normal flow curve.

5*C*). The explosive flow pattern is commonly seen in women with stress urinary incontinence, but it is also noted as a variant of normal.

Cystometry

The cystometrogram (CMG) is the cornerstone of urodynamic investigation. It is a graphic representation of bladder function comparing volume and pressure. Cystometry is performed by measuring pressure in the bladder, which is filled with carbon dioxide or a liquid (e.g., sterile water, saline solution, or radiographic contrast solution).

The CMG is best obtained by inserting two catheters—one is used to fill the bladder and the other to measure pressure within the bladder (intravesical pressure) (Fig. 3–6). A tube is then passed into the lower portion of the rectum for abdominal pressure measurement. The catheter used to fill the bladder is connected to a fluid reservoir. The two pressure monitoring tubes are connected to a chart recorder by pressure transducers (Fig. 3–6), which convert pressure into electricity and produce a tracing.

CMG is divided into two phases, filling and emptying. Bladder filling is assessed by infusion of a liquid or gas at a continuous rate. Three infusion rates (defined by the International Continence Society, 1984) can be used; a rapid infusion is greater than 100 ml/minute, a medium fill rate is 30 to 100 ml/minute, and a slow fill rate is lower than 30 ml/minute. The patient is asked to report the first sensation of filling, strong urge to urinate, and sensation of bladder fullness. Functional capacity is determined by filling the patient to the maximum

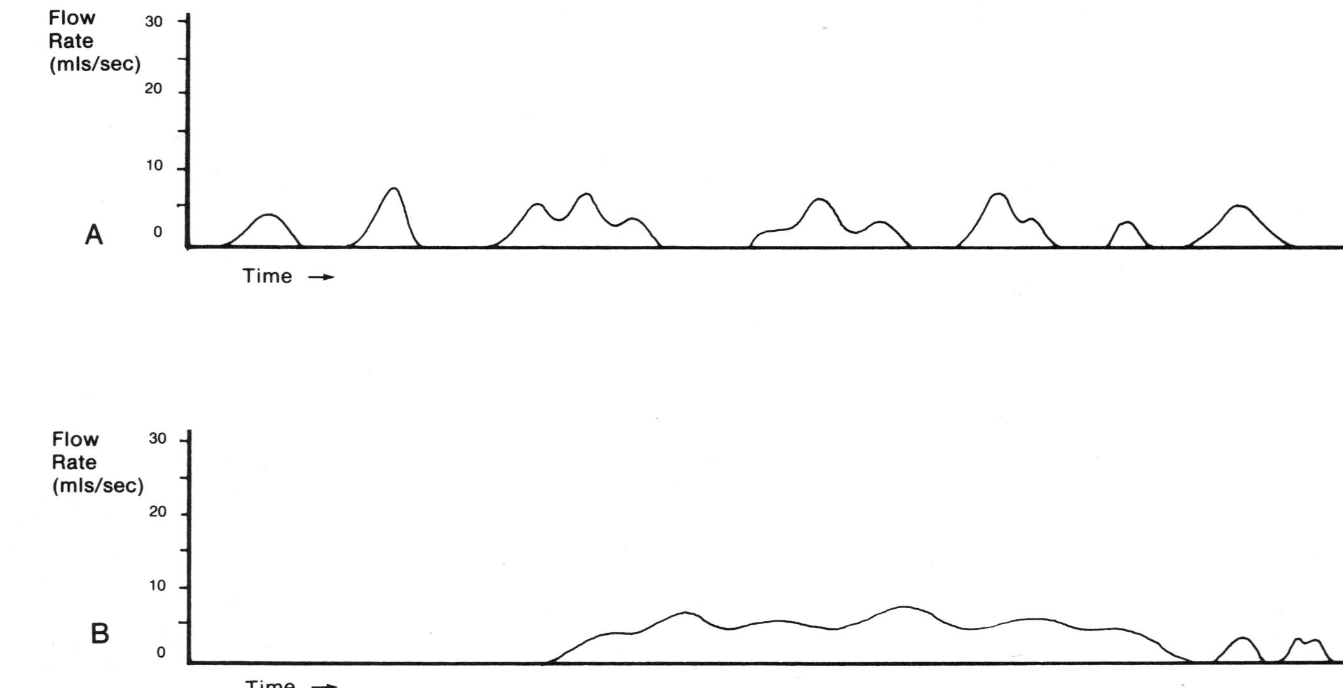

Figure 3–5. A, *Intermittent flow pattern interpreted as deficient detrusor function versus bladder outlet obstruction.* B, *Poor flow pattern interpreted as bladder outlet obstruction versus deficient detrusor function.*

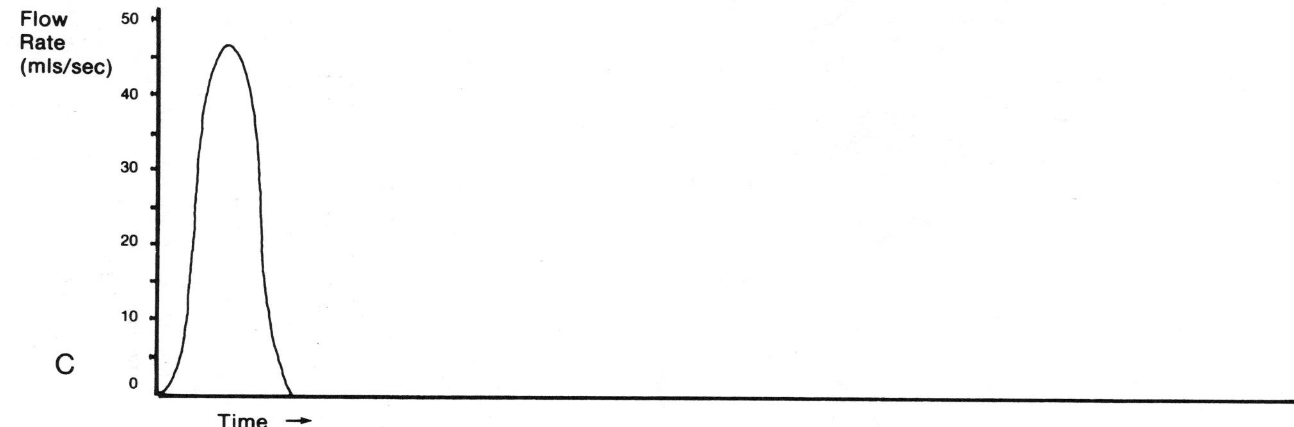

Figure 3–5 Continued C, *Explosive flow pattern commonly found in women with stress urinary incontinence, but could be variant of normal.*

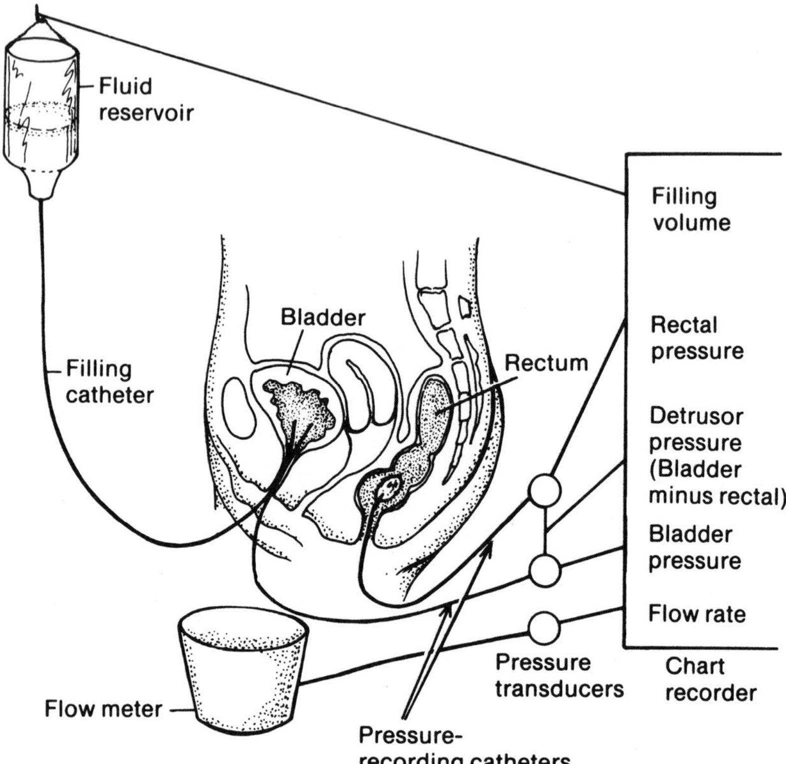

Figure 3–6. *Schematic representation of cystometry.*

capacity that can be tolerated without undue discomfort. The patient is instructed to refrain from voiding until asked to do so. Micturition is assessed by removing the filling catheter and asking the patient to urinate.

The goal of filling cystometry is to provoke dysfunctional bladder behavior by reproducing stressors that commonly affect the urinary tract. To be diagnostic this test must reproduce the voiding symptoms a patient commonly experiences without producing artifactual findings. Bladder filling is often sufficiently provocative to reproduce a dysfunctional voiding condition. If expected symptoms are not reproduced by bladder filling other provocative maneuvers, such as running a faucet, coughing, walking, or jumping, are used to provoke the patient's voiding dysfunction.

The goal of voiding cystometry is to assess bladder emptying. Micturition is best assessed by comparing detrusor contractions with urinary flow and the sphincteric response to contraction. After the filling catheter is removed the patient voids into a uroflowmeter with an intravesical pressure tube, abdominal pressure tube, and electromyography apparatus in place. These parameters are often combined with electromyography of the pelvic floor and can be done under fluoroscopic monitoring to assess bladder morphology during micturition.

Interpretation of the CMG reflects the two phases of bladder function, filling and voiding. A CMG produces three recordings used to make an interpretation. The intravesical catheter detects all pressures reflected in the bladder. Because the bladder is an abdominal organ it is subjected to pressure produced by the bladder muscle (detrusor pressure) and pressure from the abdomen. The rectal catheter detects abdominal pressure. Urodynamic strip chart recorders can subtract abdominal pressure from intravesical (bladder) pressure. The resulting parameter is called the detrusor pressure, which represents the pressure that the bladder muscle exerts against intravesical contents during filling and voiding. Measurement of all three pressures allows the tester to distinguish bladder pressure created by movement and abdominal straining from pressure created by detrusor muscle contraction.

Figure 3–7 is a schematic representation of a normal urodynamic study. The cystometrogram is interpreted by four main parameters. Capacity represents the volume that the patient can hold while fully awake without undue discomfort or bladder contraction. Bladder wall compliance represents change in bladder pressure as a function of volume. The normal bladder can fill from 0 to 300 ml or more, with little change in detrusor pressure. This is represented by the nearly flat nature of the detrusor pressure line throughout bladder filling, despite steadily increasing bladder volume.

The sensations of filling represent the patient's subjective reports of bladder fullness. The first sensation of bladder filling (first urge) usually occurs between 90 and 150 ml; feelings of bladder fullness occur between 300 and 600 ml. It is important to attempt to distinguish between feelings of urgency and abdominal fullness. Sensory urgency is typically perceived at the glans penis or clitoris; abdominal fullness is centered above the symphysis pubis (Mundy, 1985).

The concept of detrusor or bladder instability is central to an understanding of urinary incontinence and urodynamic testing. The normal bladder should not contract at any time during filling or storage, despite provocative maneuvers such as coughing, physical exertion, or taking a warm shower. The stable bladder contracts only when the person wishes to urinate. In contrast, the unstable bladder experiences uninhibited or inappropriately timed contractions in response to provocative maneuvers such as bladder filling or coughing. The International Continence Society (1984) has limited unstable contractions to those that meet or exceed 15 cm H_2O assessed as detrusor pressure.

Figure 3–8 shows a schematic of common urodynamic abnormalities diagnosed by cystometry combined with a urinary flow study and electromyography. Figure 3–8*A* shows an unstable bladder. The ab-

Text continued on page 62

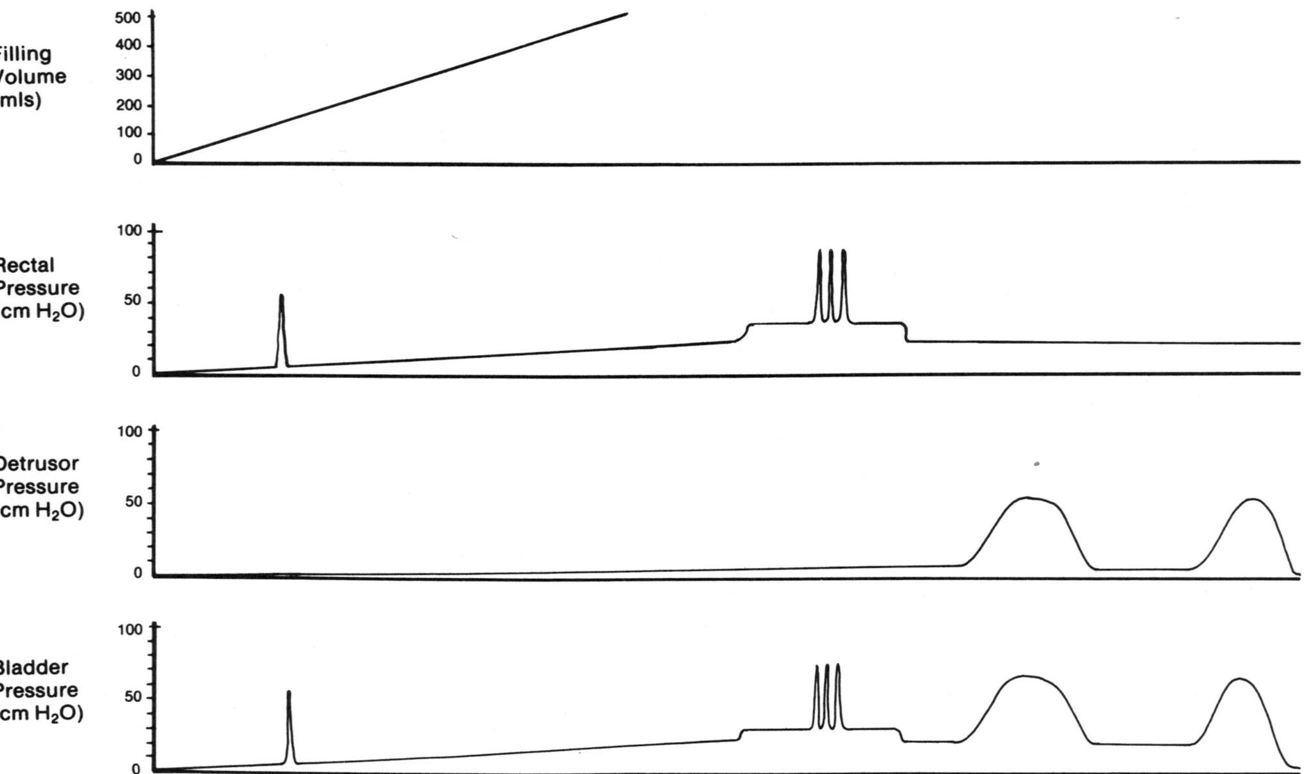

Figure 3–7. *Normal urodynamic study.*

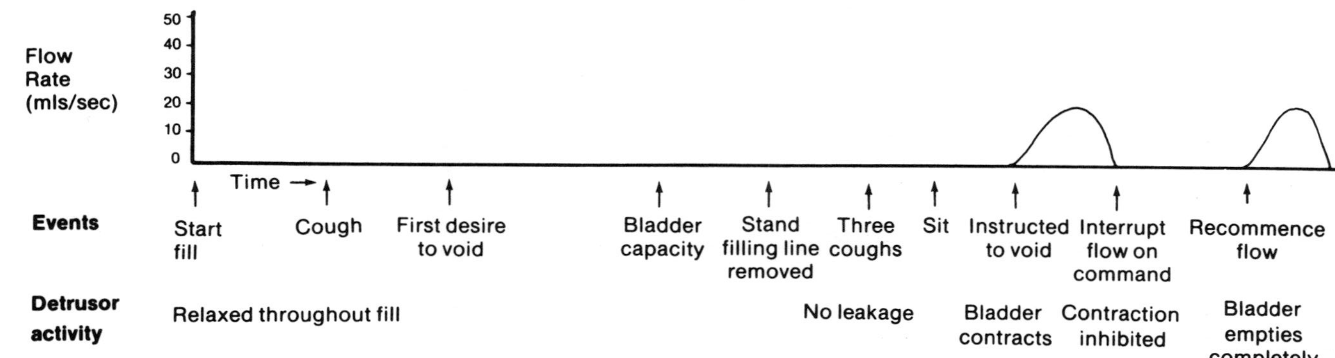

Figure 3–7 Continued *Normal urodynamic study.*

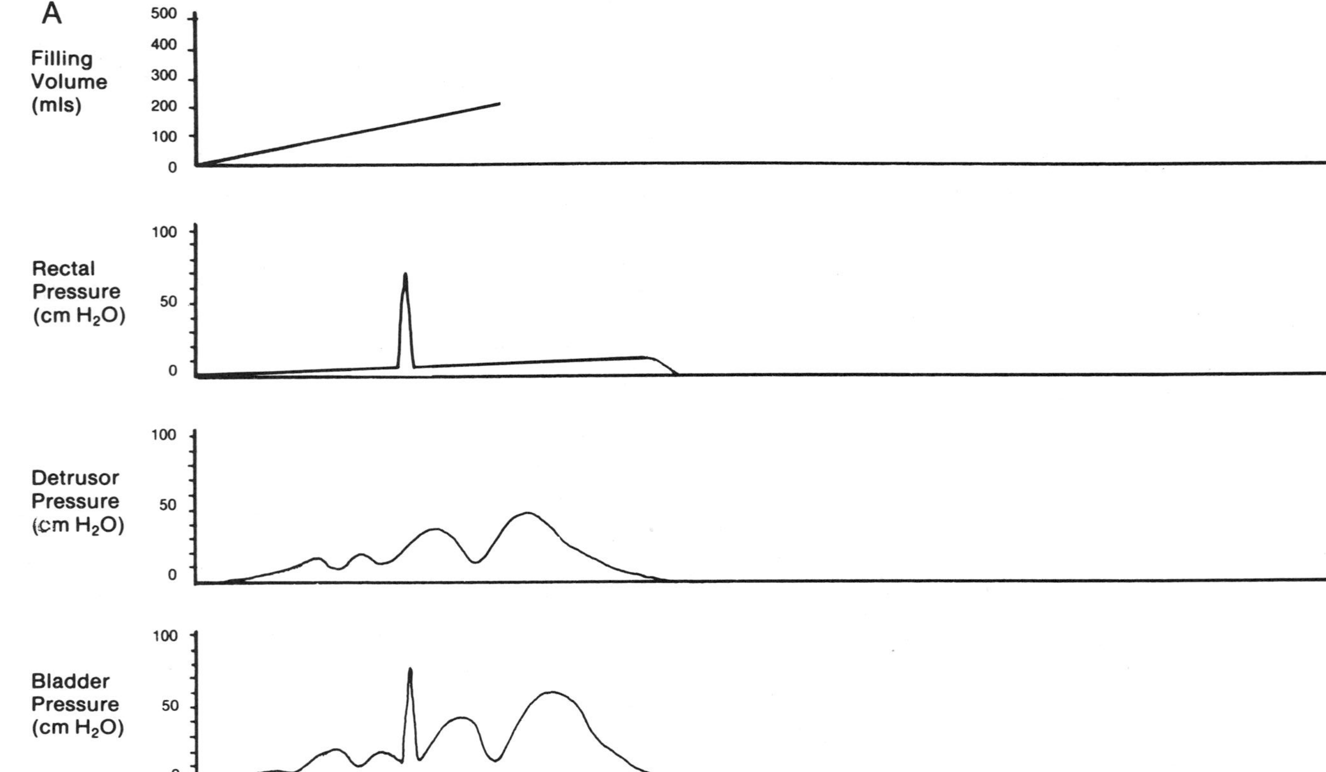

Figure 3–8. *Urodynamic studies.* A, *Detrusor instability.*

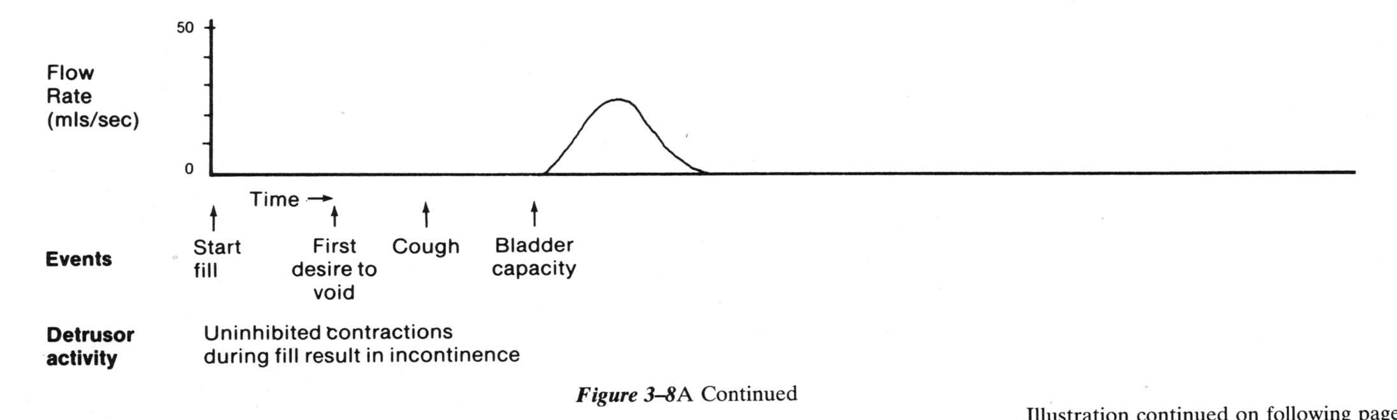

*Figure 3–8*A Continued

Illustration continued on following page

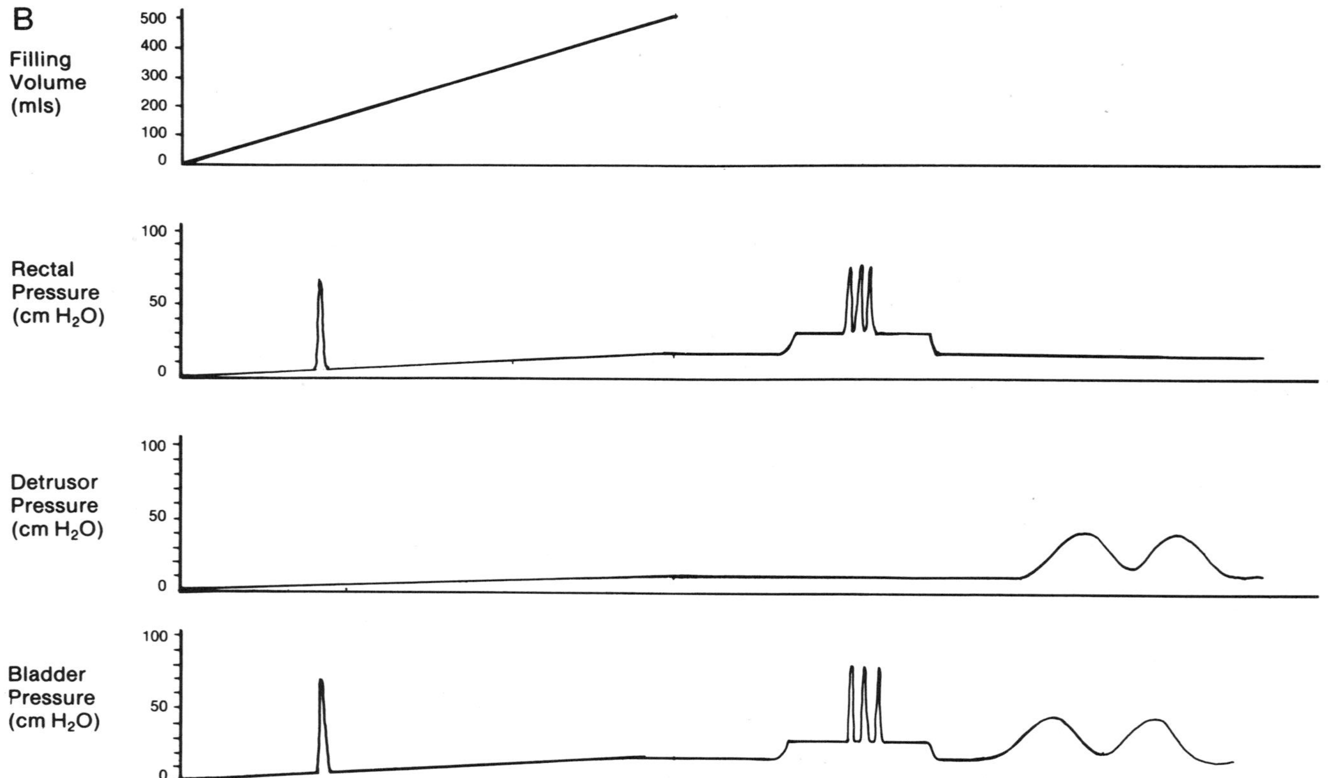

Figure 3–8 Continued B, *Genuine stress urinary incontinence.*

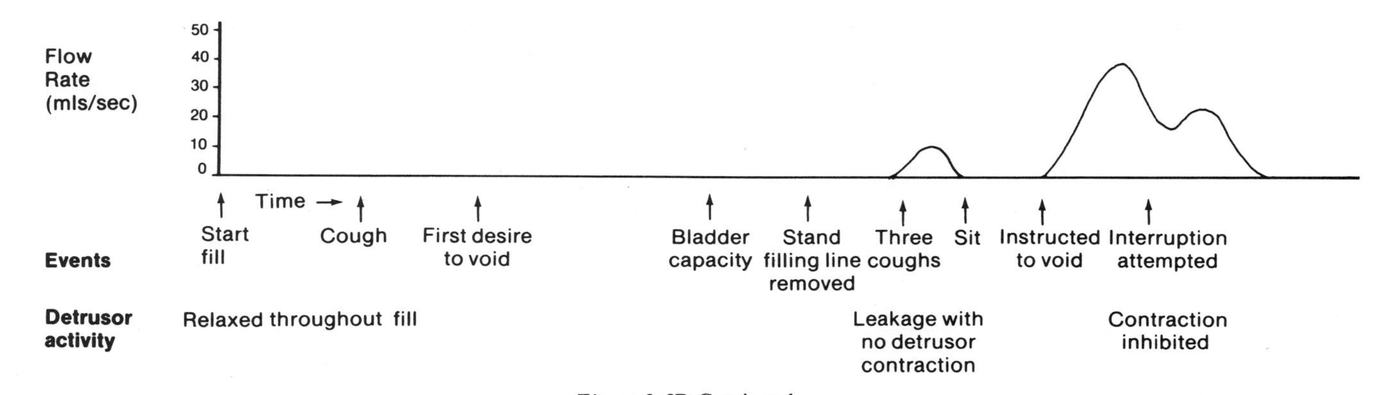

*Figure 3–8*B Continued

Illustration continued on following page

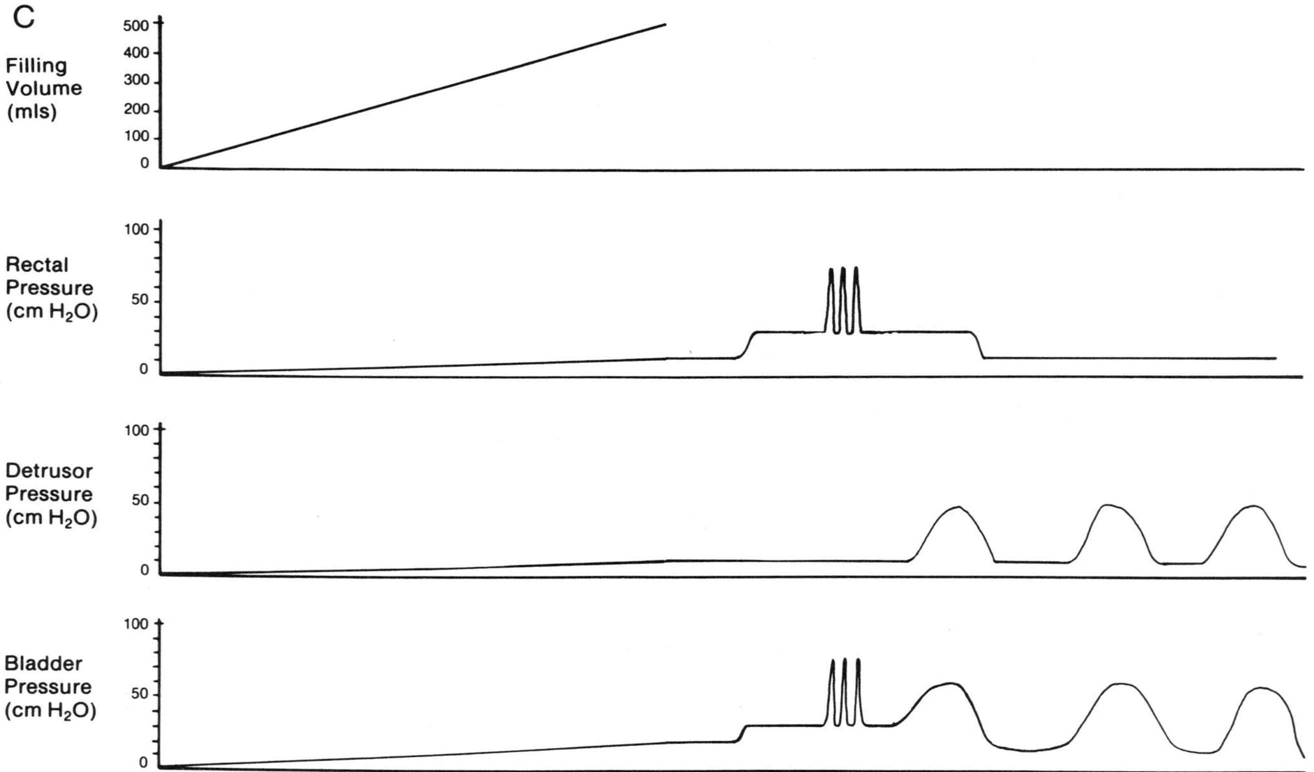

Figure 3–8 Continued C, *Mixed stress and urge incontinence.*

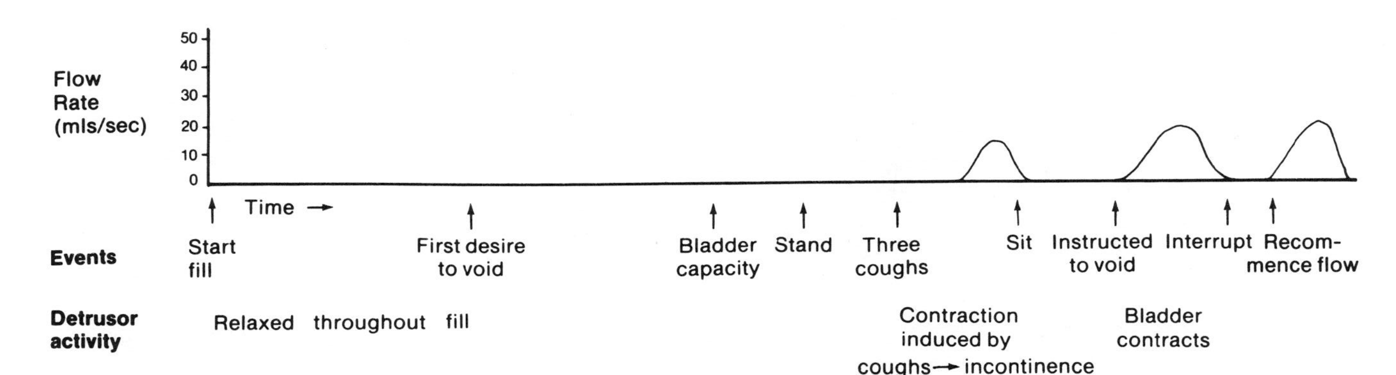

Figure 3–8C Continued

Illustration continued on following page

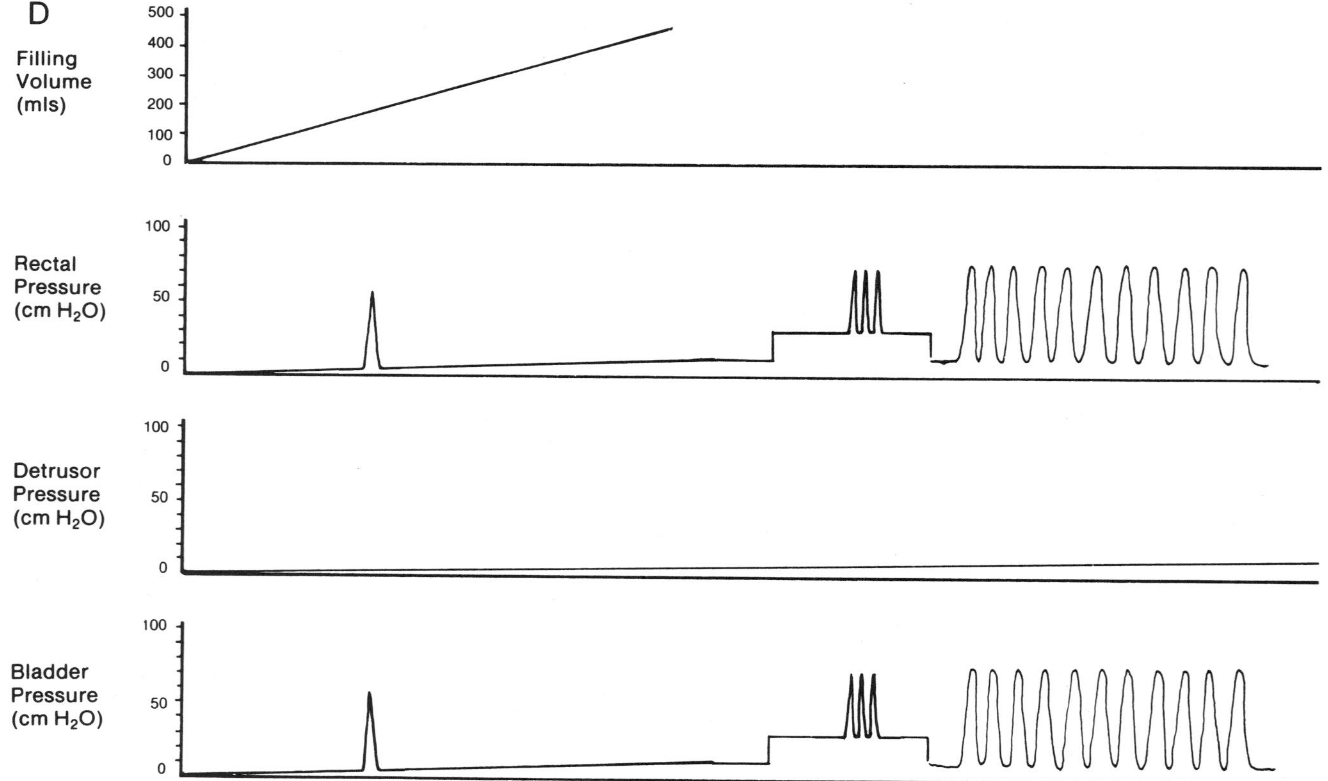

Figure 3–8 Continued D, *Large-capacity bladder with absent detrusor muscle function.*

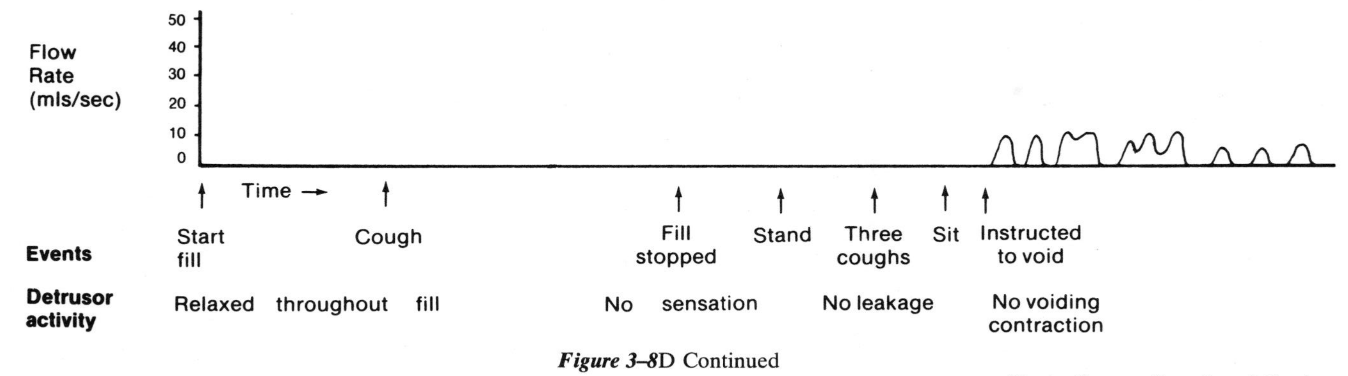

Figure 3–8*D* Continued

Illustration continued on following page

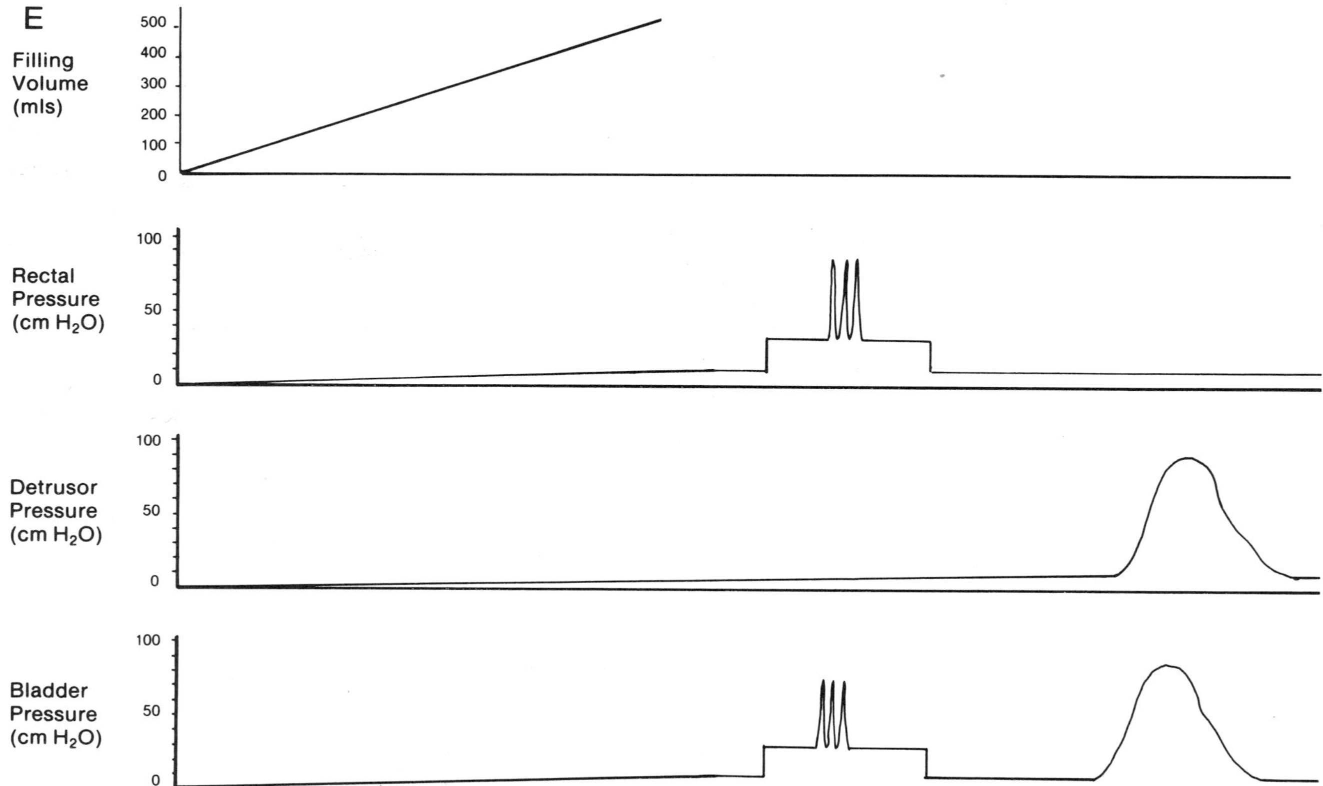

Figure 3–8 Continued E, *Bladder outlet obstruction.*

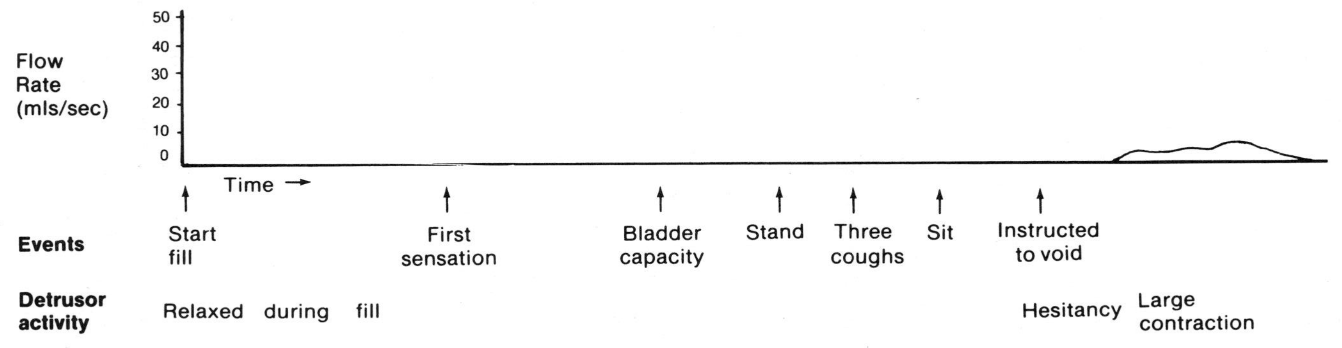

*Figure 3–8*E Continued

normality is noted in the detrusor and intravesical pressure tracings of the CMG. The upward slope of the bell-shaped curve in the detrusor and intravesical pressure channels represents contraction of the bladder muscle followed by muscle relaxation. Small functional capacity, sensory urgency, and urge incontinence are common associated findings.

Figure 3–8*B* illustrates common urodynamic tracings associated with genuine stress incontinence. The CMG and electromyogram are entirely normal. The flow pattern is explosive and contraction pressure during voluntary voiding is often quite low (<30 cm H_2O). Incontinence can be measured by a uroflowmeter or observed by the tester in association with physical exertion such as coughing or laughing. Leakage is not associated with a detrusor contraction.

Figure 3–8*C* demonstrates mixed stress and urge incontinence. The abnormality is noted during bladder filling when coughing produces stress urinary incontinence followed by an unstable contraction with urge incontinence. Urge incontinence occurs because of an unstable bladder contraction, which can result from urine entering the posterior urethra during an episode of stress incontinence (Gray and Dougherty, 1987). There is a close temporal relationship between leakage associated with physical stress and onset of an uninhibited contraction.

Figure 3–8*D* illustrates urodynamic findings associated with deficient detrusor contraction. The filling cystometrogram typically shows an enlarged capacity with delayed sensations of filling. Analysis of the pressure flow study demonstrates intermittent flow pattern with absent contraction; voiding occurs by abdominal strain.

Figure 3–8*E* demonstrates urodynamic findings typical of bladder outlet obstruction. Filling cystometry can be normal or can demonstrate detrusor instability (Anderson, 1982). The diagnosis of obstruction is made by analysis of the pressure-flow study. The flow pattern is typically poor or intermittent, with abdominal enhancement of the voided stream. The voiding pressure is high (>60 cm H_2O). Obstruction can also be evaluated with a computer-generated plot of pressure versus flow or by calculation of a Bernoulli resistance factor.

Urethral Pressure Studies

Urethral pressure studies are designed to measure intraurethral pressure during bladder filling or during micturition. The goal of any urethral pressure study is objective assessment of the function of the urethral sphincteric mechanism. The urethral pressure profile is a static measurement of urethral closure pressure and functional urethral length during bladder filling. During the procedure a catheter is slowly pulled through the urethra and pressure is measured by microtip or by an external dome transducer. The clinical relevance and usefulness of the urethral pressure profile remains unclear.

Dynamic urethral pressure studies are designed to measure urethral sphincter responses to stress or micturition. A stress urethral pressure study or cough profile measures the urethral response under conditions similar to those that produce stress urinary incontinence. A catheter is withdrawn slowly through the urethra or placed at the point of maximum urethral closure pressure while the patient is asked to cough. Intraurethral pressure and intravesical pressure are measured simultaneously and a third recording is made that subtracts intravesical pressure from intraurethral pressure.

In the normal person, intraurethral pressure remains consistently higher than intravesical pressure, even under physical stress such as coughing, and urinary leakage is prevented. The tracing produced by subtracting intravesical from intraurethral pressure reflects this maintenance of positive closure pressure. When stress urinary incontinence occurs, intravesical pressure briefly exceeds intraurethral pressure, causing the sphincter to open briefly so that urinary leakage occurs. The tracing produced by subtracting intravesical pressure from intraurethral pressure reflects this loss of positive closure pressure.

References and Further Reading

Anderson, J.T.: Prostatism: Clinical, radiological, and urodynamic aspects. Neurourol. Urodynamics, *1:*241, 1982.

Clay, E.C.: Incontinence of urine. Nurs. Mirror, *146:*No. 9, 14; No. 10, 36; No. 11, 23; No. 12, 23; 1978.

Gray, M.L., and Broadwell, D.C.: Genitourinary system. *In* Thompson, J., et al. (eds.): Clinical Nursing. St. Louis, C.V. Mosby, 1986, pp. 1283–1299.

Gray, M.L., and Dougherty, M.C.: Urinary incontinence—pathophysiology and treatment. J. Enterost. Ther. *14:*152, 1987.

Griffiths, D.J.: Urodynamics: The Mechanisms and Hydrodynamics of the Lower Urinary tract. Bristol, England, Adam Hilger, 1980.

Incontinence Action Group: Action on Incontinence. London, Kings Fund Center, 1983.

International Continence Society Committee on Standardization of Terminology: The Standardization of Terminology of Lower Urinary Tract Function. Glasgow, Scotland, International Continence Society, 1984.

Krane, R., and Siroky, M.B.: Clinical Neurology. Boston, Little, Brown, & Co., 1979.

Mandelstam, D. (ed.): Incontinence and its Management. Breckenham, England, Croom & Helm, 1980.

Mundy, A.R.: The unstable bladder. Clin. Obstet. Gynecol., *12:*431, 1985.

Mundy, A.R., Stephenson, T.P., and Wein, A.J.: Urodynamics: Principles, Practice and Application. London, Churchill-Livingstone, 1984.

Norton, C.S.: Assessing incontinence. Nursing, *1:*789, 1980.

Norton, C.S.: "The promotion of continence." Nurs. Times (Suppl.), *80:*4, 1984.

Stanton, S.L. (ed.): Gynecologic urology. Clin. Obstet. Gynecol., *5:*1, 1978.

Stanton, S.L. (ed.): Clinical Gynecologic Urology. Part 2: Investigation. St. Louis, C.V. Mosby, 1984.

Turner-Warwick, R.T.: Foreword. *In* Mundy, A.R., et al. (eds.): Urodynamics: Principles, Practice and Application. London, Churchill-Livingstone, 1984.

Webster, G.D.: Urodynamics. *In* Resnick, M.I., and Older, R.A. (eds.): Diagnosis of Genitourinary Disease. New York, Thieme-Stratton, 1982, p. 173.

Katherine F. Jeter, EdD, ET

4 Treating and Managing Incontinence

The general principles involved in treating and managing urinary incontinence and that pertain to any incontinent person are presented in this chapter (Table 4–1). Subsequent chapters will discuss specific types of incontinence and specific groups of incontinent people.

All interventions must take into consideration information gathered during the assessment and investigation of the individual's incontinence (Chap. 3). Treatment aims to alter factors that have been causing incontinence. Management, on the other hand, aims to ameliorate the effects of being incontinent on individuals and their caregivers. Obviously, *treatment aimed at cure and management aimed at improved coping* cannot be separated completely. Both are usually implemented at the same time.

Sometimes only one intervention is indicated—this tends to be the case for the younger, otherwise healthy, incontinent person. In other, more complex, cases, various interventions will be required, and several

Table 4–1. *TYPES OF URINARY INCONTINENCE, CHARACTERISTICS, AND TREATMENT*

Type	Characteristics	Definition	Usual Causes	Diagnostic Procedures	Possible Treatment
Stress	Common in women; loss of urine, usually in small amounts, with increases in intraabdominal pressure (e.g., coughing, laughing, lifting, exercise)	Involuntary loss of urine when intraabdominal pressures increase	Weakness of pelvic floor muscles (e.g., because of childbirth); bladder neck descension; sphincter weakness; obesity may exacerbate; iatrogenic; sphincter damage	Marshall test; cystoscopy; cystometry; StressCath; urethral pressure profile; sphincter electromyography; Q-Tip test; pad test	Pelvic floor exercises (Kegel); biofeedback; electrical stimulation; alpha-adrenergic agonists (e.g., pseudoephedrine, phenylpropanolamine, imipramine); conjugated estrogens (oral, topical); bladder neck suspension surgery; artificial sphincter; vaginal pessary; pads, diapers
Urge	Urgency; frequency; nocturia; suprapubic discomfort; loss of urine in any position; loss of entire bladder volume	Spontaneous contraction of the bladder on provocation when the patient is attempting to inhibit contraction	Genitourinary abnormalities; neurologic conditions (e.g., stroke, multiple sclerosis, spinal cord injury); bladder inflammation (e.g., bladder infection); functional	Cystometry; uroflowmetry; cystoscopy	Anticholinergic or antispasmodic drugs; biofeedback; bladder retraining; habit training; scheduled toileting; electrical stimulation; estrogen; removal of obstruction; removal of irritating agent; antibiotic (if caused by infection); external collection device
Overflow	Frequent to nearly continuous dripping of urine; small amounts lost (frequently); large residuals; bladder is overdistended; diminished stream; impaired sensation of bladder fullness	Leakage of small amounts of urine caused by mechanical forces on an overdistended bladder	Bladder outlet obstruction because of enlarged prostate, urethral stricture, or cancer; deficient detrusor function because of medications or neurologic lesions (e.g., multiple sclerosis, myelomeningocele, diabetes, trauma); large prolapse (e.g., cystocele in females); detrusor-sphincter dyssynergia	Uroflowmetry; cystoscopy; cystometry	Surgical removal of obstruction; intermittent catheterization; cholinergic agonists; alpha-adrenergic blockers; indwelling catheter
Functional	Voiding at inappropriate times; usually, loss of full bladder volume; norml muscle and sphincter function	Urinary leakage caused by inability to reach toilet on time	Impaired mental status (e.g., Alzheimer's, retardation, closed head injury, emotional illness); unfamiliar environment; inaccessible facilities	Cystometry; uroflowmetry	Habit training; scheduled toileting; external collection device; environmental manipulation

From Wheeler, J. S., Niecestra, R. M., and Coggins, S. J.: Urinary incontinence: Diagnosing the problem. J. Enterost. Ther., *6*:242, 1988.

different team members will be needed. There are few people for whom attempt at cure is inappropriate—usually only the critically or terminally ill and the profoundly retarded. For most patients cure or considerable improvement is possible and should be attempted. For those with intractable incontinence, efficient and appropriate management methods are essential so that incontinence does not itself become a handicap.

NURSING MANAGEMENT AND ADVICE

Nurses play a key role in providing advice and support to incontinent individuals and their families. Minimizing the effect of incontinence on patients and their surroundings means that most can lead a relatively normal life, despite their bladder dysfunction. Whenever nurses advise patients and family the basic principles of teaching should be respected, with due consideration of the readiness and ability to learn. Information should only be given a little at a time, and repeated often. Written information is essential, because it can be reviewed at a later time.

Explaining the Problem

Many people are ignorant about how their body functions, and their understanding of incontinence might be based on common misconceptions. A clear explanation of the normal lower urinary tract and how it has *not* functioned can help patients to participate in their own therapy. Patients who understand their condition can be more active in tackling their problems, but the tendency of many nurses and physicians has been to remove that responsibility from individuals by not imparting sufficient information. Even if patients are incapable of learning, the rest of the family can benefit from teaching.

Providing information can also help patients and their families to make decisions about treatment options when alternatives exist. For example, if surgery is suggested, patients must be told what is involved with the operative procedure, the chances of success, and possible risks and side effects. Of course, the surgeon will discuss these, but often patients ask a nurse for detailed information. Many people are reluctant to ask what they think are obvious questions and to reveal their fears and ignorance. Nurses should allow time for this, and should offer encouragement to patients and help them make informed decisions.

Psychologic Support

Nurses' attitudes toward incontinent patients should demonstrate that they do not regard incontinence as a stigma, but rather as a symptom of an underlying condition. The guilt, shame, and embarrassment felt by many incontinent people (and by their relatives) can be lessened by caregivers who treat patients with respect. This is vital, because so many incontinent people can lose all self-esteem and confidence and become pessimistic about the possibilities of improvement. Nurses should be comfortable about discussing intimate details if patients are to express their fears and worries. It might be tempting to dismiss unfounded fears quickly, but a brusque statement such as "Of course you don't smell," "Nobody thinks you're a baby," or "Of course your husband [or wife] still finds you attractive" does little to provide reassurance. Nurses who can develop a close and trusting relationship with their patients can empathize more closely with their problems and can be in a better position to help them with their needs.

Support takes different forms. Sometimes just listening is enough. Acting as a sounding board for the expression of feelings, especially frustration and anger, can be useful in defusing tensions within a family. Often, individuals can be helped to reach their own solutions with the help of a nurse who listens and encourages them to express their problems, rather than a nurse who talks continually and leaves no room for response.

Improving their self-image is an essential part of enabling incontinent people to cope with incontinence. If interpersonal or sexual relationships have suffered because of the incontinence, considerable encouragement is needed before patients will attempt to resume normal relationships. Fear of rejection is powerful and restricting. Relatives who care for an incontinent person at home need as much support as the patient. It is easy to see how relatives might come to feel inadequate, hopeless, and guilty about not doing all that they could, especially if they compare themselves to professional caregivers who appear to be competent and able to cope. Under such circumstances, home health nurses might find themselves spending as much time reassuring and listening to caregivers as they do providing nursing care to the patient.

Some incontinent people need more formal psychologic help; in situations in which the nurse does not have the appropriate training or expertise, it might be better to refer to a counselor, psychiatrist, psychologist, or sexual dysfunction counselor. Nurses must be able to recognize their own limitations and the point at which another professional would be of greater help to patients.

Skin Care

Proper skin care is essential for anyone who is incontinent. Patients who are incontinent and immobile are at higher risk of developing pressure sores (Willington, 1975; Allman, 1986). Urine and feces can both irritate the skin, and also provide a damp, warm environment that is ideal for the proliferation of pathogenic microorganisms. Healthy skin depends on the general state of the patient, especially in regard to a balanced diet and adequate fluid intake, and on impeccable skin care. Sick or debilitated patients are more vulnerable to skin breakdown. Nurses can provide useful advice on diet, general health care, and the prevention and treatment of skin problems.

The most important element of skin care is thorough cleansing of the entire genital area (and any other skin in contact with urine or feces) at least twice daily, and every time an absorbent product or device is changed. Ideally, a bath or shower should be taken daily, but this is not always practical and a sponge bath must sometimes suffice. Elderly people should bathe less frequently to avoid drying their skin. Warm water and a cleanser specifically formulated for those who are incontinent should be used. Heavily scented soaps can provoke a skin reaction, and could cause discomfort if the skin is already sore. After washing, the skin must be gently and thoroughly dried with a soft towel. When the skin is dry, a moisture barrier cream or film should be applied. The cream should be used sparingly, because too much can make the skin surface soggy and actually increase the risk of problems. Talcum powder should be avoided, because it can irritate the skin, especially if it is strongly perfumed. Powder tends to form lumps when dampened by urine or sweat and can cause moisture to be trapped in the groin skin folds.

A skin rash that is fiery red, itches, and burns is usually of fungal origin. The nurse should request an order from the patient's physician for an antifungal cream or powder. The skin should be treated with the antifungal prescription two or three times daily, after it has been washed with the incontinence cleanser.

If the skin is becoming sore, causes other than the incontinence should be kept in mind. A collection device or absorbent product could be the cause. A diaper might have a rough surface or might be trapping moisture next to the skin, or a device might be too tight. Plastic in contact with wet skin is a particular source of trouble, and plastic pants should be avoided. Some patients' skin is sensitive to the materials used in absorbent products or devices, and inflammation might be caused by an allergic reaction. In some cases pressure and friction are more significant causes of skin problems than urine. In elderly women a sore vulva might be caused by atrophic vaginitis, rather than by incontinence.

In rare cases the only viable method of healing damaged skin is the temporary placement of an indwelling catheter to control the incontinence. This should never be used solely for nursing convenience (Chap. 13), but might be unavoidable for the relief of skin problems or pressure sores.

Controlling Odor and Soiling

Odor is one of the greatest fears of incontinent people. They might restrict their activities and social contacts, not because of obvious leakage, but because they worry that their smell will be offensive to others. In our society natural odors are taboo, and a great deal of money is spent on disguising everyday smells in the home and on the body. If ordinary perspiration odors are considered unacceptable, consider that this is more true for bowel and bladder contents. People who smell of urine or stool are considered to be socially unacceptable, and are avoided. Most people assume that those who smell bad must neglect themselves and be unclean.

For most incontinent people the worry is unfounded, because the odor that they perceive is not noticeable to others. Freshly voided urine has only a faint odor, provided it is not concentrated and is free of infection. If attention is paid to personal hygiene, even those with a total lack of bladder control should not smell. Odor becomes offensive only if urine is allowed to linger because of the breakdown of urine components on contact with air. If possible, soiled pads and clothing should be changed as soon as incontinence has occurred. Appliances are less of a problem, because urine is contained in a collection device. Washing the skin might not be feasible after each episode of incontinence, but it must be done regularly. Fecal incontinence presents a more difficult problem (Chap. 14).

If urine odor is particularly offensive, the patient should be encouraged to increase fluid intake and the urine must be tested for evidence of infection. A most effective method of preventing odor is ensuring that the incontinence is well contained by an absorbent product or appliance and that clothing and home furnishings are protected from wetness. When a pad is removed, it should immediately be put into a sealable plastic bag or a container with a tight-fitting lid. Appliances should be washed thoroughly each day. They can be soaked in a commercial cleanser or in a solution of equal parts of white vinegar and water. The appliance should be rinsed with cool water to dispel the pungent odor of the cleanser.

Soiled cloths, beds, chairs, and carpets are often the source of lingering smells. Some materials, notably wool, seem to exacerbate the problem. Furniture can be difficult to clean when soiled, but this problem can be overcome by the use of a plastic cover. This can make the bed or chair uncomfortable and hot, however, and many people do not wish to live in an environment in which everything is plastic-covered. It can be difficult to strike a balance between adequate protection and an acceptable environment.

Slippers are often a particular source of odor. Shoes that can be wiped easily are preferable to nonwashable bedroom slippers. It should be stressed to nursing personnel and to people who are incontinent and their families that incontinence is to be managed at the level of the bladder, rather than at the feet and ankles.

Not all incontinent people can maintain high standards of hygiene, especially those who live alone, those who are disabled, or both. Some people have difficulty in washing soiled clothing and bedding. The problem can be eased by advising the person to buy clothing and bedding made of materials that are easily laundered and quick-drying. Dark clothing tends to show wet spots less, and can be helpful in lessening embarrassment when the incontinent person is careless about using an absorbent product.

Some people seem unconcerned about odor and cleanliness. In extreme cases they are excluded from activities and are banned from social, family, and even work settings. It might be a visiting nurse or office nurse who is called on to discuss the situation frankly with the patient. Of course, the main focus of every nurse's attention should be treating the incontinence, rather than disguising wetness and banishing odor.

When odor is a problem (real or imagined), several types of deodorizers can be helpful. Some preparations can be taken orally to deodorize the urine as it is expelled from the body. Some absorbent products have deodorizing agents incorporated within their layers. Room deodorizers are available that eliminate odor, rather than masking it, without leaving a smell more pungent than the offending one.

Fluid Intake

Many incontinent people restrict fluid intake in an attempt to control incontinence. If taken to extremes, however, this practice can lead to dehydration—even to electrolyte imbalance—and confusion, especially in older persons. Others can suffer almost continuous thirst, which can become unpleasant. Fluid restriction should usually be discouraged, and can actually be counterproductive, for several reasons. Low urine production combined with frequent voiding means that the bladder is never fully expanded. Although this might not physically reduce bladder capacity, it is likely to make the bladder sensitive to a smaller habitual volume. Low fluid intake can worsen any tendency to constipation. Also, concentrated urine might actually irritate the bladder mucosa and trigone and aggravate feelings of urgency and frequency. In those prone to cystitis, a bladder that is only irregularly or infrequently emptied and flushed can encourage reinfection.

Incontinent people should be encouraged to consume reasonable amounts of fluid. The timing of fluid intake is important. If patients are troubled by incontinence while they are out during the day, they may wish to consume most of their fluid after returning home. If nocturia or nocturnal enuresis are the main problem, fluid restriction beginning in the afternoon might be advisable.

Drinking certain beverages can create problems. Some people find that tea and coffee have a rapid diuretic effect. Others say that white wine is fine, but red wine is not, and still others implicate all alcoholic beverages as troublesome. It is not uncommon for milk and sugar to be a problem for a few individuals. Even decaffeinated coffee is irritating to the bladder. Highly spiced foods, citrus juices, and tomato-based products can also cause bladder discomfort and exacerbate urgency and incontinence.

A voiding diary, coupled with a record of fluid and food intake, is invaluable for helping to reveal a person's idiosyncrasies. Nurses are well advised to look out for those who complain of urgency and frequency and who are compulsive drinkers of fluids, usually water or soft drinks. Many extreme diets require people to drink several quarts of liquid each day. This can become habitual, even when such a diet has long been abandoned, and frequent voiding is the normal result of a voluminous fluid intake.

Bowel Management

Poor bowel function can affect bladder control and is often the major problem in fecal incontinence. Nurses should encourage patients to establish a program of good bowel habits, and teach them and their families how to maintain such a regimen (Chap. 14).

The Environment and Physical Activities

An environment geared to personal needs, especially if someone is physically disabled, can encourage continence. Chapter 9 includes suggestions about how the environment can be modified to improve continence and ways in which the individual's physical abilities can be maximized to help cope with bladder function problems.

MEDICAL AND SURGICAL INTERVENTION

Drug Therapy

Many drugs can be prescribed to help those with urinary incontinence. Often the results are disappointing, and certainly there is no "wonder drug" for any of the types of incontinence. Some can be useful, though, for carefully selected and accurately diagnosed patients (Wiggins et al., 1985).

Detrusor Instability

The control of unstable bladder contractions and urge incontinence, by the use of drugs to relax the detrusor muscle and inhibit reflex contractions is often attempted. Sometimes this therapy is helpful but in some patients, when the drug is given in large enough doses to be effective, side effects are so troublesome that drug therapy must be abandoned (Table 4–2).

Anticholinergic and antispasmodic drugs reduce bladder contractions so they should be used carefully in patients who have voiding difficulty, because urinary retention can be precipitated. Careful assessment should include a measurement of residual urine. Drug therapy should be used with caution in patients with a residual volume of over 100 ml.

Genuine Stress Incontinence

Some drugs are used in an attempt to prevent stress incontinence by increasing urethral tone. Phenylpropanolamine and ephedrine are used most often, and are thought to act on the alpha receptors in the urethra.

Estrogen replacement therapy to improve urethral resistance in the atrophic urethra might not be as effective as it was once thought, and further research is indicated (Cardozo, 1988).

Outflow Obstruction

Drug therapy can be used to relieve outflow obstruction. Phenoxybenzamine is the most commonly used, but can have troublesome side effects (e.g., tachycardia, postural hypotension). It should be used with great caution.

Atonic Bladder

If the bladder does not contract sufficiently to ensure complete bladder emptying, drug therapy can be tried to increase the force of

Table 4–2. *DRUG THERAPY FOR THE UNSTABLE BLADDER*

Drug Name	Usual Dose	Method of Action	Common Side-effects	Comments
Imipramine (Tofranil)	10–25 mg nightly initially Up to 25–50 mg t.i.d.	Anticholinergic (blocks reflex contractions) + alpha agonist (increased urethral resistance) + ? central effect	Dry mouth Constipation Drowsiness Postural hypotension (possible falls in the elderly)	Tricyclic antidepressant. Use with great care in glaucoma and *never* with monoamine oxidase inhibitors.
Propantheline (Pro-Banthine)	15 mg t.i.d.	Anticholinergic	Dry mouth Blurred vision Constipation	
Flavoxate hydrochloride (Urispas)	200 mg t.i.d.	Smooth muscle relaxant	Nausea Dry mouth Blurred vision	
Oxybutynin (Ditropan)	5 mg t.i.d.	Anticholinergic Antispasmodic	Very dry mouth Constipation	

the voiding contractions. Carbachol, bethanechol, and distigmine bromide have all been used, with limited success.

Other Types of Drug Therapy

Other drugs might be useful in treating factors affecting incontinence—for example, antibiotics to treat a urinary tract infection, or laxatives to treat or prevent constipation.

Many drugs can exacerbate a tendency to incontinence, and caregivers should be aware that drugs prescribed for other conditions might be affecting bladder function adversely (see Table 2–2). For those who are prone to incontinence, care should be taken to choose medications and dosage schedules that will have a minimal effect on bladder control. For example, a slow-acting diuretic, in a divided dose, can help someone with urgency and weak sphincter tone to avoid incontinence. An analgesic might be preferable to night sedation for those who need pain relief but who wet at night if they are sedated.

Surgery

Detrusor Instability

None of the several surgical approaches that have been used in an attempt to treat an unstable bladder has gained widespread use. Cystodistention (stretching the bladder under general anesthesia), bladder transection, and selective sacral neurectomy are all presumed to act by disturbing the neurologic pathways that control uninhibited contractions.

Genuine Stress Incontinence

Many vaginal and suprapubic procedures are available to help correct genuine stress incontinence in women (Chap. 6). Advocates of each make a convincing case for the particular technique they favor.

Outflow Obstruction

Surgery can be used to relieve outflow obstruction—for example, to remove an enlarged prostate gland (Chap. 7), divide a stricture, or widen a narrow urethra. If such procedures are done by an inexperienced surgeon, there is the risk of rendering the patient permanently incontinent.

Severe Intractable Incontinence

Some people with severe intractable incontinence might wish to consider major surgery. For those with a damaged urethra, a neourethra can be constructed (Chap. 6). For those with a nonfunctioning sphincter, an artificial sphincter can be implanted (Chap. 7). In some patients, a urinary diversion with a stoma is the only and best alternative for continence. Although a drastic solution, a urostomy might be easier to cope with than an incontinent urethra, because an effective appliance will contain the urine. Extensive preoperative counseling is essential for people considering this option and, if possible, an experienced ET (enterostomal therapy) nurse should become involved with the patient and family. A visit with another person who has had a urostomy, of similar age and background and of the same sex, is particularly helpful for a patient considering elective urinary diversion.

Iatrogenic Incontinence

Urinary incontinence is occasionally the result of surgery, usually urologic or gynecologic, but it could also be a major pelvic or spinal procedure. Iatrogenic incontinence can be caused by neurologic or sphincter damage, leading to various dysfunctional voiding patterns. As with pharmacologic therapy, the type of surgery required is dictated by the dysfunction to be corrected.

CONTRIBUTIONS OF OTHER HEALTH PROFESSIONALS

In a well-integrated multidisciplinary team, each member has a role to play in helping to relieve the problems of those who are incontinent.

The physical therapist, whether from the hospital or the community, can assess the patient's mobility and dexterity and offer valuable suggestions. Extending the range and strength of movements can make it easier for a person to get to and onto the toilet. A demonstration of safe lifting techniques can help prevent accidents or strains if a caregiver is involved in aiding transfers. If a cane, walker, or wheelchair is used, the physical therapist can ensure that these are optimal for the individual's needs.

An occupational therapist can help the individual achieve independence in activities of daily living, including personal hygiene and toileting. Techniques can be taught to improve function and aids can be provided to maximize existing abilities. Modifications to clothing, grab bars beside the toilet, elevated toilet seats, and implements to assist with washing or dressing can all be tailored to individual needs.

Social workers are ideal to help mobilize and coordinate resources in the community, because of their extensive knowledge of local facilities. They can help the incontinent person obtain modifications in the home, attend a day care center, and receive other forms of assistance, such as Meals on Wheels, a home health aide, financial help, and transportation (Chap. 11).

A psychologist can be particularly helpful for handicapped or demented patients and for those in whom incontinence is thought to be a behavioral problem. If incontinence is suspected to be the source of depression, or depression the cause of incontinence, a detailed psychologic assessment can enable an appropriate treatment plan to be formulated.

Other health professionals, such as a podiatrist to enhance mobility, an optician to improve the patient's vision, and a dietician or dentist to help the patient eat properly, can be important in patient care. Often restoration of continence is only one aspect of a comprehensive rehabilitation program designed to achieve maximum independence for each person.

BLADDER TRAINING

"Bladder training" or "retraining" are much misused and misunderstood terms. If asked, most nurses who care for incontinent patients will claim to practice "bladder training." They rarely elaborate on what is meant, on how such training is to be carried out, or on the goal of bladder training. Often the training amounts to nothing more than reminding patients to use the toilet or taking them to the toilet every 2 hours.

Bladder training is a useful nursing tool, but only when used appropriately by someone who understands the techniques. Several different types of toileting programs are distinguishable and can be used in different circumstances. The most important element for success is that the correct regimen be selected for each patient and situation. Success will not be achieved if all incontinent people are treated alike. A thorough assessment identifies those patients who will benefit from bladder training and determines the most appropriate method. Other factors that contribute to the incontinence should also be treated (e.g., a urinary tract infection or constipation), because ignoring them will certainly impair the success of a program.

Bladder training is most suitable for people with the symptoms of frequency, urgency, and urge incontinence (with or without an underlying unstable bladder), and for those with nonspecific incontinence that seems to "just happen." Elderly people in institutions often have these symptoms. The following discussion outlines bladder training for the mentally alert. (Programs for the elderly, mentally infirm, and mentally retarded are discussed in Chapters 8 and 12.)

Patients with voiding dysfunction, other than an unstable bladder, are unlikely to benefit from bladder training. A woman with an incompetent urethral sphincter, and consequent stress incontinence, cannot regain continence by manipulating her toileting schedule. By excessive voiding frequency, she might be able to keep the bladder relatively empty so that it contains only a little urine, but her underlying problem will still remain. Even if she has just passed urine, the next time she coughs she is likely to leak. Similarly, the person with urinary retention and overflow incontinence cannot be helped by such training. The importance of thorough assessment and of accurate diagnosis prior to the use of any behavioral management techniques cannot be overemphasized.

Bladder Training for Urge Incontinence

The aim of bladder training is to restore the patient with frequency, urgency, and urge incontinence to a more normal and convenient micturition pattern. Ultimately, voiding should occur at intervals of 3 to 4 hours (or even longer) without any urgency or incontinence. Drug therapy can be combined with bladder training for the person with an unstable bladder.

The key to success is accurate record keeping and frequent professional contact and support. Bladder training can be successful for both inpatients or outpatients.

The patient must fully understand and enthusiastically participate in this treatment. It can be difficult for the patient to follow the regimen. Initially, a clear description of normal bladder function, and why and how it has gone wrong, should be given. If the patient cannot or will not cooperate, for any reason, there is little point in attempting this type of bladder training.

It must be explained to the patient that the bladder has become overactive and oversensitive. The individual might have experienced urge incontinence. The natural reaction to this embarrassing experience is to try to prevent it from happening again. Usually the patient develops the habit of rushing to the toilet at the first hint of bladder filling to avoid an accident. Because the bladder is filling continuously (and most people can sense some urine in the bladder if they think about it), it is easy to see how a vicious cycle of passing urine more and more frequently can develop. The person who is anxious about incontinence is likely to interpret any type of bladder sensation as an urgent need to pass urine. Anxiety or worry merely exacerbates the sensation of urgency. In extreme cases, people's lives can become completely taken over by the need to pass urine every 10 or 15 minutes. Few people reach this unhappy state, but might use the toilet every hour or half-hour throughout the day. Despite this level of frequency they might also experience urge incontinence—especially if they have an unstable bladder. When people get up and rush to the toilet while the bladder is contracting, they are likely to be incontinent. Women are more vulnerable than men because of lower urethral resistance. "Key-in-the-lock" incontinence can develop, in which someone can hang on while rushing urgently home, but might wet on the doorstep while fumbling to get the door unlocked or begin passing urine while trying to remove clothing in the bathroom.

Bladder training aims to restore an individual's confidence in the bladder's ability to hold urine, and to re-establish a more normal pattern. Initially, a patient should keep a baseline chart for 3 to 7 days, recording how often urine is passed and when incontinence occurs. This is then reviewed with the program supervisor and an individual regimen is developed. The purpose is to extend the time between toileting gradually, encouraging the patient to practice delaying the need to void, rather than giving in to the feeling of urgency. Initially, the times chosen should not be difficult for the patient to follow. These can be at set intervals throughout the day (e.g., every 1 or 2 hours) or can be variable, according to the individual's pattern as indicated by the baseline chart. For example, someone taking a diuretic in the morning might need to go hourly in the morning, every 1½ hours in the middle of the day, and every 2 hours in the evening. It is important to work around fixed time commitments (e.g., working or taking children to school). The more convenient the program, the more likely it is to be followed. When the baseline chart reveals a definite pattern to the incontinence, it might be possible to set toileting times to anticipate this. If someone is usually wet at 3:30 PM, a good time to void is 3 PM.

A pattern of toileting should be set for patients throughout the day. Usually no pattern is set at night, even if nocturia or nocturnal enuresis is a problem. Patients are instructed to pass urine as necessary during the night. Sometimes it is useful for people to set their alarm to anticipate a known peak wetting time. Usually this is unnecessary, because nocturnal problems often resolve themselves once daytime frequency has returned to normal.

Patients are instructed to pass urine at the set times and to attempt to delay voiding in between. Sometimes the provision of a suitable pad or appliance helps to increase confidence and means that, if incontinence does occur, the results will not be too disastrous. If urgency is experienced patients are taught to sit or stand still and try to suppress it, rather than to rush immediately to the toilet. A normal fluid intake is encouraged, because the goal is to have the patient continent and be able to drink adequately.

As patients achieve the target intervals without having to go prematurely or leaking, the intervals can gradually be lengthened. The speed of progress in this depends on the individual and on other variables, such as the initial severity of symptoms, motivation, and the amount of professional support. Patients usually remain at one time interval for 1 to 2 weeks before it is increased by 15 to 30 minutes for another 2 weeks. Again, this varies considerably among individuals. Any times that seem particularly difficult should be adjusted to suit individual needs—for example, someone who habitually drinks four cups of tea or coffee at breakfast will probably never achieve a 4-hour voiding interval in the morning. Intelligent patients who fully understand the purpose of the program can often adjust their own time intervals and will progress considerably between office visits.

Once the target of 3- to 4-hour voiding without urgency has been achieved, it is useful to maintain the charts and set times for at least another month to prevent relapse. Some people take several months to achieve this, whereas others might need only a few weeks. There seems to be no way of predicting how long bladder training will take for each individual. Figure 4–1 shows a series of charts that monitor the progress of a woman with an unstable bladder. Filling in the charts consistently is vital in assessing progress and in giving the patient encouraging feedback when the results are positive.

An alternative to bladder training by preset time intervals is to instruct the patient to extend the time interval between the first sensation of urgency and actually passing urine gradually. Instead of setting a pattern to aim for, the patient tries to delay voiding for increasing intervals after feeling the need to go. For example, someone with severe urgency could be asked to count to 10 slowly before starting for the toilet. Once this is achieved, the count should be increased to 20, then 30, and then 60. If urgency is less severe the patient might start by waiting 5, 10, 20, and then 30 minutes. Highly motivated patients often see for themselves on their charts that they are reaching their goal.

Some people find that practicing pelvic muscle exercises helps to suppress urgency. It is important not to underestimate how difficult it is for people to ignore the sensation of urgency when they are afraid that they might wet themselves. Many patients will be tempted to give up the bladder training or will refuse to push themselves. Bladder training may contradict other advice they have been given—for example, many children are taught that it is bad to wait too long to go. It is one of few hopes that people with urge incontinence have of regaining

Text continued on page 87

Continence Chart

Week beginning ______________ Name Mrs Bell

Please put a check in LEFT column each time urine is passed

Please put a check in RIGHT column each time you are wet

	Monday		Tuesday		Wednesday		Thursday		Friday		Saturday		Sunday	
6 am	✓				✓					✓	✓	✓✓		
7 am	✓	✓	✓	✓	✓	✓	✓		✓	✓	✓		✓	
8 am			✓		✓				✓✓					✓
9 am	✓		✓				✓	✓			✓		✓	
10 am		✓	✓✓		✓				✓	✓	✓		✓	
11 am	✓				✓		✓					✓		
12 pm	✓✓		✓	✓	✓	✓	✓		✓		✓		✓	
1 pm			✓		✓✓		✓						✓✓	✓✓
2 pm	✓				✓				✓		✓✓		✓✓	✓
3 pm	✓	✓✓	✓				✓			✓	✓		✓	✓
4 pm		✓		✓	✓		✓		✓				✓	
5 pm	✓		✓✓								✓	✓		
6 pm							✓		✓				✓	
7 pm	✓		✓		✓	✓				✓	✓			
8 pm			✓						✓					
9 pm	✓						✓		✓		✓		✓	
10 pm			✓		✓				✓					
11 pm								✓	✓					
12 am	✓		✓		✓		✓				✓		✓	
1 am											✓			
2 am	✓	✓												
3 am														
4 am													✓	✓
5 am														
Totals	13	6	14	3	13	3	10	2	12	5	13	4	14	6

A

Special Instructions:

Baseline charting. Please record your pattern of visits to the toilet and wetting, without intentionally changing them this week.

Figure 4–1. *Series of charts showing the progress of a patient on a bladder training program.* A, *Baseline week. The patient is asked to record micturition and incontinence.*

Illustration continued on following page

Continence Chart

Week beginning Week 1 Name Mrs Bell

Please put a check in LEFT column each time urine is passed

Please put a check in RIGHT column each time you are wet

	Monday		Tuesday		Wednesday		Thursday		Friday		Saturday		Sunday	
6 am				✓										
(7 am)	✓		✓		✓		✓		✓					
(8 am)	✓		✓		✓	✓	✓		✓		✓		✓	
9 am		✓			✓									✓
(10 am)	✓		✓				✓	✓	✓		✓		✓	
(11 am)	✓		✓		✓		✓				✓		✓✓	
12 pm	✓	✓			✓	✓			✓	✓				
(1 pm)	✓		✓	✓	✓		✓		✓		✓		✓	
(2 pm)	✓		✓		✓		✓		✓		✓		✓	
3 pm													✓	✓✓
(4 pm)	✓		✓		✓		✓		✓		✓			
5 pm													✓	
(6 pm)	✓		✓		✓		✓		✓✓	✓	✓			
7 pm														
(8 pm)	✓	✓	✓		✓		✓		✓		✓		✓	
9 pm														
(10 pm)	✓		✓				✓		✓		✓		✓	✓
11 pm					✓								✓	
(12 am)	✓		✓		✓		✓		✓					
1 am											✓			
2 am														
3 am														
4 am							✓							
5 am														
Totals	12	3	11	2	12	2	12	1	12	2	10	0	11	4

B

Special Instructions:

Pass urine only at the times indicated at left. Try to hold on in between. If you have to make additional trips to the toilet, record these also.

Figure 4–1 Continued B, *The nurse and patient review the baseline chart and work out a pattern of visits to the toilet (times circled in left-hand column).*

Continence Chart

Week beginning Week 2 Name Mrs Bell

Please put a check in LEFT column each time urine is passed

Please put a check in RIGHT column each time you are wet

	Monday		Tuesday		Wednesday		Thursday		Friday		Saturday		Sunday	
6 am			✓											
7 am	✓		✓		✓		✓		✓		✓			
8 am									✓✓	✓				
9 am	✓		✓		✓		✓						✓	
10 am					✓				✓		✓	✓		
11 am	✓		✓		✓		✓		✓		✓		✓	
12 pm														
1 pm	✓		✓		✓		✓		✓		✓		✓	
2 pm	✓	✓✓												
3 pm	✓		✓		✓		✓		✓		✓		✓	
4 pm									✓				✓	
5 pm			✓		✓	✓✓					✓	✓		
6 pm	✓		✓		✓		✓		✓	✓	✓		✓	
7 pm														
8 pm	✓												✓✓	✓
9 pm	✓		✓		✓		✓		✓		✓		✓	
10 pm														
11 pm					✓	✓			✓				✓	
12 am	✓		✓		✓		✓		✓		✓			
1 am														
2 am														
3 am							✓							
4 am											✓			
5 am														
C Totals	10	2	10	0	11	3	9	0	12	2	10	2	10	1

Special Instructions:

Pass urine only at the times indicated at left. Try to hold on in between. Try to delay voiding in between.

Figure 4–1 Continued C, *At the weekly review the patient agrees to try to extend the time interval slightly between visits to the toilet.*

Illustration continued on following page

Continence Chart

Week beginning Week 4 Name Mrs Bell

Please put a check in LEFT column each time urine is passed

Please put a check in RIGHT column each time you are wet

	Monday		Tuesday		Wednesday		Thursday		Friday		Saturday		Sunday	
6 am														
7 am	✓		✓		✓		✓		✓		✓			
8 am														
9 am	✓		✓		✓	✓	✓		✓		✓		✓	
10 am					✓	✓								
11 am	✓		✓	✓	✓		✓				✓		✓	
12 pm									✓	✓				
1 pm	✓		✓		✓		✓		✓		✓		✓	
2 pm														
3 pm	✓		✓		✓		✓		✓		✓		✓	
4 pm														
5 pm									✓					
6 pm	✓		✓		✓		✓		✓		✓		✓	
7 pm										✓				
8 pm													✓	
9 pm	✓		✓		✓		✓		✓		✓			
10 pm														
11 pm							✓							
12 am	✓		✓		✓		✓		✓		✓		✓	
1 am														
2 am														
3 am														
4 am														
5 am														
D Totals	8	0	8	1	9	2	9	0	9	2	8	0	7	0

Special Instructions:

Pass urine only at the times indicated at left. Try to wait in between.

Figure 4–1 Continued D, *By the fourth week the patient is usually managing to wait until the set time, and incontinent episodes have become rare.*

Continence Chart

Week beginning Week 5 Name Mrs Bell

Please put a check in LEFT column each time urine is passed

Please put a check in RIGHT column each time you are wet

	Monday		Tuesday		Wednesday		Thursday		Friday		Saturday		Sunday	
6 am									✓	✓				
7 am	✓		✓		✓		✓		✓		✓			
8 am													✓	
9 am	✓								✓					
10 am	✓		✓		✓		✓		✓		✓		✓	
11 am														
12 pm			✓											
1 pm	✓		✓		✓		✓		✓		✓	✓	✓	
2 pm											✓	✓		
3 pm		✓												
4 pm	✓	✓	✓		✓		✓		✓		✓		✓	
5 pm														
6 pm														
7 pm	✓			✓			✓	✓✓						
8 pm	✓		✓	✓	✓		✓		✓		✓		✓	
9 pm														
10 pm														
11 pm		✓		✓							✓			
12 am	✓		✓		✓		✓		✓				✓	
1 am														
2 am														
3 am														
4 am														
5 am														
Totals	8	3	7	3	6	0	7	2	8	1	7	2	6	0

E

Special Instructions:

Pass urine only at the times indicated at left. Try to hold it in between.

Figure 4–1 Continued E, *Extending the time interval still further to achieve a "normal" micturition pattern causes a slight relapse of incontinence.*

Illustration continued on following page

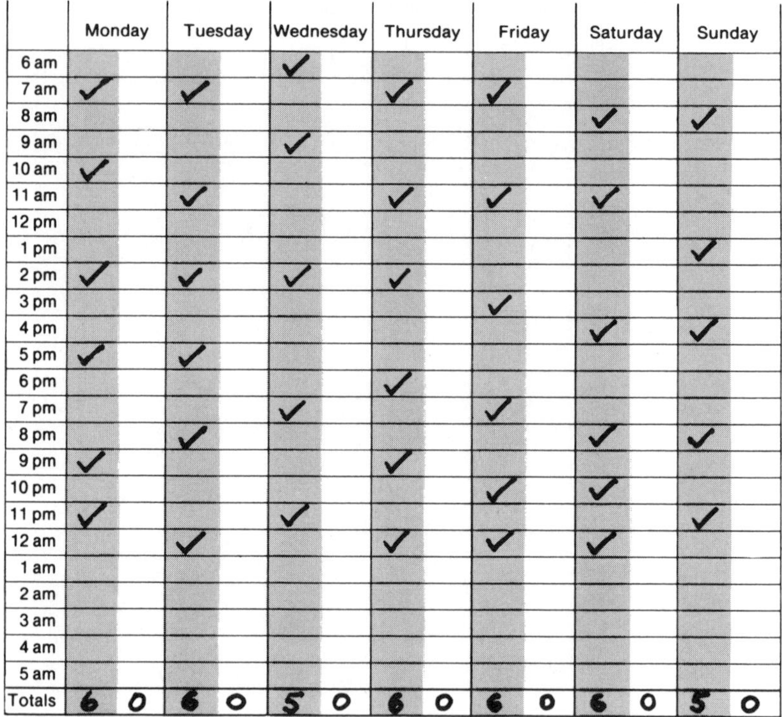

Continence Chart

Week beginning Week 8 Name Mrs Bell

Please put a check in LEFT column each time urine is passed

Please put a check in RIGHT column each time you are wet

	Monday		Tuesday		Wednesday		Thursday		Friday		Saturday		Sunday	
6 am					✓									
7 am	✓		✓				✓		✓					
8 am											✓		✓	
9 am					✓									
10 am	✓													
11 am			✓				✓		✓		✓			
12 pm														
1 pm													✓	
2 pm	✓		✓		✓		✓							
3 pm									✓					
4 pm											✓		✓	
5 pm	✓		✓											
6 pm							✓							
7 pm					✓				✓					
8 pm			✓								✓		✓	
9 pm	✓						✓							
10 pm									✓		✓			
11 pm	✓				✓								✓	
12 am			✓				✓		✓		✓			
1 am														
2 am														
3 am														
4 am														
5 am														
F Totals	6	0	6	0	5	0	6	0	6	0	6	0	5	0

Special Instructions:

Try to wait at least three hours between visits to the toilet.

Figure 4–1 Continued F, *Incontinence has disappeared again by the eighth week. By now the patient need not stick rigidly to set times. She merely ensures that she always waits at least 3 hours between toileting.*

continence, though, and every attempt must be made to encourage and support their efforts.

More use could be made of mutual support between patients than is currently practiced.

Scheduled Toileting

Much of what goes under the name of bladder training actually does nothing to train the bladder, and consists solely of reminding patients or taking them to pass urine at set intervals. This is most commonly practiced in extended care facilities. The intervals chosen might be time-related (e.g., every 2 or 4 hours) or related to events (e.g., before or after taking meals, drinks, or drugs.) Often such programs are used indiscriminately for all residents, or at least for all incontinent patients. Because everyone's bladder function is different, such programs will, at best, eliminate some incontinence before it occurs. Usually the "success" is unrelated to individual needs. Hopefully, with the advent of more individualized patient care, such rigid regimens for whole groups will be recognized as time-consuming and ineffective.

Scheduled toileting is useful for selected patients. Those with a poor memory, who simply forget about their bladder until it is too late, might benefit from a fixed time or full reminder or from a standing instruction always to visit the toilet after meals. Sometimes an alarm clock or set interval timer can serve as a reminder if no one is around. Patients with impaired bladder sensation might also need to be instructed to urinate by the clock, rather than to wait for sensation if they are to avoid overflow incontinence. Patients with advanced dementia, for whom all attempts at incontinence have failed, may be kept drier by scheduled toileting (Chap. 8).

Habit Retraining

Habit retraining has been described as a method of training the elderly in the hospital. A baseline chart is kept to determine the individual's pattern of continence and incontinence. A program of toilet times is then worked out to anticipate incontinence. Toileting times are individualized, rather than treating everyone in the same way. Once continence is achieved the time intervals can be lengthened. In practice, such a program is much more likely to keep patients continent than scheduled toileting for all people, and it might retrain some. Possibly the biggest benefit, certainly to nursing home residents, is to "retrain" the staff to recognize individual toileting needs, rather than taking everyone to the toilet at the same time (see Chapter 11 for a discussion of toileting regimens in extended and acute care facilities.)

Biofeedback

Biofeedback is an adjunct to bladder training for patients with urgency and stress incontinence without anatomic displacement (e.g., cystocele, rectocele, prolapse). Using urodynamic equipment or devices made especially for the treatment of incontinence, patients are given direct feedback through manometry or electromyography in regard to the strength and duration of pelvic muscle contractions. No consensus has been reached about the efficacy of biofeedback-assisted pelvic muscle training, but those who have reported success with it are unswerving in their enthusiasm and commitment (Burgio et al., 1986). Usually 6 to 10 1-hour treatments with a skilled trainer are needed. This might be a nurse, physician, occupational therapist, or clinical psychologist. Further research is warranted to make this technique available to more people.

It is clear from the various measures highlighted in this chapter that incontinence has many forms of treatment, from simple dietary modification to lengthy and creative surgical procedures. Nurses might be called on to discuss alternative therapies with patients. Since nurses carry out nonsurgical treatments, they may disparage attempts at surgical correction. Every nurse has the responsibility to understand accepted and emerging solutions for voiding dysfunction.

References and Further Reading

Allman, R., et al.: Pressure sores among hospitalized patients. Ann. Intern. Med., *105*:337–342, 1986.

Burgio, K.L., Robinson, J.C., and Engel, B.T.: The role of biofeedback in Kegel exercise training for stress urinary incontinence. Am. J. Obstet. Gynecol., *154*:58, 1986.

Cardozo, L.D.: The role of estrogen in the treatment of female urinary incontinence. Programs and abstracts from National Institutes of Health Consensus Conference, Bethesda, MD, October 3–5, 1988, pp. 75–77.

Hadley, E.C., et al.: Bladder training and related therapies for urinary incontinence in older people. J.A.M.A., *256*:372, 1986.

Kegel, A.H.: Progressive resistance exercise in the functional restoration of the perineal muscles. Am. J. Obstet. Gynecol., *56*:238, 1948.

Mandelstam, D.: Incontinence. London, William Heinemann, 1977.

Norton, C.S.: Training for urinary continence. *In* Wilson-Barnett, J. (ed.): Patient Teaching. London, Churchill-Livingstone, 1983.

Palmer, M.: Urinary Incontinence. Washington, DC, National Gerontological Nursing Association, 1986.

Urinary Incontinence in Adults: Program and Abstracts from National Institutes of Health Consensus Conference, Bethesda, MD, October 3–5, 1988.

Wiggins, et al.: Pharmacotherapy in urinary incontinence. J. Urol. Nurs., *4*(2):315–318, 1985.

Willington, F.L.: Management of urinary incontinence. *In* Caldwell, K.P.S. (ed.): Urinary Incontinence. New York, Grune and Stratton, 1975, pp. 129–167.

Nancy Faller, RN, BSN, CETN

5 Incontinence in Childhood

The achievement of continence is an important developmental milestone. Society places responsibility for this achievement on a child's parents. The mother who has failed to "potty train" her infant by the expected age will often feel either that she has somehow failed in her maternal duties or that her child is backward or retarded. Child-rearing practices vary over time and fashions tend to go in cycles, alternating between starting training as early as possible and using almost no training at all.

The incontinent child is often the recipient of hostility and may feel rejected. Once past the crucial age at which continence is expected, it is no longer acceptable to crouch in a gutter or urinate against a wall in public view. What was once "quaint" behavior becomes "incontinence" as the toddler approaches school age. The child comes to realize that it is considered shameful to lack bladder control. Parents might react with anger in an attempt to disguise their own guilt and embarrassment. If the child really has no control, punishment cannot be avoided. Shyness, anxiety, and withdrawal can result.

At school the child with incontinence often suffers ridicule and humiliation at the hands of classmates. During the course of toilet training, continent children often adopt attitudes that wetting is infantile and naughty. Having shown that they have acquired grown-up habits and left behind such baby-like behavior, they may tease their less fortunate peer mercilessly. Some parents might lack understanding and tolerance, instructing their child not to play with the "smelly" or "dirty" child who is incontinent. The parents of the child might be blamed for negligence in not bringing their child up properly or not bothering to start toilet training. Most teachers and schools are more enlightened, but some make life difficult for the child with incontinence. Strict routines that only allow toilet visits during official breaks might make a child incontinent who simply has a limited ability to hang on. Such a situation will certainly increase a child's anxiety. Some nursery schools do not take children until they are reliably continent. Occasionally a child with a handicap is obliged to attend a special school, not because of intellectual ability, emotional needs, or the handicap, but only because of incontinence.

TOILET TRAINING

Training probably does more to teach the child socially acceptable toileting behavior and recognition of allowable places, than to train the bladder itself. The complex neuromuscular control necessary for continence and voluntary micturition cannot be taught. Natural maturation, especially of the central nervous system, is the most important factor in acquiring control. Even with no training at all a child may eventually control micturition, although not necessarily using the "correct" receptacle. One consequence of neuromuscular immaturity is that continence at birth is impossible. Mothers who start potty-training their child at 3 months might catch some urine in the potty, but fail to realize that this is purely by chance, and the baby cannot do this reliably at this age. Up to 80% of parents attempt some sort of toilet training by their child's first birthday. This is too early for most babies, and it is hardly surprising that so much anxiety is aroused over what must inevitably become a prolonged battle.

The optimum time to begin training is probably around the second birthday, depending on developmental achievements. Ideally the child should be able to walk, follow simple instructions, and have some speech and basic feeding skills. At this point the training is most likely to be easy and rapid, although the prospects of dispensing with diapers and gaining social approval for early achievement are powerful temptations for the parents to start much sooner.

Most children are toilet-trained without professional intervention. Many nurses are asked for advice, however, either officially as a public health, office, or clinic nurse or socially as a relative or friend. The best advice is to wait until the child is ready and then to train fairly intensively. If possible, a time should be chosen when little else is going on (e.g., avoiding Christmas or family vacations.) This is preferable to random and premature attempts over a long period. The child should be taken out of diapers and put into dry pants so that the difference betwen wet and dry can be appreciated. Clothing and underwear should be easily removable by the child. Frequent prompts and pottying are combined with immediate reward (physical or verbal) for urinating and disapproval or rebuke for accidents. Excessive punishment is counterproductive, because it raises anxiety and decreases the learning potential. Mild reprimands are not harmful, provided that the child can learn to avoid them in the future. The child should be given clear and repeated explanations of what is required. It might be useful to increase fluid intake temporarily to increase the number of learning opportunities available.

Some intensive toilet-training methods have been devised—for example, in less than a day (Azrin and Foxx, 1974). These techniques, however, are difficult to implement without experienced professional supervision.

If a planned attempt conducted at an appropriate time fails it is best to stop trying, put the child back in diapers, and try again after 2 or 3 months. By this time the child might be ready. A parent or sibling can sometimes help the child to learn by demonstrating appropriate toileting behavior.

Adults can take continence so much for granted that it is easy for them to forget how many different skills are involved. It is not simply a matter of urinating while sitting on the potty. The child must learn to recognize the need to void consciously and be able to monitor the state of the bladder, both asleep and awake. Once the need is appreciated, micturition must be postponed until an appropriate receptacle can be reached. It is not always easy to know what an acceptable place is, especially if the surroundings are unfamiliar. For example, boys learn to recognize a urinal as appropriate, as well as a toilet. They go in front of other boys, but not in front of girls, and prefer to defecate in private. Girls learn to go behind a closed (preferably locked) door, except in outdoor settings, where they can go behind a bush. The preliterate child naturally cannot read signs on public toilets. The child must learn how to open doors, remove clothing, use toilet paper, flush the toilet, and wash up. Once in position the stream must be started voluntarily. Not until all these skills have been mastered can the child be independent at toileting.

The final skill in the sequence is not gained until the child is about 5 years old, when the ability to urinate in the absence of any sensation of needing to do so is perfected. This is most important socially, because it enables anticipatory micturiton: being able to empty the bladder "just in case" (e.g., prior to a class or a trip). This is vital for the prevention of inconvenient interruptions to activities, and makes everyday life more orderly.

If professional help is sought for the child's failure to become dry, an initial assessment is done to exclude serious pathology. It is best to reassure parents that there is probably nothing wrong and that the child is not stupid or naughty. They should be advised to give up and try again in a few months. Explanation of a simple reward system to the parents (e.g., a cuddle immediately after performance) can be helpful. If repeated attempts fail, it is useful to keep a chart to monitor progress and put the problem into perspective (see Fig. 3–2). Sometimes established points of conflict can be changed—for example, buying a new potty, using a different room, or having someone else do the training. Confidence and optimism, with emphasis on positive achievements rather than failures, usually resolve most problems.

PERSISTENT DIURNAL INCONTINENCE

Daytime wetting sometimes persists until the child reaches school age. It is less common than bed-wetting and the two often go together. If the child is continuously dribbling this should be fully investigated, because there might be a urologic abnormality. Wetting usually takes the form either of urge or stress incontinence. Many children wet on the odd occasion when they have been so engrossed in playing that they repeatedly ignore warnings from the bladder. This can be safely dismissed as having no pathologic significance.

Most children grow out of daytime wetting eventually, without any formal intervention. Because incontinence can be such a nuisance and embarrassment, however, both to the child and parents, it is usually worth trying to hasten continence, especially if both the child and the parents want help and are eager to cooperate.

If the problem is frequency, urgency, or urge incontinence, treatment is similar to that for adult toilet training (Chap. 4.) A time should be chosen when full attention can be devoted to the training program (e.g., during a school vacation). The training can either be strictly by the clock or by delaying micturition once sensation is felt. With the former method, the child is reminded to urinate once every half-hour. This interval is increased by a half-hour each day until voiding is occurring every 2½ to 3 hours. With the latter method, after feeling the need to go, the child must count to 10 before setting out for the bathroom. On day 2 the count is increased to 20 and on day 3 to 30. The count should be lengthened gradually until 10 minutes elapse between the onset of sensation and going to urinate. With both these methods some accidents must be expected and tolerated. A chart should be kept throughout the training period to monitor progress and to provide both the child and parents with feedback about success. A parent or other trainer must be enthusiastic and willing to devote about a week to the program, giving maximum encouragement and positive reinforcement to the child throughout. It is vital that any program be carried out consistently by all concerned. Frequent small rewards can be offered during the training period, but the promise of one big reward for success should be avoided. It can put considerable stress on the child to know that there will be no new bicycle if failure occurs, and this might even be counterproductive. Fluids should not be restricted during the training period. Usually the child is well motivated by the desire to be rid of the problem.

A different but complementary approach to controlling urgency is having the child practice when actually at the toilet. This is useful for the child who tends to wet at the last moment. The child should get into position, ready for micturition, and then count to 10 before allowing the stream to start. When this can be done comfortably the count of 10 is also done at the door. Once this is mastered the count of 10 is done before starting out for the bathroom, as well as at the door and in position. This is aimed at increasing confidence in the ability to control the bladder. Nothing exacerbates urgency as much as the fear that it will lead to wetting.

Sometimes a pants alarm (Fig. 5–1) is useful in toilet training, especially if the child is unaware when incontinence is occurring. These alarms have the dual function of interrupting the stream, because the child is startled when the alarm sounds, and of alerting the child to wetness. A sensor is worn inside or outside the child's underpants and is connected to an alarm worn on the collar or wrist. This is obviously unsuitable for use anywhere but at home.

Occasionally persistent urgency and frequency can be caused by a urinary tract infection, especially in girls. If the child has dysuria, smelly urine, or fails to respond to toilet training, it is always useful to have a urine specimen tested for evidence of infection.

Although training should always be started with an optimistic attitude, the child should not be blamed or punished if it fails. Instead, the child should be reassured that the problem will be under control soon and that the training can be tried again at the next feasible opportunity.

Stress incontinence—leakage on physical exertion—is usually caused by a weakness of the pelvic floor component of the urethral sphincter. The treatment of choice is pelvic muscle exercises (Chap. 6). The child should be taught to interrupt the urine midstream at every micturition and to practice pelvic muscle contractions regularly throughout the day. A few girls seem to be born with a congenitally weak or open bladder neck. For a few this resolves spontaneously at

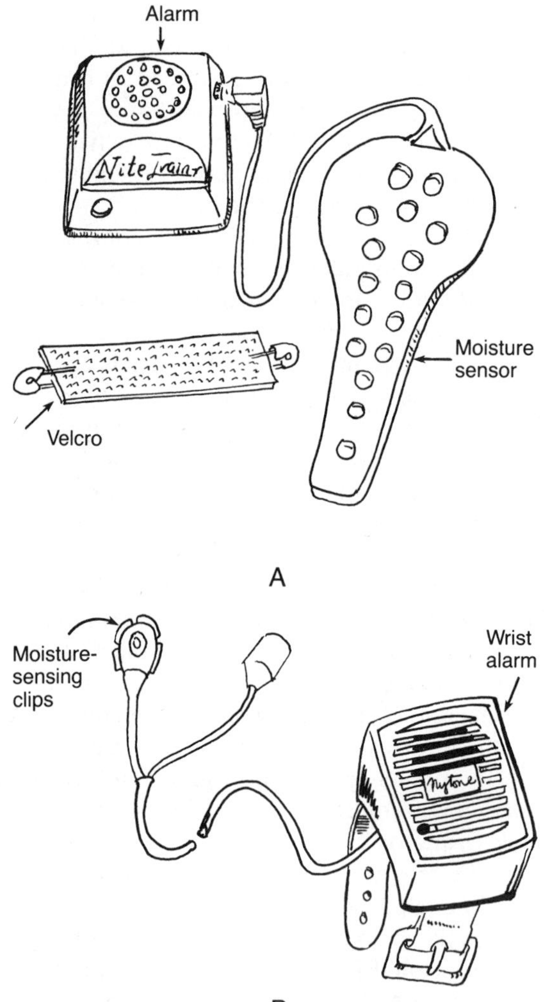

Figure 5–1. *Various types of pants alarms.* A, *Nite Train-r: The alarm is attached to the pajama shoulder or collar by Velcro; the moisture-sensing pad is worn in the underpants.* B, *Nytone: The alarm is attached to the wrist; the moisture-sensing clips attach to the outside of the underpants.*

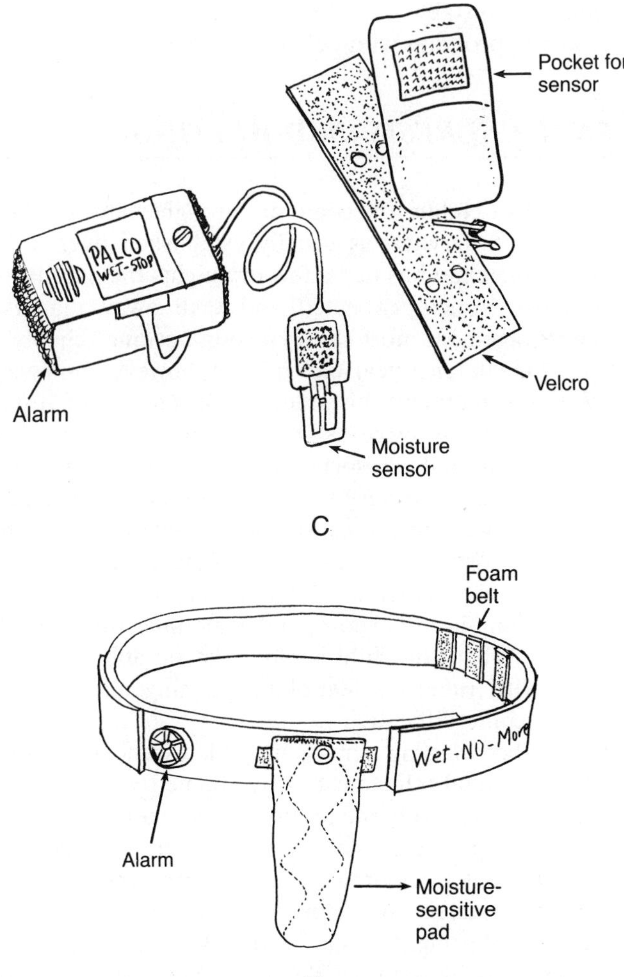

Figure 5–1 Continued C, *Palco: The alarm is attached to the pajama shoulder or collar with Velcro; the moisture-sensing pad is worn in the underpants (the pocket for the sensor attaches to the underpants with Velcro).* D, *Wet-No-More: The alarm is worn on a belt around the waist; the moisture-sensing pad is worn in the underpants.*

puberty, but corrective surgery is sometimes required if incontinence is troublesome.

Some girls suffer "giggle incontinence," in which they start to leak when they laugh and sometimes continue to leak until the bladder is completely empty. This is probably a combination of stress incontinence and an unstable bladder. It can be treated by combining a toilet-training program with pelvic muscle exercises.

NOCTURNAL ENURESIS (BED-WETTING)

Most children become dry at night between their third and fourth birthdays. Dryness is usually established over a fairly short period. Once the child has had a few dry nights the parents should explain that dryness is now expected and take away diapers. With plenty of encouragement most children soon become reliably dry.

One in ten 5-year-old children, however, still wet the bed regularly. With no treatment this gradually falls to 5% of 10-year olds and to 2% of adults. It is twice as common in boys as girls, has strong familial tendencies, and is associated with stressful events in the third or fourth year of life. A urinary tract infection might be the cause.

Bed-wetting can cause considerable distress. The sheer volume of dirty laundry is great, especially if more than one child wets or laundry facilities are inadequate. Parents might think the child is just lazy or even doing it on purpose, and sometimes this can actually lead to child abuse. When the child is older the situation often prevents overnight stays with friends for fear of it happening, and school or family vacations can become difficult.

If bed-wetting persists into adolescence and adult life, it can make the individual reluctant to leave home or to form long-lasting relationships. Occasionally the problem is not mentioned, even to a prospective marriage partner, and the adult with enuresis might break off an engagement rather than face the embarrassment of telling a partner. In fact, enuresis often stops spontaneously on change of circumstances, such as starting to share a double bed. Many adults with enuresis, however, will not take this risk. Attitudes of partners or roommates might lead to repeated rejections. Imagine how unpleasant it would be to share a bed with someone who has enuresis and why it is a major deterrent to forming long-term relationships.

Simple Treatment Measures

Treatment for nocturnal enuresis is usually delayed until it becomes enough of a problem for both the child and parents that action is requested. Seldom should it be considered before the age of 5. The child should be able to take responsibility for the program.

Sometimes simple remedies are effective. A clear explanation of bladder function should be given to the child and the parents. Popular myths, such as laziness or intentional wetting, should be dispelled. It is common for a child to wet only at home, not when sleeping elsewhere (e.g., at the grandparents' house). Parents might interpret this as the child being able to control it at will. Every attempt should be made to put the problem into perspective if the situation has become tense and wetting is a point of conflict. For example, most children do not realize that there is likely to be at least one other child with enuresis in their class at school. They are not alone or a freak. Many do not know that they have an excellent chance of growing out of it and probably will not continue bed wetting for much longer.

Sometimes an obvious mistake can be identified, such as failing to urinate before going to bed or having inadequate lighting. If the child also has daytime frequency and urgency, the training programs and exercises discussed earlier are useful for increasing functional bladder capacity and attentiveness to bladder cues. Some parents wake their child to urinate when they go to bed. This does not always prevent wetting, but probably does no harm, although it does little to train the child. Occasionally it can be counterproductive, because the child will come to expect it and might never develop the ability to hold urine all night. The child could even become conditioned to wet at the sound of footsteps coming up the stairs. If the child is awakened at a regular time, this might become the time at which wetting occurs when not awakened. If this practice is used it is wise to vary the time and who does it, so that it does not become a trigger for wetting.

Practice and imagery are additional adjuncts (Scharf, 1986; Faller, 1987). With practice, the child goes through the steps for toileting, starting from bed. With imagery, the child visualizes the steps, rather than actually acting through them.

Dietary modifications can be helpful (Scharf, 1986). Some children with a milk allergy improve if milk or a milk product is eliminated in the evening. It is wise to reduce salty snacks at bedtime that increase fluid intake. Additionally, sodas, caffeinated drinks, and chocolate should be discouraged, because of their diuretic effect.

Star charts (Fig. 5–2) can be useful. The child is encouraged to take responsibility for the chart. A common system is for the child to get one star (say, a blue one) for each dry night. For three consecutive dry nights a gold star can be given. Emphasis should be on positive achievements and "black marks" should not be used for wet nights. Care should be taken to explain to parents that success with the use of a star chart does not mean that the child simply wasn't trying hard

Name ______________________________

Date commenced ______________________________

Remember: Always go to the toilet before going to bed. In the morning stick on a blue star for a dry night. For the third dry night in a row stick on a GOLD star.

	1st Week	2nd Week	3rd Week
Monday	☆	☆	☆
Tuesday	☆	☆	☆
Wednesday	☆	☆	☆
Thursday	☆	☆	☆
Friday	☆	☆	☆
Saturday	☆	☆	☆
Sunday	☆	☆	☆
	4th Week	5th Week	6th Week
Monday	☆	☆	☆
Tuesday	☆	☆	☆
Wednesday	☆	☆	☆
Thursday	☆	☆	☆
Friday	☆	☆	☆
Saturday	☆	☆	☆
Sunday	☆	☆	☆

Figure 5–2. *Star chart.*

enough before. Response to a reward does not imply that the same results could have been obtained by effort alone.

Medication (Table 5–1) is sometimes used in conjunction with a star chart, but not all pediatricians agree. Some argue that enuresis is benign and should be treated as such. Medication given to decrease bladder contractions (e.g., oxybutynin, imipramine) usually allows a rapid cure, but relapse is common when the medication is withdrawn. Drug therapy should be tapered gradually after the desired effect has been obtained to prevent rebound enuresis. It can also cause or aggravate a tendency to constipation. Imipramine can be used to decrease the level of sleep, but it has major drawbacks. Side effects and accidental poisoning have been noted, with one reported death. Obviously this provides a strong contraindication to its use. In addition, it has a high relapse rate when discontinued and a decreased response rate if restarted. Antidiuretics and diuretics are generally not used in treatment. They might be used by some physicians on special occasions, however, such as participation in overnight activities.

Enuresis Alarms

If bed-wetting is problematic and does not respond to simple measures, the treatment of choice is an enuresis alarm. This is an extremely effective method if well supervised and will cure 80% of children who are bed wetters. Unfortunately, in practice, it is often used improperly and poorly supervised. Many pediatric departments, health clinics, public health nurses, and surgical suppliers have a stock of alarms that can be borrowed or rented. Usually, though, the alarm is given to the family with little explanation of how or why it should work, with the only instruction being to come back in 3 months. Understandably, few children are cured and treatment is often abandoned before becoming effective. An alarm works better for the older child, who can take responsibility for its use.

The amount of disruption and extra work occasioned by the use of an alarm should not be underestimated. It is essential for the child and parents to be well motivated for success. If there is any suspicion

Table 5–1. *MEDICATIONS FOR ENURESIS*

Drug Class	Example	Mechanism of Action
Antispasmodic	Oxybutynin	Reduces uninhibited bladder contractions
Anticholinergic	Imipramine	Reduces uninhibited bladder contractions
Antidepressent	Imipramine	Decreases level of sleep
Antidiuretic	Desmopressin	Induces temporary water retention
Diuretic		Induces moderate dehydration

From Faller, N. A.: Enuresis. J. Enterost. Ther., *14*:66, 1987.

of child abuse the treatment should be particularly closely supervised and supported.

The use of the alarm must be explained in language appropriate to the child's level of understanding. It can be described as a helper for learning bladder control. There are two types of alarms, the modern pants system (see Fig. 5–1) and the older bell-and-pad device. The former is compact, discreet, lightweight, easy to assemble, and sensitive to a few drops of urine. The latter consists of a pad with connecting leads to an alarm (Fig. 5–3.)

Most alarms can be tested, and this should be done nightly. Normal (unrestricted) fluid intake should be allowed and the bladder emptied before the child goes to bed. When feasible, sleeping in a room alone is ideal so that siblings are not disturbed. This is not crucial, however, and an older brother or sister might even assist the child.

When the child wets, the presence of urine completes a transistorized circuit, which causes the alarm to sound. The usual response is interruption of micturition and the child waking up. Often the child has difficulty in waking, especially during the first week. Sometimes the alarm can initially cause panic or fright and, if possible, the parents should sleep within earshot. If the child does not awaken the parents should wake the child while the alarm is still sounding. It is important for the child to learn to wake up at the sound of the alarm. Once awake the child should get up and attempt to finish urinating in the toilet. Younger children might need help to remake the bed and reset the alarm. Older children can usually manage alone. A night-light is especially helpful. Resetting the alarm is important in case of a second wet. In the morning a chart should be filled in to record the size of the wet patch and whether the child has urinated in the toilet (Fig. 5–4).

Most children need 15 to 20 nights before they learn to wake up

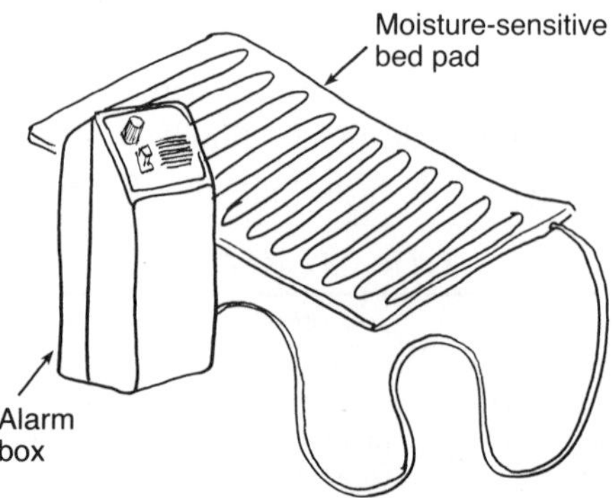

Figure 5–3. *Bed alarm. The alarm is placed on a bedside table; the moisture-sensing pad is placed on the bed beneath the sheet.*

Name .... **Week Commencing** ....

Please fill in this chart each morning

	Was the bed wet? (Yes or No)	Did the child wake to pass urine in the night? (Yes or No)	Fill in this section if alarm sounded in the night			
			At what time(s) did the alarm sound?	Did the alarm wake the child? (Yes or No)	Size of wet patch S = small, M = medium, L = large	Did the child have more urine to pass in the toilet? Write no, small, or large amount
Monday						
Tuesday						
Wednesday						
Thursday						
Friday						
Saturday						
Sunday						

Figure 5–4. *Detailed treatment record chart.*

prior to bladder emptying (and get up to urinate) or to hold urine all night. Either is a sign of success. Progress is usually indicated by the wet patch getting smaller and more urine being left in the bladder.

Some common problems can lead to the failure of therapy. The equipment itself might be faulty, especially if frequently on loan. Each user will need new batteries and sensors or mats. Sometimes the connector leads can become loose or the batteries weaker during treatment. A false alarm can occur if the wires become frayed or touch each other. Sweating can cause a false alarm, but a cooler bedroom can remedy this. Nylon sheets should be avoided. If the child fails repeatedly to wake to the sound of the alarm, models are available with louder signals or the alarm can be put into a cookie tin to amplify the sound. The child can be conditioned to wake to the alarm by using it for waking in the morning. The child can also be taught to interrupt micturition at the sound of the alarm if it is sounded during the day.

Vibrating alarms that can be placed under the pillow or against the collarbone are available for children with a hearing impairment or for those who sleep in a dormitory or with siblings.

It is not clear why the enuresis alarm is effective. Some professionals claim that it is classic conditioning—the child learns to pair the sensation of a full bladder with the conditioned response of waking and voiding. Others suggest that it might be avoidance learning; the child learns to avoid the unpleasant event of being awakened by the alarm. It is difficult to prove either theory.

An enuresis alarm can be used for children with both mental and physical handicaps. Obviously, more parental supervision will be required in such cases. Care must be taken with the mentally handicapped that the alarm is not seen as pleasurable, so that wetting is intentional to trigger the alarm. It sometimes happens that a child will sit on the bed in the daytime and wet on purpose just to create the buzz.

Treatment with the alarm usually takes 3 to 4 months. During this time it is prudent for the nurse to keep a regular check on the family to iron out any problems as soon as they arise and to keep motivation high. A home visit to check the equipment is useful if problems do occur. Once the bed has been reliably dry for 4 weeks the use of the alarm can be discontinued.

Roughly one-third of children relapse at some time after the conclusion of successful treatment. This relapse rate can be lowered considerably by using "overlearning" (Smith and Smith, 1987). This means that once the child has been dry for 14 consecutive nights, 1 to 2 pints of extra fluids should be given before going to bed. This often results in a recurrence of wetting for a few nights, but the child usually becomes dry again soon and now has a margin of error. Once there have been 2 dry weeks with the high fluid intake, the extra fluid and alarm are discontinued. If wetting does not start to diminish after 2 weeks of use of the overlearning method it should be abandoned and the child put back to normal fluid intake, with the alarm, until dry again.

Relapse does not mean that the alarm will not work a second time, and it should be used again. The child who has relapsed once does, in fact, have the same chance as first-timers of becoming dry and not relapsing again.

The enuresis alarm has been extensively used and researched with childhood bed wetters (Smith and Smith, 1987). Its use for adults with enuresis, however, has not been well documented. It is certainly worth trying with life-long bed wetters. Whether it has any role to play with the elderly who develop secondary enuresis remains to be seen.

CONGENITAL ABNORMALITIES

Certain congenital abnormalities of the urinary tract can be the underlying cause of incontinence in childhood. Minor abnormalities might be overlooked unless a careful physical examination is carried out on a child presenting with continuous or frequent wetting, day or night. Occasionally, congenital abnormalities are not picked up in childhood and persist undiagnosed into adult life.

Epispadias and Hypospadias

Epispadias is a condition in which the urethra opens onto the upper surface of the penis (Fig. 5–5*A*). It can vary from an abnormally wide meatus to a complete split of the penis. Rarely, it is seen in females in whom the clitoris and pubic bone are split. Treatment is surgical repair, but only 50% of boys treated surgically achieve complete continence.

Hypospadias, an opening of the urethra onto the undersurface of the penis, is more common, affecting 1 in 600 boys (Fig. 5–5*B*). These boys tend to have a "hooded" foreskin, no normal erections, and a urinary stream that is passed backward, between the legs. Again, treatment is surgical. It usually provides good results in regard to continence and sexual function.

Ectopic Ureter

The ureter, instead of inserting into the bladder at the trigone, may enter the urethra directly. If this occurs below the sphincteric level

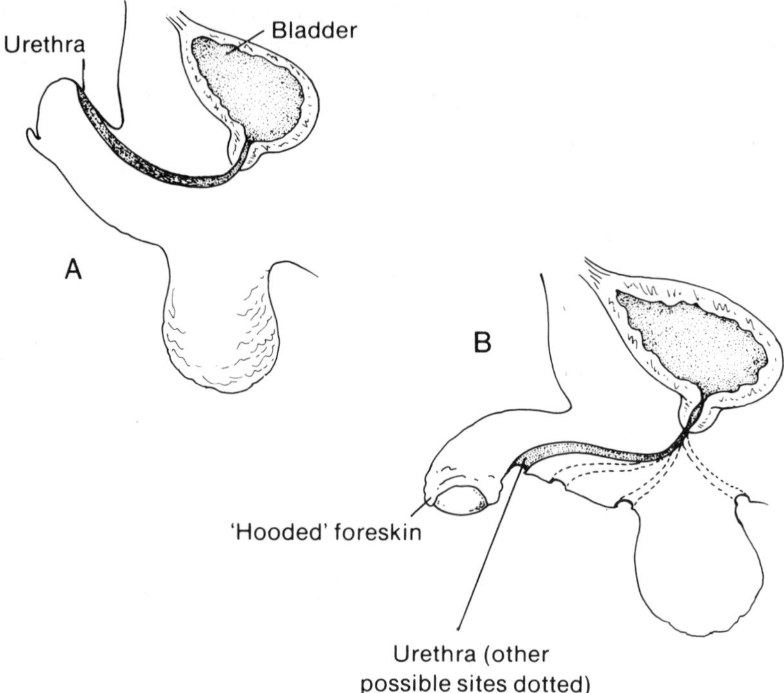

Figure 5–5. A, *Epispadias.* B, *Hypospadias.*

a continuous dribbling incontinence results. Usually this is associated with duplication of the upper urinary tract, with one ureter in the correct place and the second being ectopic. In such a case the child can urinate normally but also has dribbling.

Urethral Valves

Some boys are born with urethral valves that prevent proper bladder emptying, leading to retention with overflow incontinence. Usually diagnosed early in life, the baby often presents in renal failure with a poor urinary stream and a urinary tract infection. This serious condition must be corrected surgically. Occasionally, boys who have had this surgery later develop continence problems.

Ectopia of the Bladder

This is a rare and obvious condition in which the abdominal wall fails to develop over the bladder and consequently opens directly onto the skin at birth. The bladder has to be reconstructed surgically or the ureters diverted into an ileal conduit.

Parents of children with congenital abnormalities usually need a great deal of support. They often feel guilty for somehow having caused the abnormality and usually worry that the child will never be "normal." They fear for later sexual identity and function. A careful explanation and realistic reassurance are vital. Some repairs are done in several stages, involving the child in repeated hospital admissions at a vulnerable stage. The child and siblings can suffer emotionally, whether or not the parents stay in the hospital with the child. If the condition is not urgent, repair is often left until the child can cope better psychologically (e.g., after school age), but this might result in several years of both incontinence and feeling abnormal. Although long-term physical results are often excellent, the nurse has an important contribution in ensuring that the child makes a satisfactory psychologic adjustment.

References and Further Reading

Azrin, N.H., and Foxx, R.M.: Toilet Training in Less Than a Day. New York, Pocket Books, 1974.

Faller, N.A.: Enuresis. J. Enterost. Ther., *14*:66, 1987.

Meadow, R.: Patient Handbook: Help for Bed-Wetting. Edinburgh and London, Churchill Livingstone, 1980.

Morgan, R.T.T.: Childhood Incontinence. London, William Heinemann, 1981.

Scharf, M.B.: Waking Up Dry: How to End Bedwetting Forever. Cincinnati, Writer's Digest, 1986.

Schmitt, B.D.: Daytime wetting (diurnal enuresis). Pediatr. Clin. North Am., *29*:9, 1982.

Schmitt, B.D.: Nocturnal enuresis: An update on treatment. Pediatr. Clin. North Am., *29*:21, 1982.

Smith, P.S.: Questions mothers ask about toilet training. Nursing, 1:800, 1980.

Smith, P.S., and Smith, L.J.: Continence and Incontinence: Psychological Approaches to Development and Treatment. London, Croom Helm, 1987.

Brenda Donovan, RN, BSN

6 Female Incontinence

Although men and women can be incontinent for all the reasons outlined in Chapter 2, there are a few conditions specific to females that are discussed in this chapter. Stress incontinence is particularly common among women. All nurses have an important role in teaching preventive measures, counseling, and providing care. It is often a nurse who teaches and supervises a program of pelvic muscle exercises or the use of an occlusive device. For women who choose surgery, preoperative counseling and postoperative care and support comprise a major contribution that nurses can make to ensure a successful outcome. Also, the nurse will encounter many women with incontinence problems in pregnancy and immediately after childbirth.

GENUINE STRESS INCONTINENCE

There is much confusion about the term "stress incontinence." In fact, it can be used to describe a symptom or it can be a medical diagnosis. As a symptom it denotes the experience of leaking urine on physical exertion (physical, not emotional, stress). As a diagnosis it refers to incontinence caused by incompetence of the bladder neck and urethra—a failure of the urethra to maintain continence when aggravated by increased intra-abdominal pressure.

The symptom and diagnosis do not always coincide in one person.

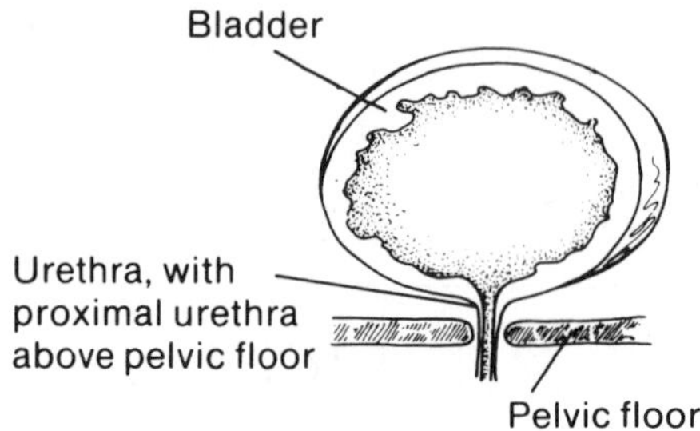

Figure 6–1. *Normal anatomic relationship of bladder, urethra, and pelvic floor: at rest.*

Leakage on exertion could be caused by an unstable bladder—for example, a cough might trigger a bladder contraction, thus mimicking an incompetent sphincter. Similarly, people in retention might experience overflow incontinence with exertion. Conversely, a patient whose underlying urinary problem is an incompetent bladder neck might complain of symptoms more suggestive of bladder instability, including frequency and urge incontinence. Thus, a history can be misleading in diagnosing the cause of incontinence, and often urodynamic investigation is required (Chap. 3).

In the remainder of this chapter the term "stress incontinence" is used to refer only to incontinence caused by a weak sphincter or incompetent bladder neck. The International Continence Society (1984) has defined this as genuine stress incontinence.

Mechanism

It is thought that stress incontinence in women is caused by an altered anatomic relationship between the bladder and urethra and their muscular supports, notably the pelvic floor. Normally the bladder and proximal urethra sit well supported above the pelvic floor (Fig. 6–1). The intravesical (bladder) pressure is below maximum urethral pressure at rest—a pressure gradient that maintains continence. Because the bladder is situated inside the abdominal cavity, any increase in intra-abdominal pressure (e.g., on coughing) raises the intravesical

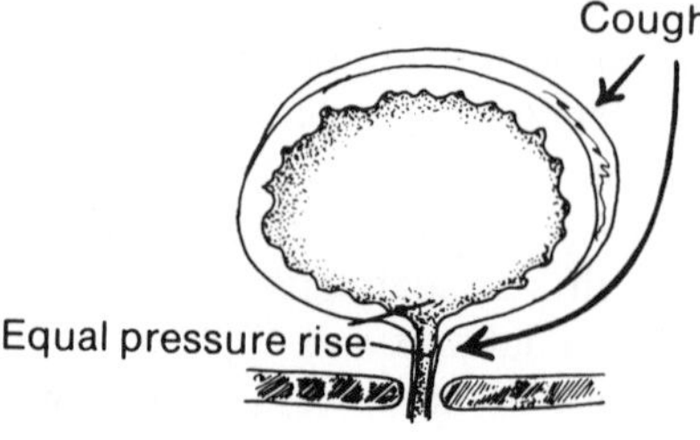

Figure 6–2. *Normal anatomic relationship of bladder, urethra, and pelvic floor: during a cough.*

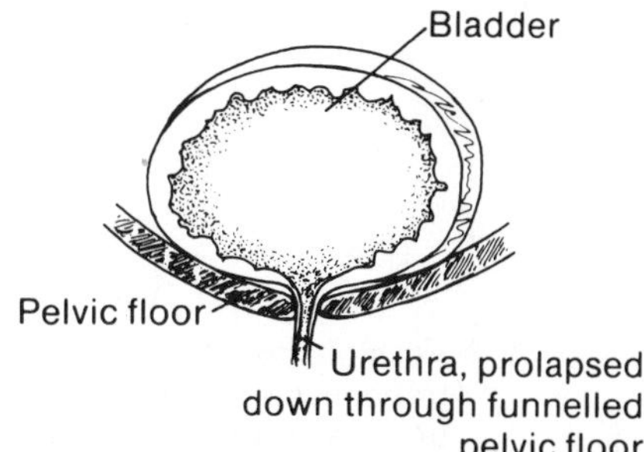

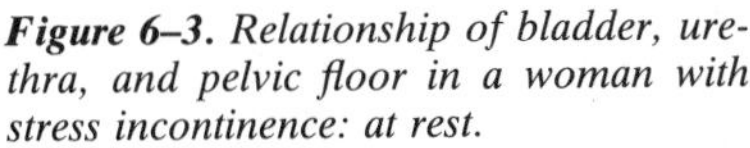
Figure 6–3. *Relationship of bladder, urethra, and pelvic floor in a woman with stress incontinence: at rest.*

pressure accordingly, which tends to squeeze urine out of the bladder. The upper (proximal) urethra is well supported and is also inside the abdominal cavity, so it is subject to the same rise in pressure, which can squeeze it shut. The pressure gradient is thereby maintained (Fig. 6–2). As long as urethral pressure is above bladder pressure at some point along the length of the urethra, continence is maintained.

Figure 6–3 depicts the relationship of the bladder and urethra to the pelvic floor in a woman with stress incontinence. The bladder has prolapsed through the pelvic floor. At rest this woman will be continent, because the urethral pressure is greater than the bladder pressure. Bladder pressure is raised when she coughs, but this pressure increase is only partially transmitted through the pelvic floor to the urethra, and sometimes not at all (Fig. 6–4). If the increase in intra-abdominal pressure is high enough for the pressure gradient to be lost, incontinence is the inevitable result.

Stress incontinence usually occurs immediately and coincidentally with the onset of effort, and ceases promptly when the activity ceases. It can be mild, only occurring with extreme physical exertion, such as jogging or playing tennis, or it can be severe with minor effort, such as walking, talking, or changing position causing leakage. In premenopausal women it tends to be worse in the week before a menstrual

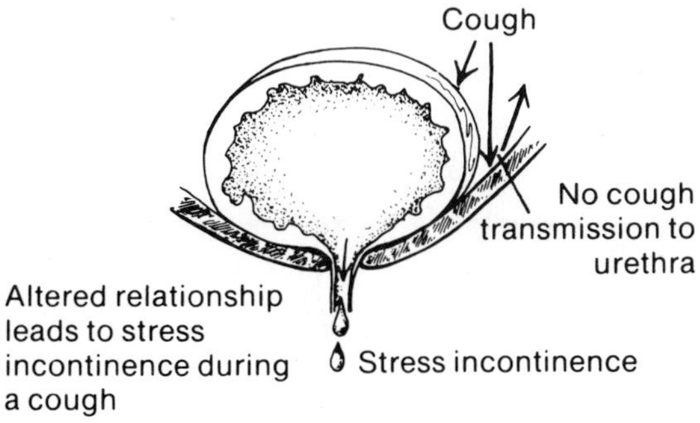

Figure 6–4. *Relationship of bladder, urethra, and pelvic floor in a woman with stress incontinence: during a cough.*

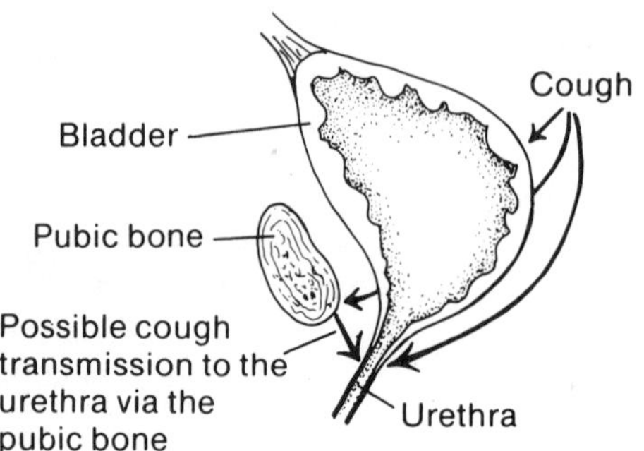

Figure 6–5. Possible cough transmission to the urethra by way of the pubic bone.

period, because the resting urethral pressure decreases with estrogen withdrawal. Similarly, menopausal women with a decreasing estrogen level experience an increased tendency to stress incontinence (Chap. 8).

It has been hypothesized that the relationship of the urethra to the pubic bone is important to continence. A urethra that is firmly supported up behind the pubic bone might have transmission of an increase in intra-abdominal pressure augmented by reflection from the bone (Fig. 6–5). This theory, however, remains unproved.

The pelvic floor contracts by reflex as the abdominal pressure is raised (Fig. 6–6), which also adds to the urethral closure pressure at the crucial time. If the pelvic floor is at an oblique rather than a right angle to the urethra, however, the efficiency of this extra margin for continence is impaired (Fig. 6–7).

Causes

Stress incontinence as described above does not occur in men (who could, however, have sphincter incompetence caused by direct trauma to the sphincter, such as postprostatectomy), which highlights the vulnerability of the female anatomy. With such a short urethra and a

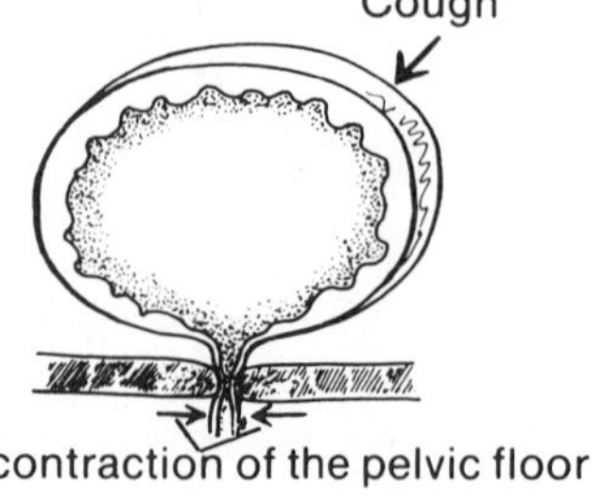

Figure 6–6. Normal contraction of the pelvic floor with raised abdominal pressure.

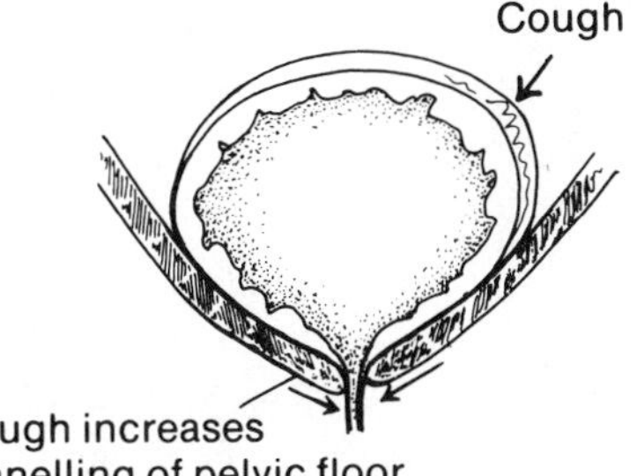

Figure 6–7. *Contraction of the pelvic floor with stress incontinence.*

relatively weak sphincteric mechanism, women are more susceptible to stress incontinence. Some surveys suggest that over 50% of all women experience stress incontinence at some time in their lives. For many it is a regular occurrence that can lead to considerable social restriction: the woman becomes unwilling to dance or even to laugh in public, and comes to dread colds, hay fever, or lifting.

Some females are born with a congenitally weak sphincter mechanism, and even an open bladder neck at rest. This is probably the cause of incontinence in girls who wet when they laugh or giggle ("giggle incontinence"). For some this resolves at puberty, but a few women have never known what it is like to have a good laugh without ending up soaked.

The process of childbirth is without doubt the most important factor underlying stress incontinence. Even though nulliparous women do get stress incontinence it is more likely to occur after childbirth, and multiparous women have a greatly increased chance of developing it. Improved obstetric care, especially that which does not allow a prolonged second stage of labor with consequent prolonged stretching of the pelvic floor, might decrease the incidence of the problem in the future.

After menopause many women experience atrophy and sagging of the pelvic supports. It is common for stress incontinence to start around menopause. This laxity, added to the previous trauma from childbirth, can allow the bladder and urethra to prolapse down through the pelvic floor. The uterus can also prolapse.

Other factors have been implicated in the cause of stress incontinence, but none with totally convincing evidence. Obesity is said to aggravate it, with some women experiencing improvement in their symptoms after weight loss. Repeated heavy lifting can cause trauma to the pelvic floor (although if done correctly this might actually strengthen rather than weaken the muscles). A chronic cough can put repeated stress on the pelvic floor. Habitual straining during defecation could cause eventual prolapse. The fact that slim, young, childless women experience stress incontinence, however, suggests a basic design flaw in the female anatomy.

Prevention

Research studies on the value of preventive health measures are both difficult and expensive to conduct. They have not yet been attempted in relation to the nonfatal condition of stress incontinence, so what follows is conjecture rather than proved fact.

Probably one of the most effective protective measures is conscientious practice of prenatal and postnatal exercises. Many women regard such exercises as designed to ease delivery and restore their figure after childbirth, as indeed they are. But their value in preventing pelvic floor laxity has not been emphasized enough. With the excitement of having a new baby and the exhaustion of sleepless nights, exercise programs are often deferred or forgotten completely. Many women either do not appreciate or are not properly taught about the risk to continence presented by childbirth. Many obstetric units now have a clinical nurse specialist who emphasizes postnatal pelvic muscle re-education. In the absence of such a specialist staff nurses should take on the responsibility for teaching and, more importantly, for reinforcing the importance of these exercises, especially in the difficult period after hospital discharge.

Greater health awareness might also help to prevent stress incontinence in more general ways. Regular bowel habits, aided by a balanced, high-fiber diet, an interest in fitness, and increased use of hormone replacement therapy for postmenopausal women, might all lead to future generations of women having a lower incidence of stress incontinence. Some exercise classes now include pelvic muscle exercises as part of the routine. Awareness that the pelvic muscles exist should be taught as part of basic health education, ideally beginning in middle school.

Treatment

The best time to begin treatment for stress incontinence is when the problem arises. Unfortunately, many women tolerate it for a considerable length of time or until it becomes really troublesome. Those involved in public health education could do more to make women realize that they should not expect to leak after having a baby or as they get older, and that they should seek help for this curable condition. The choice of treatment depends on the severity of symptoms, the degree of concomitant uterine prolapse, and the individual's personal preference.

Pelvic Muscle Exercises

Re-education of the pelvic muscles by regular exercise is the best form of therapy for mild to moderate stress incontinence in the absence of severe uterine prolapse. The patient needs to be well motivated and sufficiently alert to cooperate intelligently and to remember to carry out the exercise program, if it is to be successful. The exercises can be taught by a nurse or other trained specialist.

There are three groups of muscles comprising the pelvic floor—the levator ani, the urogenital diaphragm, and the outlet muscles. For the purpose of these exercises the levator ani are the most important. These have three components, the pubococcygeus, ileococcygeus, and ischiococcygeus muscles. The pubococcygeus forms a sling with an interior gap through which the urethra, vagina, and rectum pass (Fig. 6–8). This striated muscle constitutes the voluntary component of both bladder and bowel control.

Preventive and remedial pelvic muscle exercises are essentially identical, although once stress incontinence has occurred they must be done more frequently and persistently. Before starting the exercises a careful history should be taken and a thorough explanation of the aims of the exercises given. The following explanation can be adapted to the individual's level of understanding.

It is useful to describe the pelvic floor as a "hammock" that is suspended between the pubic and tail bones. When this muscle is young and healthy it lies fairly flat and keeps the body's orifices firmly closed. After childbirth (or menopause, or whatever is appropriate to the patient) the hammock sags and can no longer hold these openings tightly closed, especially when additional stress is put on it. With a cough it just gives way and lets a little urine out. The aim of the exercise is to bring the pelvic muscle back to where it should be. Using two cupped hands this explanation can be clearly illustrated to the patient.

The patient should then be examined in the supine position, with her knees bent up and abducted laterally. The presence of a cystocele (prolapse of the anterior vaginal wall) or rectocele (prolapse of the posterior vaginal wall) should be noted. If either of these is severe, or if the uterus itself descends down the vagina, the chance of success from these exercises is probably diminished. They might still be worth a try, though, especially if the patient is motivated. Even if surgery becomes necessary these exercises improve muscle tone and local blood flow, thus aiding in the postoperative healing process.

The instructor should insert two fingers into the vagina and instruct

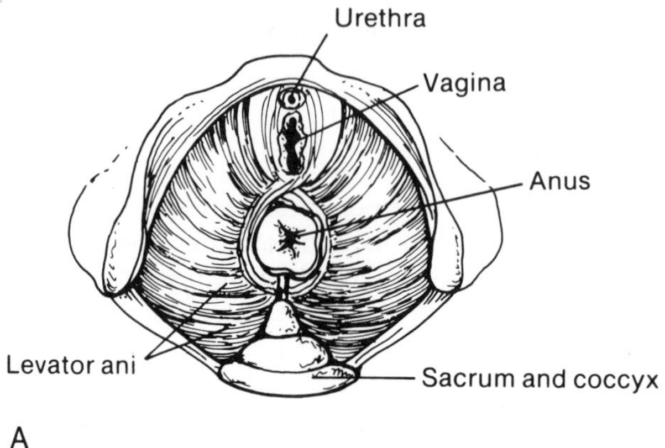

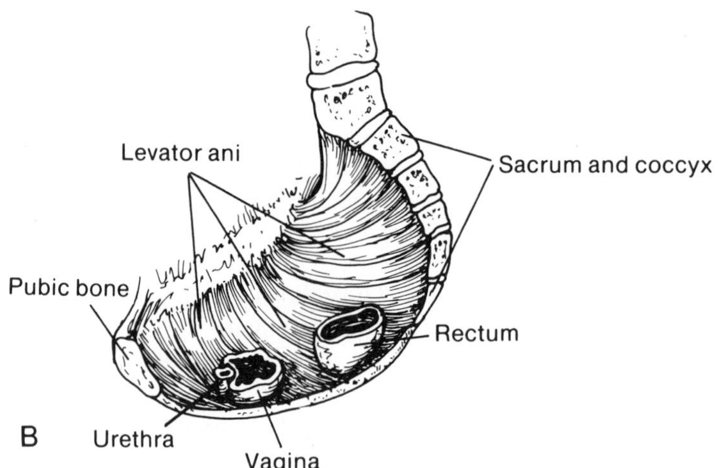

Figure 6–8. *Muscles of the pelvic floor.* A, *Levator ani muscles viewed from below.* B, *Side view.*

the patient to squeeze. Many women cannot do so or do something else, such as bearing down or contracting the buttocks or abdominal muscles. The muscle tone should be carefully assessed, and it is best for the examiner to persist until the patient can identify the correct action or at least stop using the wrong muscles. A gentle squeeze can be felt about two finger joints inside the introitus if the patient is doing it correctly. It can help to ask the patient to imagine that she is attempting to control severe diarrhea in public to locate the muscle. Some women can distinguish a contraction of the anterior portion of the pelvic muscle (around the urethra and vagina) from a posterior contraction (around the anus), and can exercise either separately. If this is so the patient can concentrate her efforts anteriorly. This is beyond most women, however, who are best advised to contract the entire pelvic muscle during these exercises. The exercise program includes interruption of micturition midstream to identify the muscles and regular practice of the same action. Interruption midstream uses the muscles effectively and helps to identify what a pelvic muscle contraction feels like. The patient is instructed to sit on the toilet with her knees apart, to start passing urine and then, once the stream is coming fast, to stop as quickly and completely as possible. At first she might only be able to slow rather than stop the stream, but this will come with practice. When stopping she should concentrate on the feeling produced, which is the pelvic muscle contraction. The bladder should then be emptied completely. Two or three interruptions can be done each time the woman passes urine if the bladder is nearly full.

Once the pelvic muscles have been correctly identified, either by digital examination or by interruption of the stream, the exercise can start in earnest. The patient is instructed to lie, sit, or stand with her knees slightly apart, and slowly but firmly to contract the pelvic muscles, hold the contraction for 5 seconds, and relax. This should be done five times every hour throughout each day, every day. This might sound like a lot at first, but it should be emphasized to the patient that the exercises involve minimal disruption of activities—they can be done almost anywhere without anyone else knowing. They will do no good if practiced less often and should not be done more frequently either, because the muscles will become fatigued and ache and the patient will become disinclined to continue. If an hourly program is difficult to remember, the patient can relate the exercise to regular daily activities (e.g., brushing the teeth, drinking morning coffee).

Some women like to check that they are doing the exercises correctly by inserting a finger into their vagina while exercising. They should be able to feel the gentle squeeze for themselves. A perineometer is useful for feedback. This comprises a vaginal probe with a gauge that indicates the strength of the squeeze (Fig. 6–9). This can tell the patient that she is exercising correctly and that her muscle strength is gradually increasing. This is important in the phase before symptoms actually improve—it is always tempting to give up before progress is evident.

After starting these exercises it is important for the patient to be seen regularly and to be re-examined. This provides an opportunity to check whether she is using the correct muscles, give her encouragement, sustain motivation, and discuss any worries or questions. Usually patients should be seen every 2 to 4 weeks. Few will notice any major improvement for 6 to 8 weeks. Most patients improve somewhat by 3 months if they are going to, although some take 6 to 9 months to achieve maximum benefit from the exercises. It can be difficult to keep

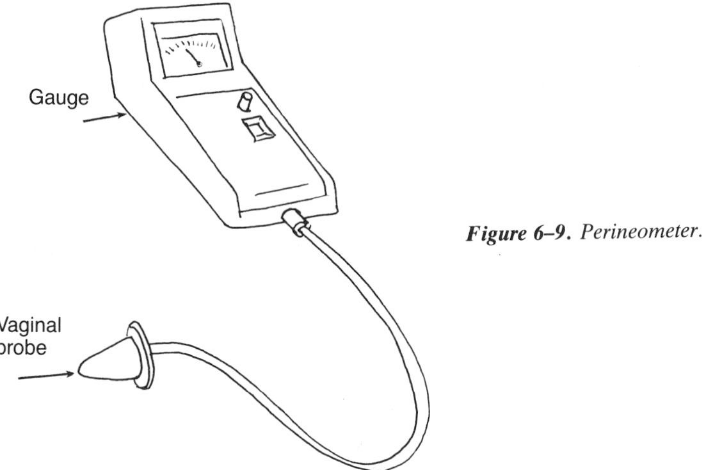

Figure 6–9. *Perineometer.*

the patient doing the exercises consistently for as long as this, although many women do find that it becomes automatic after a while.

If patients are carefully selected (i.e., a motivated woman with mild to moderate stress incontinence, without significant prolapse) many can probably be cured by doing pelvic muscle exercises. Thus, the patient can often avoid surgery and have the satisfaction that she cured herself. As an added benefit many find that their own and their partner's sexual enjoyment is increased as muscle tone improves.

Electrical stimulation can be used to assist in teaching pelvic muscle exercises. The stimulator uses a vaginal probe that induces a pelvic muscle contraction electrically. It can be useful for a patient who is totally unable to do this voluntarily to identify the correct sensation, and thereby learn how to replicate it. Electrical stimulation and biofeedback are advocated by some as an adjunct to pelvic muscle exercises.

Biofeedback is an adjunct for teaching pelvic muscle exercises. Visual or auditory feedback is provided by a gauge or monitor attached to a sensor. Some studies have shown biofeedback to be more effective than verbal feedback alone (Burgio and colleagues, 1986).

Surgery

Women with a moderate degree of stress incontinence that has not been relieved by pelvic muscle exercises, and those with a severe problem, especially if associated with considerable prolapse, often require surgery to alleviate the condition. The goal of surgical procedures for stress incontinence is restoration of the proximal urethra and bladder neck area to their normal intra-abdominal location. The choice of operation depends on the individual surgeon's expertise and the patient's preference.

Vaginal Repair. There are a great many variations on vaginal repair and needle suspension procedures. The most commonly performed are the modified Pereyra (Raz, 1981) and the Stamey (Stamey, 1980). These procedures have about a 90% success rate and facilitate simultaneous vaginal repair for associated prolapse.

Retropubic Colposuspension. The alternative approach involves an abdominal (usually bikini line) incision. Suspensory (nonabsorbable) sutures are placed in the vaginal wall lateral to the bladder neck and are fixed to the periosteum or cartilage of the symphysis pubis. Burch has described placing the sutures into Cooper's ligament (Leach and Donovan, 1985). These procedures continue to be widely employed, with an overall success rate of 85 to 95% (Raz, 1979).

Sling Procedures. In women with a severe degree of periurethral fibrosis, fixation, and possible denervation, a sling procedure can be carried out. An organic (strips of fascia) or synthetic (e.g., strips of polypropylene or polyethylene) sling is used to support and elevate the bladder neck by attachment to ligaments or the periosteum.

Other forms of surgical treatment for the denervated or severely damaged urethra include the insertion of an artificial urinary sphincter (Barrett and Furlow, 1983) and the injection of periurethral Teflon (Carrion and Politano, 1983). As with any operation, a slight risk is attached to the use of these procedures. Vaginal repair has the advantages that it is not a major procedure, there is no abdominal scar, and rehabilitation is rapid, usually with only 3 to 5 days of hospitalization required. There might be transient postoperative retention, which is easily managed with intermittent catheterization. Conversely, the retropubic and sling procedures are more extensive operations, involve an abdominal incision, and require longer hospitalization and convalescence. Candidates for insertion of an artificial sphincter should be carefully selected and advised about the possibility of mechanical difficulties and the risk of infection, which could require additional surgery. The use of Teflon remains controversial because of the concern of particle migration from the injection site.

Any type of surgery requires careful preoperative and postoperative counseling. This can help to increase both the success of the procedure and the patient's satisfaction and adjustment. The patient must be given a full explanation of the procedure and what to expect. It should be made clear that none of these operations guarantees success and the chances of cure should be honestly discussed. Patients who have an unrealistic expectation of a total cure tend to be highly intolerant and disappointed if any symptoms, however mild, persist postoperatively. If a hysterectomy is a possibility, the decision involves careful thought and discussion with spouse or family.

If the patient still intends to have children surgery should be delayed until after the final pregnancy, especially with sling operations, because vaginal delivery might be difficult and undo the effects of the surgery. All patients should be warned that stress incontinence could recur at a later date. This is especially true if vigorous exercise or heavy lifting is undertaken. Women who only leak when they lift heavy weights, or have a job that involves heavy manual labor, should probably be discouraged from choosing surgery. Because the convalescent periods are different (a few weeks for vaginal procedures, up to 3 months for slings), women with family or career commitments might prefer the former, even with the knowledge that the success rate is lower.

Postoperative advice should include instructions to limit activities during the convalescent period, especially avoiding lifting and abdominal effort. The patient should also refrain from sexual intercourse for 6 weeks to allow full healing. Many women experience problems in returning to an active and fulfilling sex life after surgery. Sometimes the reason for this is psychologic, because of a changed body image, especially after a hysterectomy. There might be physical discomfort because of incomplete healing or local infection. Usually the actual anatomy of the vagina has been altered, and it often takes both partners time to adjust to the new contours. Sometimes there is a ridge or kink in the vaginal wall. Women might be nervous or anxious in case it should hurt or the operation be "undone," and so they could be understimulated and poorly lubricated. Simple explanations, reassurances that no harm can be done, and possibly a tube of water-soluble jelly for lubrication can help to resolve the problem for some. Use of the lubricant can be made more comfortable by warming it in warm water before use. Occasionally it is advisable to experiment with new positions for intercourse to overcome problems with a taut anterior vaginal wall.

Formerly, many women underwent multiple surgical procedures for stress incontinence, with the problem remaining or recurring. Sometimes this happened because the original diagnosis was wrong, and the woman actually had detrusor instability rather than genuine stress incontinence. Hopefully, the increased use of urodynamic investigation to obtain a more precise diagnosis will help to minimize this in the future. The first operation has the highest chance of success. As more urologists and gynecologists become interested and expert in incontinence surgery, there should be fewer failures.

Construction of a Neourethra. In a few centers a technique has been developed for the construction of a completely new urethra from a flap of bladder muscle (Mundy, 1989; Blaivas, 1989; Bavendam and Leach, 1987). This can be used for women with congenital abnormalities, or for those with a urethra that has become scarred and dysfunctional from repeated surgery. It is too early to evaluate the success of this procedure, but it might hold hope for the future.

URINARY FISTULA

A fistula, or false passage, between the bladder and vagina can cause continuous, uncontrollable, passive incontinence. It is relatively uncommon in women in Western countries, where it is usually iatrogenic, a result of a mishap during gynecologic surgery or pelvic irradiation for tumor. It is more common in underdeveloped countries as a complication of obstructed delivery. Prolonged pressure of the baby's head causes tissue necrosis and the resultant sloughing leaves a fistula.

Fistulas caused surgically or during childbirth are usually repaired surgically. This is done vaginally 6 to 10 weeks after the trauma has occurred, provided that the patient is in good health. Postirradiation fistulas are more difficult to repair, because much scar tissue and an avascular zone in the vagina are usually present, and the patient is often in poor health.

There can be little doubt about the misery caused by a urinary fistula. It is difficult to cope with the constant leakage of urine. The quality of life often worsens and the patient becomes isolated and depressed. If the defect cannot be closed surgically, a urinary diversion into an ileal conduit can be performed whenever the patient's health allows it (Chap. 4). Even though a stoma means continuous incontinence, this is at least controllable with a urostomy pouch. If the patient is not a surgical candidate, absorbent products or a female external collection device can be used to manage the incontinence (Chap. 13).

INCONTINENCE AND SEXUAL ACTIVITY

Some women experience urinary incontinence during sexual activity. It is not known how common this is, but certainly any nurse working in a continence clinic is familiar with the problem. It can be difficult for a patient to talk about it and the nurse should provide an opportunity and give appropriate cues to make such a discussion possible. Women might leak urine at other times, but for some this is the only occasion in which they experience incontinence. Either way it can be a source of considerable worry and embarrassment. The patient might not have openly discussed the leakage with her partner. Other couples, on the other hand, might regard it as a minor nuisance that they can laugh about together.

Leakage usually occurs during intercourse or at orgasm (often the entire bladder contents are emptied at orgasm). The mechanism for this incontinence is unknown. Not surprisingly, it is difficult to investigate. Mechanical pressure or a detrusor contraction probably underlies the problem. Sometimes treatment for an identifiable voiding dysfunction (e.g., drug therapy for detrusor instability) cures the incontinence. Otherwise the patient needs plenty of reassurance that the symptom is of no pathologic significance and advice on learning how to live with it. The patient should, when possible and appropriate, empty the bladder fully before commencing sexual activity. The bed or other surface can be protected with a thick towel or washable drawsheet (Chap. 13) to minimize discomfort and inconvenience afterward. For couples with a close and sympathetic relationship, a postcoital bath or shower together is often the only consequence of the woman's incontinence.

INCONTINENCE IN PREGNANCY

Incontinence of urine is a common symptom in pregnancy. Probably over 50% of all primiparous women and over 75% of multiparous women experience some incontinence. Most complain of increased frequency of micturition, usually starting in the first trimester and persisting until the birth. Various causes have been proposed for this increased frequency, including polydipsia, mechanical pressure on the bladder, and the onset of an unstable bladder. None of these really explains it adequately, but each might hold true for some women. Most expect and accept frequency with only a few being unduly incapacitated by it.

Incontinence during pregnancy is usually experienced as stress incontinence. Sometimes this was present prior to pregnancy, but for many it is a new phenomenon. It is seldom severe enough to represent a significant problem. This is obviously a good time for women to be taught pelvic muscle exercises. It is important for physicians, midwives, and prenatal instructors to work together and teach women about the functioning of the pelvic muscles, and how to maintain and strengthen their vulnerable sphincter mechanism.

OCCLUSIVE DEVICES

Several devices are available that control female urinary incontinence by occluding the urethra mechanically. Although they are most appropriate for women with stress incontinence, they can be used to control any type of leakage. The aim is to restore normal pressure and anatomic relationships by lifting and supporting the bladder neck and urethra. These devices do not treat the cause of the problem, so they should not be a first choice except if the woman is not a candidate for or does not desire other therapy.

Tampons. Some women find that a large tampon worn in the vagina controls mild incontinence. This method is particularly suitable for women who are accustomed to using tampons and who have only an occasional problem. For example, a woman who leaks slightly while playing sports might choose this method to control leakage. A female who says her incontinence is better during her period should be questioned about her method of sanitary protection, because using a tampon might be the reason for improvement. She will then trust this method of control. It is unwise to use tampons continuously, because their absorbent properties can make the vagina sore and dry.

Ring Pessary. If stress incontinence is associated with an obvious prolapse of the anterior vaginal wall, a ring pessary can be fitted by a gynecologist (Fig. 6–10). The rings come in a wide range of sizes. Insertion is usually momentarily uncomfortable, but once in place the pessary is generally comfortable if the correct size has been chosen. The ring is indwelling and, in most cases, the patient can be instructed to remove and reinsert it. Careful explanation must be given before the use of a pessary is considered; some women dislike the idea and reject it. It should be carefully established that the patient is not still sexually active, because a ring pessary is unsuitable unless the patient is comfortable removing and reinserting the device. Some older women with vaginal atrophy and some nulliparous women have such a small introitus that a pessary cannot be inserted. Pessaries are best used in the older woman with stress incontinence and pelvic prolapse who does not want or is unfit for surgery. In some women reduction of a large cystocele by the pessary can actually increase incontinence. Mental and physical disabilities are not contraindications, because little management is required by the patient or caregiver.

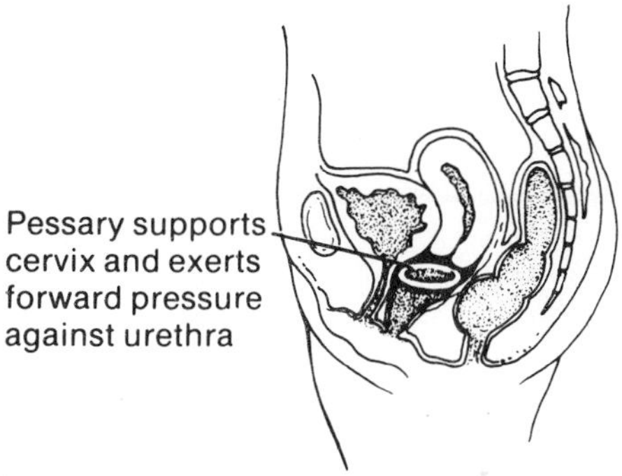

Figure 6–10. *Ring pessary. The ring stays in place, as shown here, supported by the bone and ligaments of the pelvic rim.*

References

Barrett, D.M., and Furlow, W.L.: Artificial urinary sphincter in the management of female incontinence. *In* Raz, S. (ed.): Female Urology. Philadelphia, W.B. Saunders, 1983, pp. 284–292.

Bavendam, T., and Leach, G.: Urogynecologic reconstruction. Problems in Urology, *1*(2):295, 1987.

Blaivas, J.G.: Vaginal flap urethral reconstruction: An alternative to the bladder flap neourethra. J. Urol., *141*(3):542, 1989.

Burgio, K.L., Robinson, J.C., and Engel, B.T.: The role of biofeedback in Kegel exercise training for stress urinary incontinence. Am. J. Obstet. Gynecol., *154*:58, 1986.

Carrion, H.M., and Politano, V.A.: Periurethral polytef injection for urinary incontinence. *In* Raz, S. (ed.): Female Urology. Philadelphia, W.B. Saunders, 1983, pp. 293–298.

International Continence Society Committee on Standardization of Terminology: The Standardization of Terminology of Lower Urinary Tract Function. Glasgow, Scotland, International Continence Society, 1984.

Leach, G.E., and Donovan, B.J.: Surgical correction of stress urinary incontinence. J. Urol. Nurs., *4*:306, 1985.

Mundy, A.R.: Urethral substitution in women. Br. J. Urol., *63*(1):80, 1989.

Raz, S.: Why Marshall-Marchetti operation works or does not. Urology, *14*:154, 1979.

Raz, S.: Modified bladder neck suspension for female stress incontinence. Urology, *17*:82, 1981.

Stamey, T.A.: Endoscopic suspension of the vesical neck for urinary incontinence in the female: Report of 203 consecutive patients. Ann. Surg. *192*:465, 1980.

Linda M. Duffy, RN, MS

7 Male Incontinence

Although men can be incontinent for reasons outlined elsewhere in this book, certain problems affect the male exclusively and are dealt with separately in this chapter. Prostate surgery is one of the major causes of urinary incontinence in males over the age of 40. In 1986, 319,000 prostatectomies were performed in the United States. The recorded incidence of postoperative incontinence varied from 0.1 to 22% (depending on the surgical approach, size of the gland, and definition of incontinence employed), affecting from 300 to 70,180 men.

PROSTATIC HYPERTROPHY

From the fifth decade of life onward all men have some degree of benign enlargement of the prostate gland (Fig. 7–1). About 10% will experience symptoms.

Symptoms

Symptoms caused by an enlarged prostate gland mainly involve mechanical obstruction to the passage of urine caused by the enlargement. Hesitancy, a slow, weak urinary stream, and terminal dribbling at the end of micturition are common. Often the bladder does not

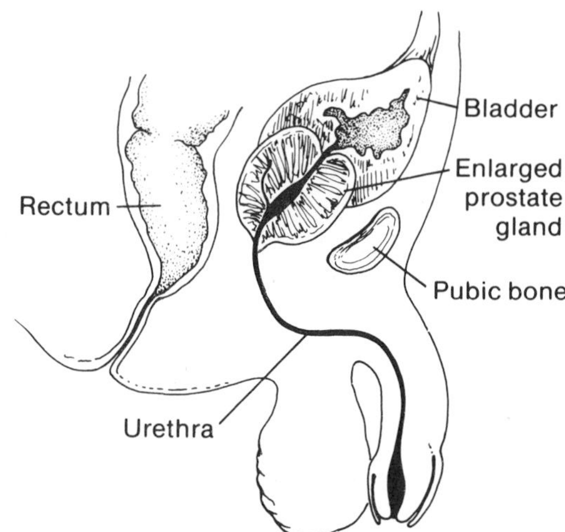

Figure 7–1. *Prostatic hypertrophy.*

empty completely and chronic residual urine is present. An unstable bladder secondary to the outlet obstruction develops in 70 to 80% of men. Symptoms of an unstable bladder include frequency, urgency, and nocturia. Approximately 60 to 75% of these bladders return to normal after the obstruction has been relieved. The presence of residual urine in large amounts can also cause symptoms of frequency and nocturia. Often nocturia is the first problem noticed by the patient. Urgency with urge incontinence or an almost continual dribbling overflow incontinence can result from overdistention of the bladder caused by large residual urine volumes. Dysuria with urgency might be seen in patients in whom the residual urine becomes infected. Sometimes rectal symptoms are troublesome—either a continuous desire to defecate caused by prostate pressure on the rectum or hemorrhoids resulting from repeated straining to void. On other occasions the first symptom the patient experiences is acute retention of urine and a complete inability to void.

Signs

The nurse might be the first person to spot the tense, distended abdomen of an elderly man who is totally unaware that his bladder is full to overflowing. If infection is superimposed, the urine can become cloudy and foul-smelling, occasionally with hematuria. A large residual volume can obstruct ureteric outflow, with consequent back pressure to the kidneys and the development of hydronephrosis. If this is the case, the patient might have symptoms of confusion, anorexia, weight loss, anemia, and dehydration resulting from the uremia.

It has been established that rapid emptying of the bladder is not dangerous to the patient if done using sterile precautions and if the bladder is not allowed to become overdistended again. No damage will be done to the kidneys and the bladder. The presence of blood in the urine should not cause alarm, because it represents only insignificant bleeding from the mucosal lining of the bladder wall. Nurses should be aware of the possibility of postobstructive diuresis during the first 24-hour period. This production of copious quantities of urine represents the kidneys' attempt to re-establish homeostasis within the body after a period of temporary shutdown caused by back pressure in the ureters from the large volume of residual urine. The patient must be carefully monitored for fluid intake and output. If large discrepancies are found, a program of fluid replacement must be initiated.

Often, by the time help is sought, the problem has been present for many years. If the detrusor muscle is repeatedly trying to overcome raised outflow resistance, the muscle tends to hypertrophy and can develop a secondary detrusor instability and trabeculation (weakened outpouchings between hypertrophied muscle bundles).

Diagnosis

Uroflowmetry of full-bladder voiding is the "essential, basic, clinical screening test for outflow obstruction" (Turner-Warwick, 1984). A careful history elicits many of the above symptoms, which are often aggravated by cold weather or alcohol. It is especially important to distinguish between symptoms of prostatic obstruction and those of a pure unstable detrusor, which more often presents as frequency, urgency, or urge incontinence, or a combination of these, with little or no voiding difficulty. The presence of residual urine can be misleading, because some patients cannot void normally unless their bladder is fully distended, they are in a familiar setting, and they are sitting or standing in their position of choice. A true postvoiding residual is not diagnostic of obstruction but indicates the need for further investigation. Digital rectal examination can reveal an enlarged prostate gland, but the palpable size of the gland bears no direct relationship to the degree of outflow obstruction. Indeed, even a minimally enlarged prostate can obstruct the urethra, whereas some large glands cause no problems.

Visualization of the prostate through a cystoscope is no longer thought to be the most reliable method of assessing size and degree of obstruction. Similarly, the presence of trabeculation of the bladder wall, once believed to relate to the degree and duration of obstruction, is now reported to correlate more commonly with unstable detrusor function, which might be associated with obstruction.

Abdominal examination can reveal bladder distention. A flow study (Chap. 3) will usually document a low, prolonged flow, sometimes interrupted or with a "tail." It is important to ensure that the patient feels the uroflowmetry record represents his usual voiding. Catheterization for postvoid residual urine volume is essential, but should be considered valid only after a full-bladder void has been perceived by the patient as adequate or usual for him. The amount of residual urine is one criterion used to decide the need for surgical intervention.

Necessary laboratory studies include taking a midstream urine specimen for urinalysis and culture and carrying out blood tests to determine renal function (e.g., BUN and creatinine). Kidney function can be investigated further by renography or intravenous pyelography. Cystometry, if performed, will show a high voiding pressure with a low flow rate and often detrusor instability during filling. Many prostatectomies are performed without prior cystometry but, if the diagnosis of an unstable bladder is suspected, the test is essential. A prostatectomy performed on a man with an unobstructed urethra and an unstable bladder merely reduces his outflow resistance and makes him even more likely to be incontinent.

Treatment by Prostatectomy

Roughly 50% of men who experience symptoms from prostate enlargement eventually require a prostatectomy. Surgery is not required unless there is residual urine and troublesome symptoms. Minor symptoms can be managed conservatively. If the gland is soft and boggy, prostatic massage might provide relief. Medication is used to reduce bladder irritation and decrease chronic congestion of the gland. Patients should be cautioned to refrain from alcohol and to avoid becoming chilled. Additionally, they should be instructed not to delay voiding once the urge is felt.

The amount of residual urine present is more important than the size of the gland in determining the need for surgery. If surgery is contraindicated for some reason, intermittent catheterization can be successfully employed to empty the bladder of all residual urine on a regular basis. If intermittent catheterization is not feasible an indwelling catheter can be used. Researchers in England recently reported on the benefits of Indoramin (an alpha antagonist used for hypertension) as an adjunct for patients unwilling or unable to undergo surgery (Stott and Abrams, 1988). The preferred surgical approach depends on the size of the gland and the preference and expertise of the surgeon.

Surgical Approaches

Transurethral Resection of the Prostate. Transurethral resection of the prostate (TUR or TURP) is performed using a specially adapted cystoscope and is a relatively safe operation. Because no abdominal incision is made, patients can ambulate comfortably soon after surgery, and this is of great benefit to older patients. All but the largest prostates can be removed transurethrally. Removal must be done by an experienced urologist, however, because it is possible to damage the external urethral sphincter, which will almost always result in incontinence.

Open Prostatectomy. Open prostatectomy is performed through a lower abdominal incision (suprapubic) and the prostate is "shelled out" of its capsule. In many ways this is a simpler operation requiring less skill than a TURP, and it can be performed on even the largest prostates. It does, however, involve an abdominal wound and general anesthesia. Ambulation can be delayed by abdominal discomfort, thus increasing the risk of respiratory and circulatory complications.

Perineal Prostatectomy. This technique is easier to perform than transurethral prostatectomy, but is more complex than using the suprapubic approach. Sexual impotence occurs more frequently as a result of this procedure than with TURP or open prostatectomy.

Complications

Roughly 20% of men experience some complications after prostate surgery. It is important to discuss these possibilities fully with the patient prior to making a decision about surgery. Unless there are urgent medical indications (e.g., imminent renal failure), the patient should be encouraged to decide whether his symptoms are troublesome enough to warrant the risk of the possible complications. It should not be forgotten that an elderly man can value his fertility and potency as highly as a younger man. Thorough preoperative counseling can reduce many later regrets and recriminations.

The most frequent complication of any approach is hemorrhage. Infection is a possibility, even with the prophylactic use of antibiotics. General anesthesia always involves a certain degree of risk, especially for those in older age groups. Thus, use of spinal anesthesia for patients undergoing TURP is common practice.

Impotence can result from prostatectomy. Men who have experienced previous erectile problems are at greater risk for developing postoperative impotence. Infertility following prostatectomy is the result of retrograde ejaculation of semen into the bladder caused by surgical alteration of the bladder neck during surgery.

TYPES OF INCONTINENCE

Postprostatectomy Incontinence

The male anatomy has two functional urethral sphincters (Fig. 7–2). The proximal (internal) sphincter includes the bladder neck and

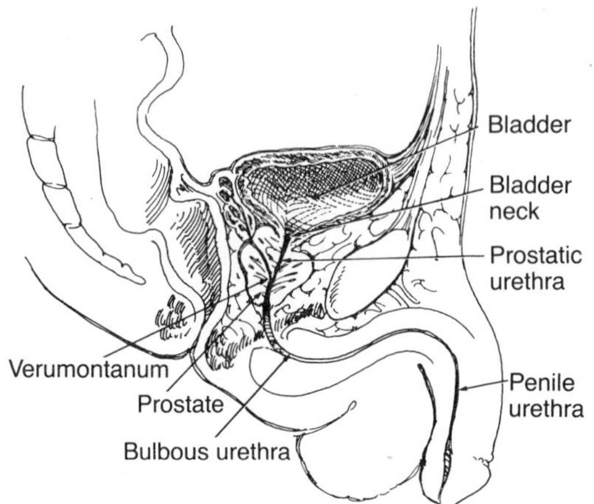

Figure 7–2. *Normal anatomic relationships of the male urethra.*

prostatic urethra, which extends down to the verumontanum. The distal (external) sphincter extends from the verumontanum to the bulbar urethra and consists of three types of muscle fibers—smooth, intrinsic, and extrinsic skeletal muscle. The bulbous urethra is not involved in continence. The proximal urethral sphincter is removed by prostatectomy. In the case of TURP and simple open procedures the distal sphincter should remain intact and maintain continence. Radical prostatectomy is associated with an increased risk of damage to the distal sphincter. The incidence of incontinence associated with TURP or simple prostatectomy is approximately 1 to 5%, depending on the definition of incontinence applied (Worth, 1984; Chilton and colleagues, 1978). Radical prostatectomy results in incontinence in 1 to 22% of patients (Lange and Reddy, 1987). The presence of an unstable detrusor combined with a weakened sphincter is more likely to result in postoperative incontinence. Both surgeons and patients should be aware of this condition preoperatively so that realistic outcomes can be anticipated.

Many men experience increased urgency and slight incontinence immediately after prostatectomy. It should be explained that time is required to adjust to the new weaker outflow resistance and that the problem is temporary and should be resolved within a few weeks. Treatment should be conservative. Pelvic muscle exercises are useful at this time. The patient is instructed to interrupt the flow of urine midstream at every void. At first he may only be able to slow rather than stop the stream. At the same time a routine of regular pelvic muscle exercises is taught. The patient is instructed to contract the pelvic muscles five times hourly throughout the day. The exercises can considerably strengthen the pelvic muscle supports to the external sphincter, on which the patient is now reliant for continence. They can also increase the patient's confidence in his ability to control any incontinence.

Those patients who had an unstable bladder prior to prostatectomy take longer to regain continence postoperatively. Instability secondary to long-standing obstruction will not disappear immediately and it can take 6 to 12 months for the detrusor muscle to adjust to the new, lower outflow resistance. For a few men the instability is persistent and troublesome, causing frequency, urgency, and urge incontinence. This generally responds to standard therapy for unstable bladder, usually drugs and bladder training (Chap. 4). Explanation, reassurance, and the provision of a suitable incontinence product, while needed, will help to get the patient through this distressing postoperative phase (Chap. 13). Few problems are more depressing to the patient than an operation that leaves his symptoms unchanged or worsened. If the patient knows this is to be expected and will be relieved, he can usually cope better.

Occasionally postprostatectomy incontinence results from inadvertent external sphincter damage at operation. If the sphincter damage has been extensive, pelvic muscle exercises will seldom effect a cure. For these men the only hope of continence is further surgery or, in some cases, Teflon or collagen injections. An implantable device can be used to correct this type of incontinence (or that caused by sphincter damage for any other reason).

Periurethral Injections. Periurethral and transurethral Teflon paste and collagen injections are currently being evaluated as an alternative to the implantation of mechanical devices. These procedures offer the advantages of a shorter hospital stay and fewer and less severe complications. The presence of the injectable material creates urethral closure with increased resistance and improved continence. Injections can be repeated if necessary. Possible complications of Teflon injections include urethritis, retention, abscess formation, and Teflon migration. Patients must be informed of these preoperatively.

Artificial Urinary Sphincter. The AMS (American Medical Systems) Sphincter 800 consists of three parts, a cuff, pump, and reservoir, all connected by silicone rubber tubing (Fig. 7–3). The cuff surrounds the urethra and is filled with fluid to exert gentle pressure, closing off the urethra. To allow urination the pump, located in the scrotum, is squeezed several times. (It can be used in women as well as men, in which case the pump is implanted in the labia rather than the scrotum). Squeezing transfers the fluid out of the cuff and into the abdominally placed reservoir. The pump feels flat when the cuff is empty. Urine is now free to exit the bladder, and the cuff automatically reinflates within 2 to 3 minutes. No action is required on the part of the patient to accomplish this return to continence. The reservoir has the unique ability to react to any increase in intra-abdominal pressure by transfer-

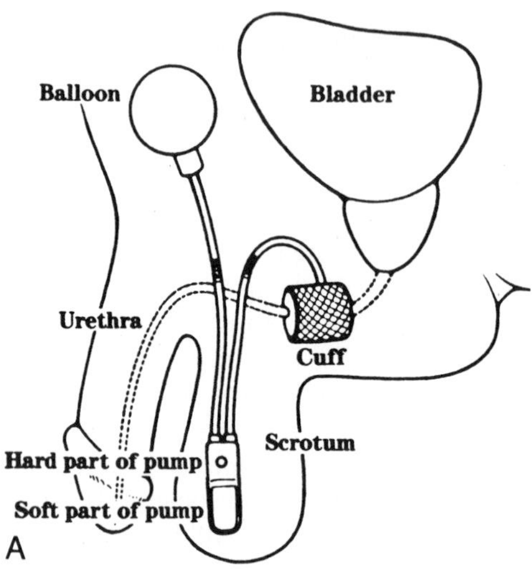

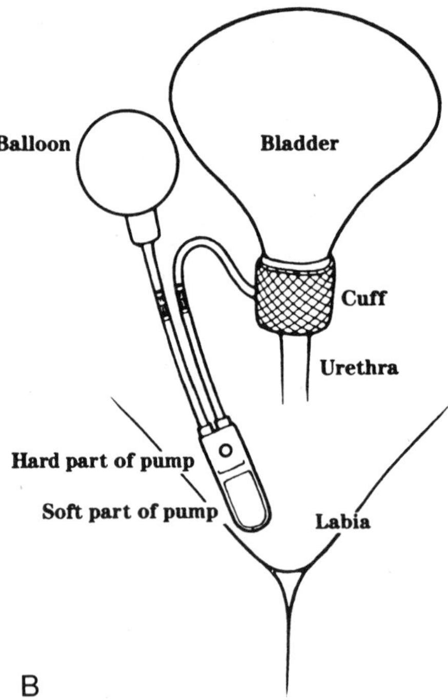

Figure 7–3. *AMS Sphincter 800.* A, *Bulbous urethra implantation, male.* B, *Bladder neck implantation, female. (Courtesy of American Medical Systems, Inc., Minnetonka, MN.)*

ring additional fluid into the cuff, which then increases urethral resistance and avoids stress incontinence during coughing, straining, or similar activities.

The long-term results with this device have been encouraging, but there are risks of mechanical failure, rejection, and erosion through the urethra, which are expensive to correct, especially the latter two. The number of surgeons experienced in the insertion of these devices is limited, but there is no doubt that many patients do benefit and experience few problems. Certainly, if the alternative is lifetime use of absorbent products or collection devices, or a urinary diversion, a prosthesis should be considered.

Surgical implantation of an artificial sphincter is generally not considered unless a minimum of 12 to 18 months has elapsed since prostatic surgery and all efforts directed toward conservative treatment have failed. Treatment goals of this type of surgery include allowing the patient to return to a normal micturition pattern while being maintained without leakage between voidings. In addition, overdistention of the bladder and ureteral reflux must be prevented. Criteria for placement of an artificial prosthesis include the documentation of unobstructed urinary flow, sterile urine, adequate bladder capacity, which would allow the patient to void only every 2 to 4 hours, the absence of bladder hyperreflexia, and the absence of reflux or residual urine (Furlow, 1981). Most of these can be accomplished by surgical or pharmacologic manipulation prior to implantation (Faller and Vinson, 1985).

Preoperative nursing assessment should ensure that the patient can understand how the device functions and can learn to operate it safely and effectively. Operating the pump of the prosthesis requires finger dexterity, which should be demonstrated by the patient or caregiver before surgery. It is helpful to have a sample device available for practice sessions; the company is happy to supply this for teaching purposes. In addition, it is important for the patient's immediate family or spouse to be included in the planning and to be supportive during this time, when all the patient's energies will be focused on bladder management. The nurse can assist the patient and family to adopt realistic expectations of what will occur postoperatively and of the anticipated surgical goal. It must be stressed that preoperative and postoperative teaching are crucial to a successful outcome.

Postvoid Dribbling

In some men incontinence takes the form of postvoid dribbling. A small amount of urine is passed, usually without much sensation, for up to several minutes after voiding is completed. This should be distinguished from terminal dribbling, which is a slow, dribbling stream at the end of the act of voiding. If clothing has been replaced, even a few drops of urine can be enough to soak through and leave an embarrassing wet patch, especially if trousers are lightweight or pale in color.

Most commonly, a postvoid dribble is caused by pooling of urine in the bulbar urethra (Fig. 7–4*A*). The reason for this abnormally lax and wide bulb is unknown. If the diagnosis is in doubt a voiding cystogram will clearly show this pool in the bulbar urethra on a postvoid film. A simple explanation of the cause, reassurance that the problem has no significance, and instruction on emptying the urine usually solve the problem. The patient is instructed to express the urine by firm upward and forward finger or fist pressure behind the scrotum at the end of voiding. The trapped urine will be milked out (Fig. 7–4*B*).

Postvoid dribble can also occur in men with prostatic enlargement, an unstable bladder (sometimes a powerful "aftercontraction" forces out a few extra drops), or an atonic bladder. In all these conditions

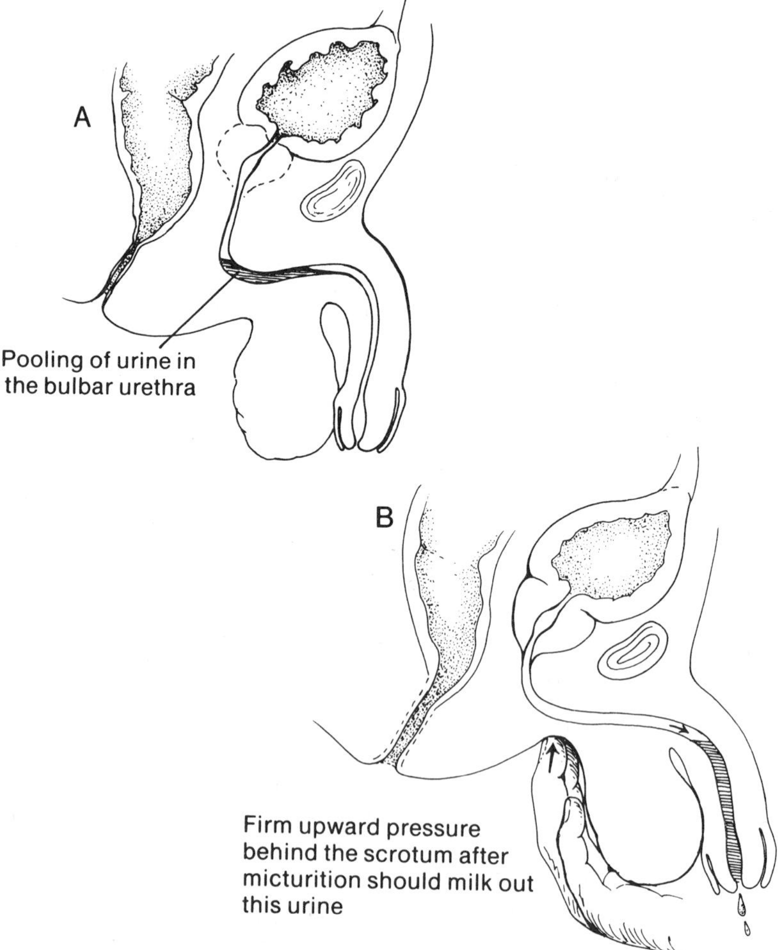

Figure 7–4. *Urine pools in the bulbar urethra* (A) *and can be milked out manually* (B).

other symptoms usually coexist and suggest the cause. The man with simple pooling in the bulbar urethra seldom has any other micturition problems. If the problem is persistent a drip collector can help to contain the leakage (Chap. 13).

CONTROL OF INCONTINENCE BY URETHRAL COMPRESSION DEVICES

A urethral compression device controls incontinence by external mechanical occlusion of the penile urethra. The two used most commonly are the Cunningham and Baumrucker clamps (Fig. 7–5*A* and *B;* also see Chap. 13). The foam-lined arms fit across the penis laterally and, when closed, exert pressure against the urethra. Clamps are available in three sizes. The Cook Continence Cuff, a newer compression device, encircles the penis with an inflatable pillow to compress the urethra (Fig. 7–5*C*).

A urethral compression device should be used with extreme caution, because it can cause considerable damage, even pressure necrosis, to the penis. It is best for specific occasions that require that it be worn only for a short time. Each device must be individually fitted by an expert. At the first wearing it should be left in place for

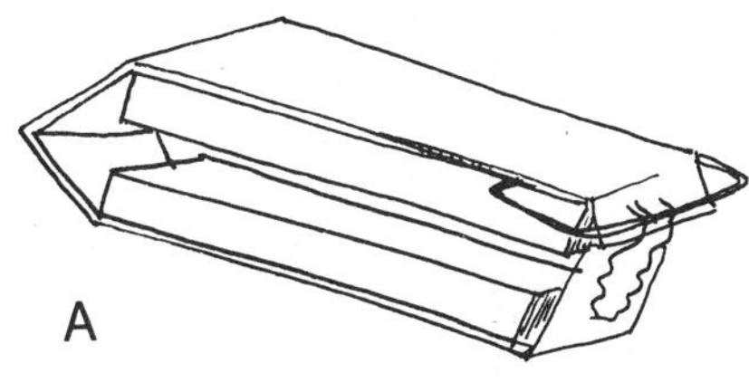

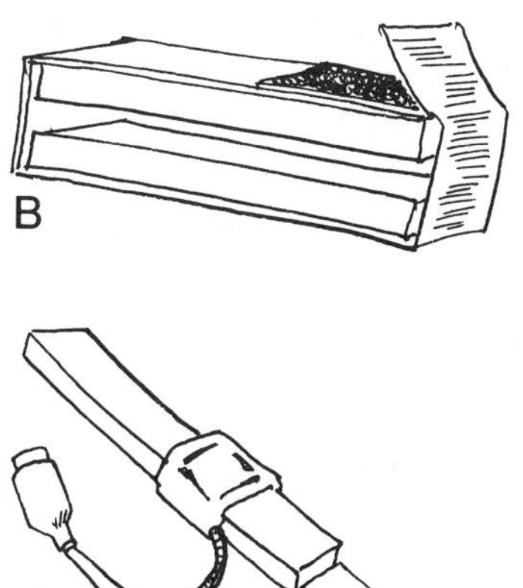

Figure 7–5. *Urethral compression devices.* A, *Cunningham clamp.* B, *Baumrucker clamp.* C, *Cook Continence Cuff.*

short periods and inspected every few minutes to check for any signs of edema, inflammation, or cyanosis of the penis. It is important to apply only as much pressure as required to stop the leakage of urine. Once in place, patients should be asked to mimic the activities that usually bring about incontinence to test whether the device will be effective and at what pressure. Some men find a device too uncomfortable or heavy to use, especially if it has to be closed tightly to control incontinence. It should not be used by patients who have high-pressure, unstable bladders, because the contractions are then against greater resistance and the instability might be exacerbated or the bladder neck damaged; vesicoureteral reflux could even occur.

To use a device the patient (or caregiver) must have manual dexterity, the ability to monitor his penis visually, some degree of sensation in his pelvis and penis, and the mental capacity to understand its use and the dangers of improper use. It can seldom be used if the penis is retracted. The patient and caregiver must be given clear instructions on its use. It is crucial that the patient release the device every 2 to 3 hours to empty the bladder and that he not wear it at night while asleep. Before being sent home with a device patients should demonstrate their ability to apply it properly. An instruction sheet sent home with the patient is useful for reinforcing teaching and reminding him of the necessity to discontinue use immediately if sores, edema, or cyanosis of the glans develop.

The use of a urethral compression device should be regarded as a last resort when all else has failed to control incontinence. It can be used by patients whose needs are not met by any of the products discussed in Chapter 13. For example, an incontinent man cannot wear a leg bag with shorts or bathing suits, but might be able to disguise a compression device under them. The sexually active man might wish to remove his external catheter and wash up prior to intercourse, using a compression device in the interim. Some men regularly do this successfully, and often it is more convenient than wearing an external catheter and leg bag all the time. The bladder is simply used as a reservoir and the clamp released at appropriate intervals. A urethral compression device should never be the first choice for management of incontinence in the male but, if fitted properly and given with adequate instruction, it can be successful in restoring a patient to continence.

References

Barnes, R.W., Bergman, R.T., and Hadley, H.L.: Urology. 3rd ed. Garden City, NY, Medical Examination Publishing, 1980.

Chilton, C.P., Morgan, R.J., England, H.R., Paris, A.M., Blandy, J.P.: A critical evaluation of the results of transurethral resection of the prostate. Br. J. Urol., *50*(7):542, 1978.

Faller, N.A., and Vinson, R.K., The artificial urinary sphincter. J. Enterost. Ther., *12*:7, 1985.

Furlow, W.L.: Implantation of a new semiautomatic artificial genitourinary sphincter: Experience with primary activation and deactivation in 47 patients. J. Urol., *126*(6):741, 1981.

Hadley, R.H., Zimmerman, P.E., and Raz, S.: The treatment of male urinary incontinence. *In* Campbell's Urology, Vol. 3. Philadelphia, W.B. Saunders, 1986, pp. 2568–2579.

Lange, P.H., and Reddy, R.K.: Technical nuances and surgical results of radical retropubic prostatectomy in 150 patients. J. Urol., *138*:348, 1987.

Mundy, A.R., and Stephenson, T.P.: The urge syndrome. *In* Mundy, A.R., Stephenson, T.P., and Wein, A.J. (eds.): Urodynamics—Principles, Practice, and Application. New York, Churchill Livingstone, 1984, pp. 213–228.

Stott, M.A., and Abrams, P.: Indoramin in the treatment of prostatic bladder outflow obstruction. Neurol. Urodynamics, *7*:217, 1988.

Turner-Warwick, R.: Bladder and outflow obstruction in the male. *In* Mundy, A.R., Stephenson, T.P., and Wein, A.J. (eds.): Urodynamics—Principles, Practice, and Application. New York, Churchill Livingstone, 1984, pp. 184–204.

Worth, P.H.L.: Postprostatectomy incontinence. *In* Mundy, A.R., Stephenson, T.P., and Wein, A.J. (eds.): Urodynamics—Principles, Practice, and Application. New York, Churchill Livingstone, 1984, pp. 205–211.

Mary H. Palmer, RN, MS

8 Incontinence in the Elderly

Incontinence becomes more prevalent with age but is not an inevitable part of growing old, as evidenced by the fact that most older adults are continent. Unfortunately, incontinence tends to be accepted far more readily in old age both by the affected older adult and health care professionals, and is less likely to receive systematic investigation or treatment than the same symptoms in a younger person. It is common for an older adult to be told or believe "It's just old age" or "What do you expect at your age?"

Devoting a separate chapter to incontinence and the elderly should not imply that older adults be treated differently from younger incontinent people. Age should not be the sole criterion on which to base assessment and treatment methods and techniques. The intent of this chapter is to highlight additional age-related conditions and issues that can influence an older adult's continence status.

Surveys of incontinence have yielded different prevalence rates. The lack of standardized terminology, differences in sampling methods, and underreporting by older adults and health care providers account for some of the differences among the survey results (Palmer, 1988). In the United States, approximately 9% of community-dwelling adults over age 65 have problems controlling urination (Harris, 1986). For those residing in long-term care facilities the rate ranges from 40 to 60% (Ouslander and Uman, 1985). Problems with incontinence are more likely to increase with age, and women are more likely than men to have these problems (Harris, 1986).

For many older adults, incontinence is not a new or even recent problem. Some have hidden it for years or decades and are only forced to reveal it when they require medical or nursing attention for some other disorder. Many learn to cope in their own way, but for others it causes a serious disruption in their lives. At the least they are uncomfortable and ashamed. At the worst they might eventually fail to cope independently at home, and either become a burden to relatives or friends or need permanent alternative care. Many relatives manage to look after severely incontinent family members at home and tolerate a considerable workload and disruption in family life. Combined incontinence (bowel and bladder) significantly contributes to perceived negative family affect and to an increase in seeking alternative care arrangements (Noelker, 1987).

The United States is experiencing an unprecedented increase in the numbers of individuals surviving into old age. The age group comprised of those 85 years old and over is the largest growing age segment of the population (U.S. Senate Special Comittee on Aging, 1984). To ensure that the elderly can live independent lives in the community with a high quality of life, it is most important that there be proper identification and effective assessment and treatment of those with bladder and bowel dysfunction. Health care professionals must focus on strategies to prevent incontinence. A change of attitude among those working with and caring for older adults is often warranted. The promotion of continence should be a priority of the caregivers. Because older adults are reluctant to seek help, health care professionals and facilities should be oriented to providing prompt, practical help involving a minimum of effort and embarrassment to the older adult.

OLDER ADULTS' ATTITUDES TOWARD ELIMINATION

Many older adults, especially those over 80 years, were born in a society with strict codes of morality and decency. Mention of bodily function was particularly discouraged. As a result, many older adults are ignorant of the way their bodies work, especially in regard to their excretory and reproductive organs. Often they either have no words to describe micturition or defecation, use words from childhood, or apply different meanings to the same words used by health care professionals. Therefore, a mutually understood vocabulary must be established early in any discussion about continence or incontinence. Older individuals can easily be upset and alienated by the use of jargon that the health care professional takes for granted, but that might be unclear or misleading to the layperson.

Incontinence has had several other meanings than the one used in this book. It was often used in nineteenth century literature to mean without any apparent control (as in "he rushed incontinently from the room" or "he talked incontinently about. . ."). The term has also been used to denote lack of moral self-control or sexual promiscuity. Webster's New Twentieth Century Dictionary lists, among its definitions of incontinence, "lack of restraint of passions or appetites; especially lack of restraint of sexual appetite; lewdness." Many older adults view incontinence as a prejudicial label, implying moral degeneracy, or at least that the individual is in some way to blame for the condition. Most wish to avoid the label incontinent at all costs, and would use it only for those who are totally unable to hold any urine or who wet openly in public without any apparent compunction. Many fear reaching this state, and a comment such as "I wet myself and I'm worried I might become incontinent" is familiar to many nurses.

Passing urine or stool is something that most older adults, particularly women, have always done behind a closed, locked door. Shyness often exists, even among long-married couples. Unwillingness to talk about elimination problems in the presence of a spouse should be recognized and respected. Many older adults, however, are expected to pass urine or stool in surroundings that are far from private. A commode in the bedroom or living room is often suggested for those with urgency and poor mobility, without considering that the individual might rather be wet than be seen (or heard) passing urine by the spouse. In the hospital lack of privacy can have an extremely inhibiting effect on bowel or bladder emptying. Curtains can hide the sight, but do not disguise the sound, smell, and knowledge of what is going on behind them. A nurse hovering outside (or even inside) the bathroom makes elimination difficult and often incomplete. Some people are embarrassed if asked within earshot of others whether they would like to use the toilet; they would rather refuse than let everyone know where they are going.

Older adults often have life-long patterns of individualistic rituals relating to elimination. Many are fastidious about personal hygiene, wash thoroughly after each bowel movement, and are meticulous about hand washing after using the toilet, but those on the nursing staff might sometimes overlook offering hand washing facilities to hospitalized patients or nursing home residents. This is often the case if a bed pan or commode is used. The older adult can, as a consequence, become unwilling to use these, especially before meals, and, in attempting to wait, become incontinent.

Some people have been raised to believe the myth that it is possible to catch a venereal disease or cystitis from toilet seats. Such individuals are reluctant to sit down on "shared" toilets, or even to use them at all. This is especially true if the facilities are unclean or are used by both sexes. Those individuals with long-standing rituals for bowel elimination often become constipated if their routine is interrupted or broken. The nurse should make every attempt to learn the preferences of the older adult, especially in the institutional setting, and to assist the older adult in attaining or maintaining normal elimination patterns.

PHYSIOLOGIC EFFECTS OF AGE ON URINARY CONTINENCE

Normal physiologic changes occur with age and affect the kidney, bladder, urethra, and micturition cycle. Pathologic changes and iatrogenic factors frequently affect older adults and have an effect on urinary continence. The effects of aging on bowel function are discussed in Chapter 14.

The Aging Kidney

There is a considerable reduction in the glomerular filtration rate with advancing age. This is caused by a combination of structural degeneration of the kidneys and diminished blood flow through the kidneys. The ability of the kidneys to rid the body of waste products is consequently decreased. The kidneys receive a smaller proportion of the cardiac output by day, although this can return to normal at night when demands of other organs are lessened. This might explain why many older adults have a disturbed diurnal rhythm of urine production. Young adults produce most urine by day and relatively little when asleep. Older adults often produce urine at the same rate day and night, or even produce more at night. Mobilization of peripheral edema caused by cardiac problems and polyuria from diabetes affect voiding patterns (Staskin, 1986). With age the kidneys concentrate urine less effectively. Although a diminished ability to concentrate urine has been implicated as a cause of nocturia, the association is not universally accepted (Staskin, 1986). Despite the loss of kidney size and nephrons with age the kidneys continue to maintain the acid-base balance of tissue fluids, although there is a prolonged response time (Steinberg, 1983).

Age Changes in the Bladder and Urethra

There is an increased tendency for the bladder to be trabeculated with age as the detrusor muscle hypertrophies and there is a loss of supporting tissue. Fibrosis becomes more common, possibly as a consequence of chronic infection or overdistention, and can result in bladder neck stenosis and voiding difficulties. With less efficient emptying of the bladder there is an increased likelihood of residual urine after voiding.

The urethral mucosa can prolapse down through the external urethral meatus and this can form a carbuncle. The significance of this condition is unknown, but it tends to be associated with incontinence. If painful and bleeding it can be treated with vaginal estrogens.

As elastic tissue and muscles weaken stress incontinence becomes more prevalent in women (Chap. 6). With atrophy of all pelvic organs the urethral meatus can recede along the vaginal wall. This causes great difficulty if a catheter is to be inserted, and the woman might have to be catheterized from behind while she is in a lateral position with her knees flexed.

The incidence of multiple dysfunctional states increases with age. Mixed pathologies should always be considered when assessing the incontinent older adult. The older individual will probably have more than one abnormality, such as an unstable bladder and stress incontinence. This indicates that, at the onset of treatment, a decision must be made regarding which dysfunction to treat first. Sometimes treatments are initiated concomitantly (e.g., bladder training for the unstable bladder combined with pelvic muscle exercises for stress incontinence). Other combinations of problems should be treated one at a time, as in the case of an unstable bladder and overflow obstruction. The instability, if the dominant problem, should be treated first, because if overflow resistance is lowered the incontinence is likely to worsen.

Hormonal Changes

The urethra and trigone in the female are formed embryologically from the same hormone-dependent tissue as the vagina. When fully estrogenized the surface of the urethral wall is soft and convoluted, forming many folds that interdigitate to form an efficient, watertight seal (Fig. 8–1).

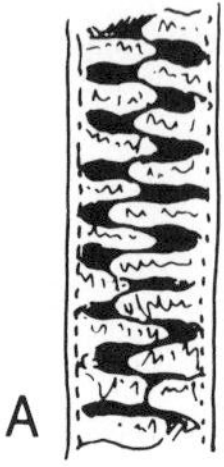

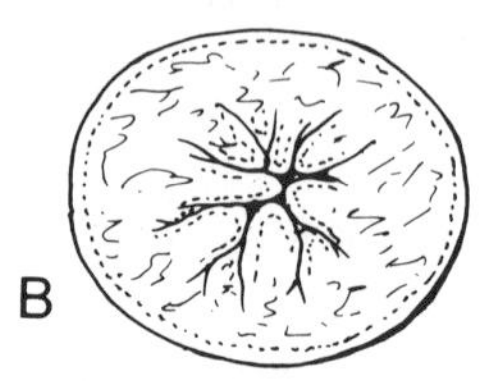

Figure 8–1. *Well-estrogenized urethra. Note the interdigitating folds, which provide efficient closure.* A, *Side view.* B, *Cross section.*

Estrogen levels do not usually drop until 10 years after menopause, and many women maintain good estrogenization well into old age. If hormone levels do fall, however, the walls of the urethra become harder and the folds become less pronounced resulting in less efficient closure (Fig. 8–2). Coupled with decreased mucus production, which lowers surface tension, both stress incontinence and leakage during uninhibited contractions are more likely to occur.

With increasing age, a larger area of the urethra and trigone become estrogen-sensitive. Lack of estrogen can cause urethritis and trigonitis. The older woman will have symptoms similar to those of cystitis, such as dysuria, frequency, and often urgency. This will be associated with a vaginitis (atrophic or senile vaginitis). This can easily be detected by looking at the vulva which will appear red, inflamed, and often dry. There can be a secondary infection. Much of the perineal discomfort commonly attributed to urine and incontinence in older women is probably a symptom of atrophic vaginitis. If diagnosis is in doubt, a histologic smear will confirm it.

Estrogen replacement therapy is the treatment of choice for these conditions. Estrogen is available in a cream, but many older women find vaginal applicators difficult or uncomfortable to use. Oral preparations (e.g., Premarin) are available for the older women who cannot use the vaginal applicator. Considerable dexterity is necessary for vaginal application and some women find it distasteful or impossible, particularly nulliparous women. Estrogen should not be used for women

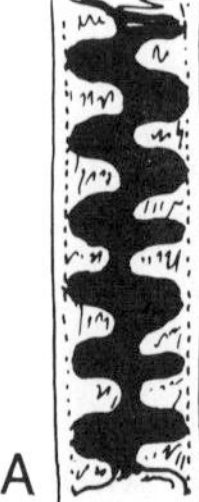

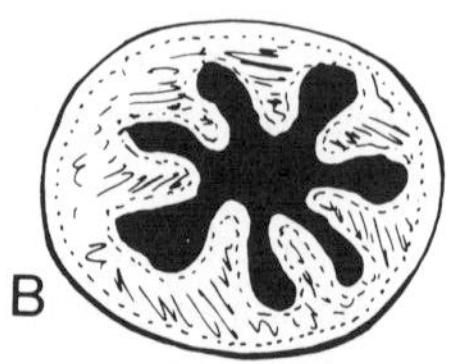

Figure 8–2. *Estrogen-deficient urethra.* A, *Side view.* B, *Cross section.*

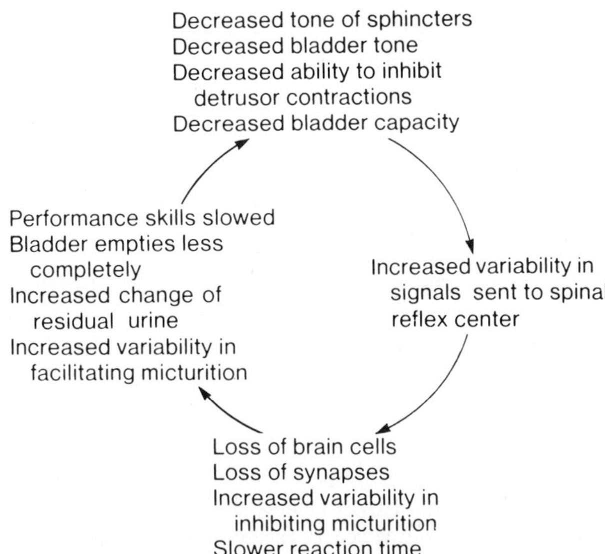

Figure 8–3. *Effects of age on the micturition cycle. (From Palmer, M.: Urinary Incontinence. Washington, DC, National Gerontological Nursing Association, 1986.)*

with a history of thromboembolic disease or malignancy of the reproductive system or breast. Optimal duration of therapy has not been determined, but Ouslander (1986) has recommended initiating treatment for a minimum of 2 months.

The Micturition Cycle

The process of micturition is complex—it involves feedback loops between the bladder and sacral reflex center in the spinal cord and between the sacral reflex center and frontal lobe of the brain (the cortical center of control). The cycle of passive bladder filling under the control of the sacral reflex center, cortical control to delay or inhibit urination, and bladder contraction and emptying is affected by age (see Fig. 8–3 for a sumary of age-related changes).

These age-related changes alone do not cause incontinence, but place the older adult at greater risk for becoming incontinent.

Pathologic Changes

The Prostate

Prostatic hypertrophy is discussed in Chapter 7. The incidence of prostatic malignancy increases with age; it is present in 30% of men 70 to 79 years of age, and there is a strong association with increasing age (Staskin, 1986). The possibility of an obstructive tumor should be considered in men who experience an altered micturition pattern, especially difficulty in passing urine.

Neurologic Conditions

Aging and neurologic disease and disorders make neurologic dysfunction more common in old age. Detrusor instability is the most common urodynamic finding (Leach and Yip, 1986). Parkinson's disease, cerebral vascular accidents, and multiple sclerosis are three causes of neurologic disability that frequently affect an older adult's continence status.

Neurogenic voiding difficulties can occur in many complex combinations (Chap. 10). It is also likely that, with the increased occurrence of autonomic neuropathy associated with aging, the number of men and women with functional (nonanatomic) obstruction from detrusor-sphincter dyssynergia will increase. The urethral sphincters do not relax completely during micturition and a degree of residual urine, possibly with overflow incontinence, can develop.

Bladder sensation can change with age. Instead of perceiving the sensation of bladder filling at about half capacity, as do younger people, many older adults first feel the need to void at, or near, bladder capacity. To an active and mobile person it can be a considerable inconvenience to locate toilet facilities immediately. To an immobile older adult or an individual with an unstable bladder or painful arthritis, this lack of time between the perception of the need to void and the actual release of urine can result in incontinence.

Diabetes

The incidence of diabetes mellitus in Western society is estimated to be 16% for those over 65 years, increasing to 25% in those 85 years and older (Williams, 1983). The presence of diabetes can have a profound effect on the bladder, especially causing atony (Chap. 10). Many of the atonic or neurogenic bladders seen in old age are directly related to diabetic neuropathy.

Undiagnosed diabetes can present as polyuria and polydipsia, vulval irritation with reddened and swollen labia, and possibly a candidal infection. An atonic bladder with overflow incontinence might also indicate the presence of undiagnosed diabetes. Screening for diabetes should be routine among older adults with urinary symptoms. If hyperglycemia is detected, a glucose tolerance test is indicated.

Urinary Tract Infections

Bacteriuria, the presence of bacteria in the urine, is common among the elderly. Bacteriuria is present in 20% of women and 10% of men over the age of 65 who live at home (Kaye, 1980). The incidence of bacteriuria in noncatheterized nursing home residents ranges from 20 to 50%, and is almost 100% in catheterized residents (Garibaldi, 1985). The presence of bacteriuria alone is not considered to be indicative of a urinary tract infection. Diagnostic criteria include complaints of dysuria, frequency, urgency, a positive urinalysis, or a urine culture of 100,000 bacteria/ml of urine (Norman and associates, 1987).

It has not been proven that urinary tract infections cause incontinence. An acute cystitis can precipitate incontinence in those already at risk and this infection should be treated. Asymptomatic bacteriuria can be transient in nature, however, and the benefits of antimicrobial therapy for asymptomatic bacteriuria in older adults have not been supported (Boscia and co-workers, 1986).

Iatrogenic Factors

Drugs

Multiple drug use is common in older adults. Many medications have side effects that cause voiding dysfunction and can result in incontinence (see Table 2–2). Eliminating unnecessary drugs, lowering the dose of a diuretic, switching to a less rapidly acting diuretic, changing the time of administration of the diuretic, decreasing sedation, or changing to an alternative medication for a specific disorder that does not cause voiding dysfunction can often improve, if not cure, the problem.

Fluids

Many older adults severely restrict their oral fluid intake in a misguided effort to control their incontinence. This habit could assume dangerous proportions in some older adults, who might drink almost nothing to prevent incontinence. Low fluid intake can actually exacerbate the problem—the signal for micturition is a full bladder, and abnormal voiding patterns can occur in the absence of this sensation. Also, many older adults suffer from precarious metabolic stability and, with low oral fluid intake, severe fluid and electrolyte imbalance can result. Dehydration, malaise, constipation, and confusion can follow.

Older people frequently find drinking large quantities of fluid to be difficult. When encouraging older adults to maintain adequate fluid intake (approximately 1500 ml in a 24-hour period), it is important to offer preferred fluids frequently and in small amounts. Those who find water unpalatable might be able to drink a noncitrus juice with little problem.

ATTITUDES AND THE ENVIRONMENT

If the environment in which the attitudes of those around the older adult (e.g., relatives, friends, caregivers) is such that continence is expected, the desired effect is often achieved. If it is expected that incontinence is inevitable past a certain age, or with a certain disease or condition, then the older adult lacks both the incentive and opportunity to be continent. If everything possible is done to prevent incontinence and to treat it when it does occur, however, then the likelihood of continence is higher.

Promotion of continence among older adults includes creation of an environment in which an optimal level of functioning, including bowel and bladder functioning, is the goal.

Independence

The greater the functional independence allowed by the environment, the greater the older adult's potential for continence. Some older adults might be reluctant to ask for assistance in going to the bathroom and assistance might not always be immediately available when needed.

The older adult should be able to get in and out of bed easily. The height of the bed must be optimized for each person. The mattress should be firm; a mattress that is soft or sags in the middle can make getting up difficult. Chairs should not be so low that rising without assistance is difficult. Arm rests at the appropriate height promote leverage.

A walking aid, such as a cane or walker, can improve mobility, speed, and confidence in ambulating to the bathroom. Attention should be paid to treatment of foot conditions that could impair mobility, such as calluses and untrimmed toenails. Properly fitting shoes that support the feet are also important.

Clothing should be attractive, easy to adjust, and any incontinence appliance should be easily removed and replaced by the wearer.

Toilet Facilities

Bathrooms and toilet stalls should have a door that is easy to open and lock. The seat must be the correct height to facilitate sitting and rising. (See Chapter 9 for a discussion of modifications that can be made and of alternatives to urinals and commodes for those who cannot get to a bathroom.)

Distance

An older adult, especially one with impaired mobility, generally needs to have faster access to a bathroom than a younger person to be reliably continent. Because many older people feel the sensation of the need to void at or near capacity, urgency is considerable. Once urgency is felt, it might not be possible for the older person to rush. Specht (1986) has provided a formula that can be used to predict incontinence. If the time from the perception of the need to void and actual micturition is exceeded by the time it takes to reach the bathroom, then incontinence will occur. Bathrooms should be situated near activity areas in nursing homes, hospitals, and day care centers. Making bathrooms accessible in the older adult's home might require structural alterations. The route should be unobstructed and without stairs if mobility is impaired.

Identification of Toilet Facilities

In unfamiliar surroundings, being able to identify the rest rooms quickly and easily is important. Legible signs in public places (including hospitals and nursing home units) and meaningful labels on doors are important. Obviously, someone who has misinterpreted an obscure symbol on a rest room door might be unwilling to enter, fearing that the same thing could happen again. Color-coded doors to rest rooms and unambiguous, well-lit signs at an appropriate height aid in the promoting of continence for older adults.

Emotional and Psychologic Factors

As with younger individuals, psychologic factors are important with older adults, although a direct causal relationship has not been proven. The onset of incontinence can be observed following a bereavement or other significant stressful event (such as admission to institutional care). Occasionally, incontinence is perceived by others as deliberate, conscious, attention-seeking behavior. This cannot be assumed; the behavior must not be dismissed. If such drastic behavior is necessary to gain the attention of others, then health care professionals must assume that the person is not receiving desperately needed human contact. If a manipulative individual discovers that incontinence achieves the attention that is craved, however, then the behavior is likely to be repeated. An individual behavioral assessment can help to determine more productive and satisfying channels to meet an individual's need for human contact.

TREATMENT

General Considerations

A proper nursing assessment (Chap. 3) will reveal many contributing factors that can be eliminated or lessened, such as impaired mobility secondary to poorly fitting shoes, sedentary lifestyle, or obesity. Concomitant assessment by a physician is also necessary to evaluate voiding function. Many frail older adults cannot tolerate the repeated catheterization that is part of urodynamic testing. Ouslander (1986) has described an algorithm using diagnostic tests to be used with older adults before referral to a urologist.

As with younger people, treatment options should be carefully explained. The benefits and risks of various treatment options must be discussed. Consideration of the older adult's current level of functioning, quality of life, expectations of treatment, and ability to participate in or cooperate with treatment is important before selecting a treatment modality.

Drug therapy requires careful monitoring. Many older adults are more sensitive to side effects than younger people. Some conditions frequently present in older adults preclude the use of certain drugs—for example, anticholinergics are contraindicated in the presence of glaucoma. With improvements in surgical techniques and safer anesthesia, surgery is an increasingly feasible option for the treatment of incontinent older adults.

Intermittent Catheterization

Voiding dysfunction with large volumes of postmicturition residual urine becomes increasingly common with advancing age. When surgical or pharmacologic intervention is inappropriate or unsuccessful, the use of intermittent catheterization should be considered (Chap. 10). Many older adults retain sufficient dexterity to catheterize themselves, although, in women, the urethral meatus can be more difficult to find if it migrates along the vaginal wall. If the older adult cannot manage, the caregiver might be able to learn the procedure. Otherwise, nursing intervention is needed. Whether in the institutional setting or in the community, if emptying the bladder by catheterization will keep the older adult continent, every effort should be made to ensure that this is done. Older people often require intermittent catheterization less frequently than younger people with voiding problems, because residual urine accumulates more slowly in the older bladder (Chap. 10). In some cases bladder function will return over a period of weeks, so that catheterization can be discontinued as residual volumes drop.

Establishing an intermittent catheterization schedule on a nursing unit or in the community requires readjustment in attitudes and nursing routines. Once the benefits of this treatment become obvious and the appropriate equipment is ordered, it is well accepted by the caregivers. Nurses quickly learn the individual's anatomic idiosyncrasies and each catheterization requires only a few minutes, especially if timing is planned around the daily routine (e.g., before dressing in the morning). Nurses performing intermittent catheterization must be scrupulous in washing their hands before and after the procedure and must use aseptic technique throughout the procedure to avoid cross infection. Clean technique by the older adult or caregiver in the home is acceptable.

INCONTINENCE IN TERMINAL ILLNESS

Many people become incontinent of urine and stool in the final stages of a terminal illness. This can be a tremendous burden on the caregivers and cause psychologic suffering to the older adult. The incontinence might be caused by physiologic reasons outlined elsewhere in this book. Most probably, however, incontinence is secondary to alterations in cognitive functioning, physical debilitation, immobility, and loss of independence. Fecal incontinence can often be prevented by bowel management techniques to prevent constipation and impaction or to regulate a neurogenic bowel (Chap. 14).

Vigorous evaluation of incontinence is seldom desirable for the terminally ill individual, but some incontinence can be reversed by the judicious use of medications for detrusor instability, the use of handheld urinals, and making caregivers sensitive to the need for regular toileting. If incontinence persists, an appliance to contain it is warranted.

If leakage is heavy or movement to a urinal or commode becomes painful and difficult, an indwelling catheter can be a positive alternative. Long-term risks can be discounted, and a catheter can enable the dying person to be comfortable during the last days. Relatives can sleep or go out without worrying that the patient might need to void or be lying in urine.

A bladder or bowel fistula, as part of a terminal illness, is most distressing and can be one of the most demanding problems. Fecal incontinence collectors or close-fitting high-quality absorbent products are effective management systems.

Uncontrolled incontinence certainly makes the development of a pressure sore more likely. In an emaciated person this risk is increased. For women, a catheter should prevent this occurring and thereby avoid extra pain and distress. Men might find a condom catheter as effective as an indwelling catheter.

COGNITIVELY IMPAIRED OLDER ADULTS

Most older adults remain cognitively intact. The prevalence of moderate to severe dementia in community-dwelling older adults is estimated to be 1% at the age of 60 and doubles every 5 years (White and colleagues, 1986). For those older adults who become impaired there is a wide continuum of impairment, from slight memory loss to severe confusion and dementia. If impairment is severe, the individual might need institutional care. Most cognitively impaired older adults, however, remain in the community and are often cared for by relatives.

Incontinence is seldom an inevitable feature of memory loss or dementia. Many people with dementia are not incontinent, and continence is so deeply ingrained in most people that it is one of the last social skills to be lost. Often other causes of incontinence are overlooked and left untreated in cognitively impaired older adults. Ouslander (1986) has discussed several causes of the sudden onset of incontinence using the acronym, DRIP (*d*elirium; *r*estricted mobility and retention; *i*nfection, inflammation, and impaction; and *p*harmaceutical and polyuria). Also, lower urinary tract dysfunction or a concomitant illness such as diabetes can be the precipitating factor. Depression, the most common affective disorder in older adults, often mimics dementia. Depression is considered to be a pseudodementia and a contributing factor in the development of incontinence.

Cognitively impaired older adults depend on their surroundings for their level of functioning. Many of those living in their own homes, with familiar people and objects, can maintain a relatively normal lifestyle, even with advanced mental impairment. Sometimes incontinence results from disorientation, especially in different surroundings. It is difficult for older adults with dementia to learn new things, and they might never become accustomed to a strange environment, even after prolonged residence. In a hospital or long-term care facility, clear signs and good lighting coupled with appropriate verbal reminders can help to prevent incontinence from occurring. Some older adults might have a reticent attitude toward elimination, however, and might deny their need to use the toilet if not asked discreetly. A nurse asking publicly, in a loud voice, can often expect to meet with refusal and even hostility.

The expectation of continence should be communicated to caregivers and impaired older adults. Cognitively impaired individuals are often assumed to be incontinent and are not given the opportunity or encouragement to be dry. In institutional settings the routine can be geared to all patients or residents being incontinent, with regular washing and changing of bed linens and clothes. It has been suggested that it could be easier for the nursing staff, in the short term, to have a monotonous, regular routine of changing sheets and patient clothing instead of struggling to rehabilitate or retrain incontinent older adults. Toileting an individual, however, has been shown to require less nursing time and cost less than an incontinent episode (Creason, 1987).

Behavioral Assessment

A behavioral assessment of each individual can help to determine why incontinence is occurring. Many psychogeriatric nursing units have a clinical psychologist or clinical nurse specialist on staff or as a consultant. These health care professionals can make valuable contributions to behavioral assessment. A simple framework for this assessment is ABC—that is, antecedent, behavior, and consequences. The behavior should first be described, objectively and specifically. Then the events and actions antecedent to the behavior should be ascertained. Finally, the consequences of the incontinent behavior should be determined.

By learning about the individual's life history (premorbid personality, interests, hobbies, pet peeves) it can be possible to determine if incontinence is a symptom of apathy, protest, or despair toward a currently unacceptable life situation. If an older adult who has always been solitary and shy is suddenly expected to become accustomed to living, sleeping, dressing, and eating with 25 strangers, it is not difficult to understand why a formerly fastidious personality might crumble under the strain. Some people do become incontinent on admission to institutional care or soon afterward. The incontinence can be related to the loss of independence, personal responsibility, and sense of self-worth. Incontinence can also occur when the older adult is obliged to sell a home and move in with a child or other relative.

Some people seem to use the defense mechanism of regression under these circumstances—becoming passive, dependent, and often incontinent. By regressing to an infantile state, they might be able to avoid facing the reality of a dismal future. Occasionally, incontinence can be interpreted as an expression of anger as one of the few weapons available against caregivers. Incontinence can occur in the presence of one particular caregiver or before or during a certain disliked activity or event (e.g., while being dressed or when rock music is on the radio), but not during preferred activities (e.g., during music therapy or watching a favorite television program). Nursing staff members often note that older adults who are considered hopelessly incontinent on the nursing unit can stay dry for an outing or during a special event.

At times, cognitively impaired older adults deny their incontinence. Although aware of the problem, they are ashamed to admit it to others. This can lead to an attempt to hide the evidence—concealing soiled clothes or pads in a closet or putting a clean sheet over a soiled one. If confronted about the behavior, the person can react with hostility or try to blame someone else. The caregiver should realize that incontinence can be so distressing that the individual denies the situation internally and is not conscious of what is happening.

Antecedents

If impaired individuals cannot communicate their needs verbally they should be monitored closely for actions and behaviors, antecedent cues, prior to micturition (e.g., getting up from a chair and wandering, pulling at clothing, and other verbal or nonverbal cues). If these are noted and communicated to all caregivers, the need for toilet facilities can be responded to quickly and appropriately.

Most people have a lifetime's conditioned reflex to pass urine into a toilet, with no clothing over the genital area, in privacy, and with the sensation of a full bladder. Cognitively impaired older adults are dependent on familiar stimuli to maintain their activities. It is easy to upset these conditioned reflexes by offering confusing stimuli (Newman, 1962). The sight of a toilet and the sensation of a full bladder act as antecedent cues to empty the bladder (Burgio and Burgio, 1986). In an unfamiliar setting such as an institution, however, the individual might be repeatedly taken to the toilet without concern for privacy. If the bladder is not full, and the person does not void, incontinence can occur later.

Paradoxic urination patterns can develop. For example, a confused individual needing to void might be seated, without underwear, in a chair in a quiet corner. Sitting with a bare bottom on underpads, the obvious message would seem to be "Go ahead—pass urine here." The individual, then, does not pass urine when taken to the toilet, but is incontinent when in a quiet place and is relaxed in a comfortable chair or bed. This can be frustrating for the caregivers. It should be understood, though, that the individual is not deliberately incontinent but is merely responding to the mixed stimuli from caregivers and the environment.

The nursing staff can determine the most likely times the older adult will need to use the toilet by keeping an incontinence chart. The structured environment in which many cognitively impaired individuals need to live usually results in meals and fluids being served at scheduled times every day. Each person's bladder reacts differently to this: no two people are likely to have an identical pattern of micturition, but the pattern for each individual is likely to be similar each day. An accurate chart can help to reveal these patterns to plan toileting schedules.

Consequences

The consequences, what happens after incontinence occurs, are also important in the behavioral assessment. Sometimes incontinence can become rewarding, because it results in attention and human contact. This is especially true if the person is in a socially impoverished situation, such as an understaffed facility. The individual might get little attention when dry or going to the toilet independently. Staff members are busy providing care to those who are more dependent, and can overlook the social needs of the more independent patients. If incontinent, however, the individual will usually gain attention; the caregiver will talk and touch and sometimes smile and offer sympathy. Even if the caregiver is angry or hostile, these reactions can be better than no reaction or communication at all. A continent person might have no human contact between breakfast and lunch; the incontinent person receives human contact with each incontinent episode. Incontinent behavior, then, is positively reinforced by the attention. Incontinence is also negatively reinforced. Negative reinforcement refers to the termination of aversive or bad effects (Baldwin and Baldwin, 1981). The aversive effects of incontinence might be the discomfort of wet clothes and the smell of urine on the body. The staff's response, exchanging wet clothes for dry ones and washing body parts, negatively reinforces the older adult's incontinent behavior.

Great care must be taken not to attribute incontinence to attention-seeking behavior automatically. It is seldom a conscious choice, especially for a confused person, but it is crucial to alert and educate staff members to the fact that some nursing practices unwittingly reinforce the least desired behavior, incontinence. The same can be true of older adults cared for in the community. The incontinent individual might benefit from increased attention, but again this should not be interpreted as the patient's conscious choices to remain incontinent. There might be few incentives for remaining dry in the environment. Reinforcement from others, whether positive or negative, strengthens the behavior, increasing its likelihood of being repeated.

Advanced Dementia

In those with advanced dementia all realization of the social desirability for continence can be absent. The individual might become completely uninhibited and, with no reason to be continent, might pass urine and stool without restraint. If the concept of the appropriate toilet receptacle becomes meaningless, nearby trashcans or other receptacles might be used indiscriminately. Urine and stool are no longer seen as unpleasant or aversive and might be played with or smeared on the body, walls, and furniture. The recognition of the toilet's purpose can be lost, so even when taken to one it might not be used appropriately. The severely confused older adult can sit and do nothing and become incontinent soon afterward, or an agitated individual might refuse to be positioned at all.

Even after all attempts have been made to maximize the individual's level of functioning (e.g., medication, reality orientation), incontinence can be inevitable. The older adult and caregiver should not be made to feel guilty or inadequate because of the inability to achieve continence. Regular toileting and attention to factors that could exacerbate the severity of incontinence are important. An adequate supply of high-quality incontinence pads or garments that are easy to use should be available. A good product will contain the urine, protect the skin, environment, and clothing, minimize odor, and maintain the dignity of the individual. (The selection and use of incontinence aids are discussed in Chapter 13.) The protection and dignity of the older adult, not convenience to the staff, should always be the primary consideration when using products to contain urine.

Nursing Interventions

Reality Orientation

It is important to maintain a reality-oriented environment for cognitively impaired older adults to keep the maximum number of conditioned responses functional. It has been noted that, if older adults are dressed in their own clothing, including appropriate underwear, have personal possessions around them, and engage in meaningful activities, incontinence is less frequent. Caregivers should speak respectfully, using the individual's preferred name often (e.g., first name, surname, or nickname). Frequent use of terms such as "honey" or "dear" are demeaning to the older adult. Conversations should include repeated uses of reality cues—about time, place, weather, family, or events. Clear, easy-to-read clocks, calendars, and signs should be at eye level to aid memory.

Most long-term care facilities are attempting to move away from the large, featureless day area in which the residents sit in plastic chairs in a large circle (making eye contact or communication difficult), with the endless drone of the television set that no one is watching. Even within the constraints of staff and resource shortages, small alterations can be directed toward individualizing care. Keeping family photographs and personal mementos and having a mirror with the individual's name clearly written near it can remind cognitively impaired individuals of their history and identity.

Although recent memory can be severely impaired, long-term memory can be intact, and old phonograph records, pictures, and photographs often bring pleasure and recognition. Seemingly confused older adults might still be able to perform a lifetime's habitual activity—for example, a former housewife could help with making her bed. Art, drama, and music therapy should be employed. Animals, such as cats and rabbits, are often kept as pets on long-term care units. Day trips and frequent visits from volunteers keep cognitively impaired older adults stimulated and in touch with humanity. By keeping the environment structured and by using carefully planned and repeated cues for reality orientation, the level of functioning of confused older adults can be maximized. Continence is often greatly improved in an environment in which the individual's worth is affirmed.

Behavioral Modification

Behavioral modification techniques can be used to help confused older adults attain continence in much the same way as for the person with mental retardation (see Chap. 12). A behavioral technique known as contingency management can reinforce the desired behavior (continence and passing urine in the appropriate receptacle) and extinguish the undesired behavior (incontinence) (McCormick and Burgio, 1984). It is often possible to use theories of operant conditioning to promote continence (Burgio, 1986).

The aim of behavioral modification is to give attention, praise, and physical contact for continence and to withdraw these when incontinence occurs. To be effective, all caregivers in contact with the individual must understand and follow the procedure. Consistency must be maintained. A caregiver should give a reward (with a smile, praise, hug—an appropriate reinforcer should be chosen for each individual). If the older adult is dry, uses the toilet facilities appropriately, or indicates the need to use the toilet, the reinforcement should be given promptly. When incontinence occurs it must be addressed, but with minimal fuss and attention—no smiles, no conversation, and minimal physical contact. Punishment is not warranted. Behavioral interventions with older adults have resulted in successful and effective restoration of continence (McCormick and colleagues, 1988).

References

Baldwin, J., and Baldwin, J.: (1981) Behavior Principles in Everyday Life. 2nd ed. Englewood Cliffs, N.J., Prentice Hall, 1981, pp. 6–34.

Boscia, J., et al.: Epidemiology of bacteriuria in elderly ambulatory population. Am. J. Med., *80*:208, 1986.

Burgio, K.: Behavioral geriatrics: Application of operant procedures to the control of urinary incontinence. Behav. Therap., *9*:67, 1986.

Burgio, K., and Burgio, L.: Behavior therapy for urinary incontinence in the elderly. Clin. Geriatr. Med., *2*:809, 1986.

Creason, N.: Costing urinary incontinence in nursing homes. Contemp. L.T.C., June:84, 1987.

Garibaldi, R.: Hospital-acquired urinary tract infections: Epidemiology and prevention. *In* Wenzel, R. (ed.): Prevention and Control of Nosocomial Infections. Baltimore, Williams & Wilkins, 1985, pp. 335–343.

Harris, T.: Aging in the eighties, prevalence and impact of urinary problems in individuals age 65 years and over. DHHS Pub. No. (PHS)86-1250. N.C.H.S. Advance Data, Number 121, 1986, pp. 1–8.

Kaye, D.: Urinary tract infections in the elderly. Bull. N.Y. Acad. Med., *56*:209, 1980.

Leach, G., and Yip, C.: Urologic and urodynamic evaluation of the elderly population. Clin. Geriatr. Med., *2*:731, 1986.

McCormick, K., and Burgio, K.: Incontinence. An update on nursing care measures. J. Gerontol. Nurs., *10*:16, 1984.

McCormick, K., Scheve, A., and Leahy, E.: Nursing management of urinary incontinence in geriatric inpatients. Nurs. Clin. North Am., *23*:231, 1988.

Newman, J. L.: Old folks in wet beds. Br. Med. J., *1*:1824, 1962.

Noelker, L.: Incontinence in elderly cared for by family. Gerontologist, *27*:194, 1987.

Norman, D., Castle, S., and Cantrell, M.: Infections in the nursing homes. J. Am. Geriatr. Soc., *35*:796, 1987.

Ouslander, J.: Diagnostic evaluation of geriatric urinary incontinence. Clin. Geriatr. Med., *2*:715, 1986.

Ouslander, J., and Uman, G.: Urinary incontinence: Opportunities for research, education, and improvements in medical care in the nursing home setting. *In* Schreider, E. (ed.): The Teaching Nursing Home. New York, Raven Press, 1985, pp. 73–196.

Palmer, M.: Incontinence: The magnitude of the problem. Nurs. Clin. North Am., *23*:139, 1988.

Specht, J.: Genitourinary problems. *In* Carnevali, D., and Patrick, M. (eds.): Nursing Management for the Elderly. 2nd ed. Philadelphia, J.B. Lippincott, 1986, pp. 447–466.

Staskin, D.: Age-related physiologic and pathologic changes affecting lower urinary tract function. Clin. Geriatr. Med., *2*:701, 1986.

Steinberg, F.: The aging of organs and organ systems. *In* Steinberg, F. (ed.): Care of the Geriatric Patient. 6th ed. St. Louis, C.V. Mosby, 1983, pp. 3–17.

U.S. Senate Special Committee on Aging: Aging America. Trends and Projections. American Association of Retired Persons. Washington, DC, U.S. Senate, 1984.

White, L., et al.: Geriatric epidemiology. *In* Eisdorfer, C. (ed.): Annual Review of Gerontology and Geriatrics, Vol. 6. New York, Springer, 1986, pp. 215–311.

Williams, T.F.: Diabetes mellitus in older adults. *In* Reichel, W. (ed.): Clinical Aspects of Aging. 2nd ed. Baltimore, Williams & Wilkins, 1983, pp. 411–415.

Marilyn Pires, RN, MS

9 Promoting Continence for the Physically Impaired

For some persons with impaired physical mobility, voiding dysfunction is part of their physical impairment. Management of incontinence caused by neurogenic bladder dysfunction is discussed in Chapter 10. For many persons with impaired physical mobility, however, the threat of incontinence is not the result of their physical impairment, but rather a consequence of environmental barriers. There are a significant number of physical impairments that affect mobility but have no effect on bowel and bladder function. This chapter discusses methods for maintaining continence and encouraging independent toileting in persons with impaired physical mobility.

Even those with the most severe impairments of physical mobility can be helped to maintain continence. Adapting home and public toilets is the optimal solution, but when this is not possible, there are many alternatives using adaptive equipment and techniques. Each person must be carefully assessed to determine the most appropriate solution. Ideally, the assessment brings the talents of rehabilitation nurses and occupational and physical therapists together with the needs and concerns of people with impaired physical mobility and their families to provide a unique and creative solution for each individual.

EQUAL ACCESS TO PUBLIC TOILETS

One of the major areas of frustration experienced by those with impaired physical mobility is the need to plan any public outing carefully. Persons with mobility impairments who have normal bowel and bladder function must consider the architectural accessibility of the event, facility, or program in which they wish to participate, as well as the availability of accessible public toilets. For example, planes and trains can often accommodate wheelchairs or ambulation aids, but the bathrooms are notoriously small and awkward to use. A person with impaired mobility might be able to get into a restaurant, but could be reluctant to do so because the toilet facilities for many restaurants are located up or down stairs and through narrow corridors, and are often very small.

Many cities offer accessibility guides that provide useful information for people with impaired physical mobility to prevent unpleasant surprises during public outings. Several consumer organizations have published guides to aid disabled travelers (App. 1). Some travel agencies specialize in assisting persons with mobility impairments who wish to go on local, regional, national, and even international trips.

In 1968 the Architectural Barriers Act set accessibility standards for buildings constructed, improved, or leased by the federal government or for buildings used for programs financed by federal grants. It was not until 5 years later that Section 502 of the Rehabilitation Act of 1973 established the Architectural and Transportation Barriers Compliance Board.

This board is responsible for the following: (1) ensuring compliance with the Architectural Barriers Act of 1968; (2) developing standards for compliance with regulations to overcome architectural barriers in public facilities and in residential and institutional housing; and (3) withholding federal funds when noncompliance exists. Section 504 of the same act prohibits discrimination and ensures equal access to education, employment, and social services to persons with disabilities. In regard to physical accessibility, Section 504 provides the following: (1) all federally assisted programs must provide facilities that are both accessible and *usable*; (2) all new facilities constructed with federal funds must be barrier-free; and (3) all existing structures must be made accessible in compliance with American National Standards Institute (ANSI) accessibility standards (Mumma, 1987).

Equal access for all citizens is improving through legislation, consumer activism, and increased public awareness, but there is still much to be done. Nurses and other health care providers need to be aware of standards and to work with patients, families, consumer groups, and public officials to encourage compliance with them.

The following is a list of design guidelines for public toilet rooms (Paralyzed Veterans of America, 1986):

Toilet rooms must have at least one toilet stall that is at least 36″ wide and 56″ deep and a door, if any, that is at least 32″ wide and swings out.

Stalls must have handrails on each side that are 33″ high, parallel to the floor and 1½″ in diameter, 1½″ clearance between rail and wall, and fastened securely at ends and center (Fig. 9–1*A*).

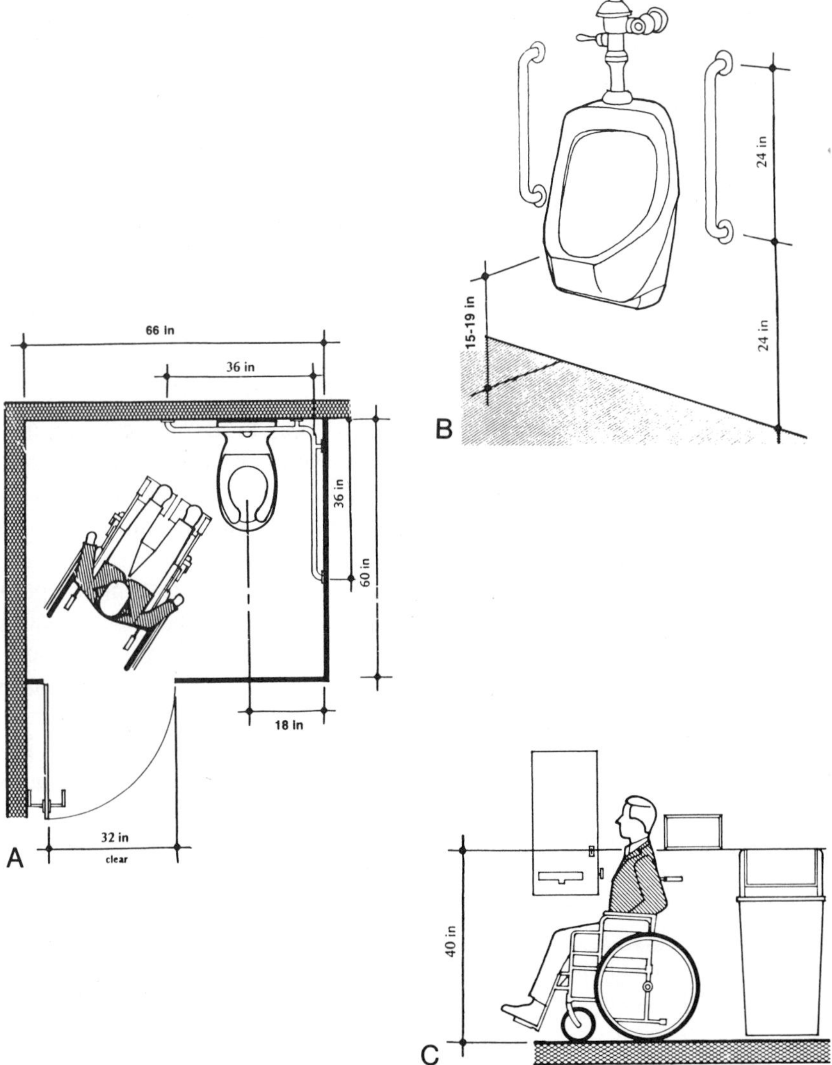

Figure 9–1. *Design guidelines for public toilet rooms.* A, *Toilet stall dimensions.* B, *Urinal dimensions.* C, *Maximum reach height. (Courtesy of the Paralyzed Veterans of America.)*

The toilet seat must be 19 to 20″ from the finished floor.

In addition to, or instead of this, a toilet room must have at least one toilet stall that is at least 66″ wide, 60″ deep, and a door, if any, that is at least 32″ wide and swings out.

If the above design is used, the toilet center line must be located 18″ from the side wall on which the handrail is located.

Wash basins shall have narrow (shallow) aprons.

Drain pipes and hot water pipes under a lavatory must be covered or insulated.

Toilet rooms for men must have wall-mounted urinals with the opening of the basin 15 to 19″ from the finished floor, or have floor-mounted urinals that are level with the main floor (Fig. 9–1*B*).

A mirror and shelf above a lavatory must be no higher than 40″ above the floor, measured from the bottom of the mirror and the top of the shelf to the floor (Fig. 9–1*C*).

Towel racks and dispensers must be mounted no higher than 40″ from the floor.

PRIVATE TOILET FACILITIES

The homes of persons with impaired physical mobility can be tailored to their particular needs. Rehabilitation nurses and other health care providers must work with patients and their families to assess each individual's unique toileting needs and to determine the most appropriate adaptive equipment or home adaptations.

If the physical impairment is severely restrictive, patients and families might need to seek architecturally accessible private or public housing. If persons with impaired physical mobility have funding available and their housing situation permits, new bathrooms, totally adapted to their needs, can be constructed. In many states the Department of Vocational Rehabilitation allocates funds to make adaptations if a patient qualifies for services and the family owns the house or has permission of the owner.

When a totally reconstructed bathroom is unnecessary, many adaptive devices are available to aid in toileting for persons with impaired physical mobility, including a wide variety of toilet frames and safety rails. These rails can provide stability for those who are unsteady on their feet and can add leverage to assist in rising from a wheelchair or the toilet. They can be attached to the toilet or fixed to the floor or walls in horizontal, vertical, or diagonal positions, depending on individual needs.

The toilet seat might need to be adapted. It should be at an optimal height to enable the individual to get up from it, down to it, or slide across it. Detachable and fixed raised toilet seats are available in various heights and some are adjustable. There are models to fit every toilet bowl contour. They are constructed of wood or plastic and some are padded to prevent excess pressure. Raised toilet seats are designed to accommodate many needs. They can have one side cut down to accommodate various limitations in lower extremity range of motion. They can have front, side, or back openings to accommodate various adaptations in wiping techniques. Raised toilet seats can be collapsible and portable, and carrying cases are available (Fig. 9–2).

The rehabilitation nurse, in cooperation with an occupational therapist, can advise the patient and family about safety techniques. These include placement of toilet paper and proper balance for wiping to prevent unnecessary reaching.

ALTERNATIVES TO TOILETS

If persons with impaired physical mobility cannot get onto the toilet, either because of the limitations of their impairment or limitations in architectural accessibility, several alternatives are available.

Commodes

The need to use a commode can be difficult for the patient and family to accept. Having a commode in a living area or bedroom is an adaptation that patients and families might resist. Pointing out the benefit of having a commode available to facilitate continence and

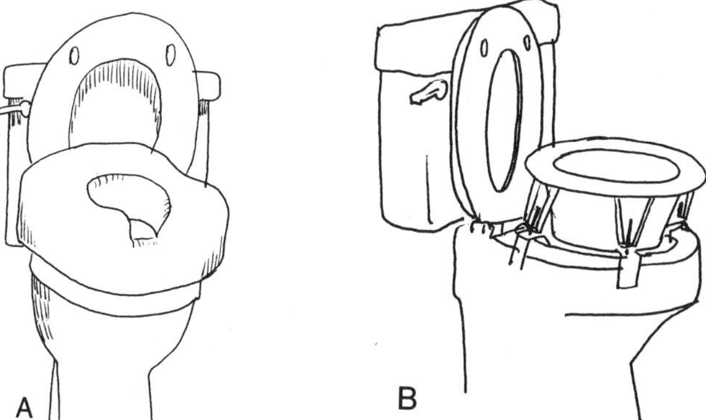

Figure 9–2. *Raised toilet seats are designed with a fixed* (A) *or adjustable* (B) *height; they can have side, back, or front openings to accommodate wiping; or they can have one side sloped to accommodate limitations of lower extremity range of motion. They can also be collapsible and portable.*

demonstrating sensitivity to the patient's and family's concerns can contribute to acceptability of its use as an alternative to the toilet.

Once the need for a commode has been determined, the correct commode can be selected from various options, depending on individual needs. Some wheelchair commodes allow the user to mobilize the commode independently. These and other wheeled commodes can be positioned over a toilet or used with a receptacle. Like wheeled commodes, stationary commodes are available with removable arms, padded seats, footrests, and front, side, and back cutout seats. Some commodes can be secured to the bed for stability, and others can be folded for easy transport. Commodes, like all other adaptive equipment, must be individually fitted to the disabled person's needs, taking into account the person's height, weight, and sitting balance (Fig. 9–3).

Male Hand-Held Urinals

Ideally, a hand-held urinal should be spill-proof and easy to use, empty, and clean independently. The standard male urinal is familiar to nurses. It is available in metal or plastic and has a capacity of 1 to 2 liters. Some urinals are equipped with snap-on lids to avoid spillage after use (Fig. 9–4*A*). Most urinals are designed with a handle or grip to facilitate holding and aid in hanging on a chair or bed when not in use. Urinals are generally designed to lay flat for use in a bed or chair and to stand upright after use. A recently developed urinal was designed specifically for use by those in wheelchairs (Fig. 9–4*B*). Men with a retracted penis might have more success using a female urinal (Fig. 9–5*A*). Because the opening covers the entire perineum, the urinal catches urine at whatever angle it emerges.

Continent men with impaired physical mobility might choose to use a condom-type external collection device attached to a leg bag when going on outings where accessible toilet facilities are not available.

Female Hand-Held Urinals

Urination for physically impaired women who cannot get to a toilet or commode is more difficult than for similarly disabled men, but various alternative urinals are available. The standard hospital bed pan is one option, but it tends to be large, cumbersome, and difficult to use independently. The fracture bed pan is smaller and easier to place, and has a grip loop handle that facilitates independent use (Fig. 9–6).

The female urinal mentioned above is an option if it can be placed properly to catch the urinary flow. There is also a newly designed

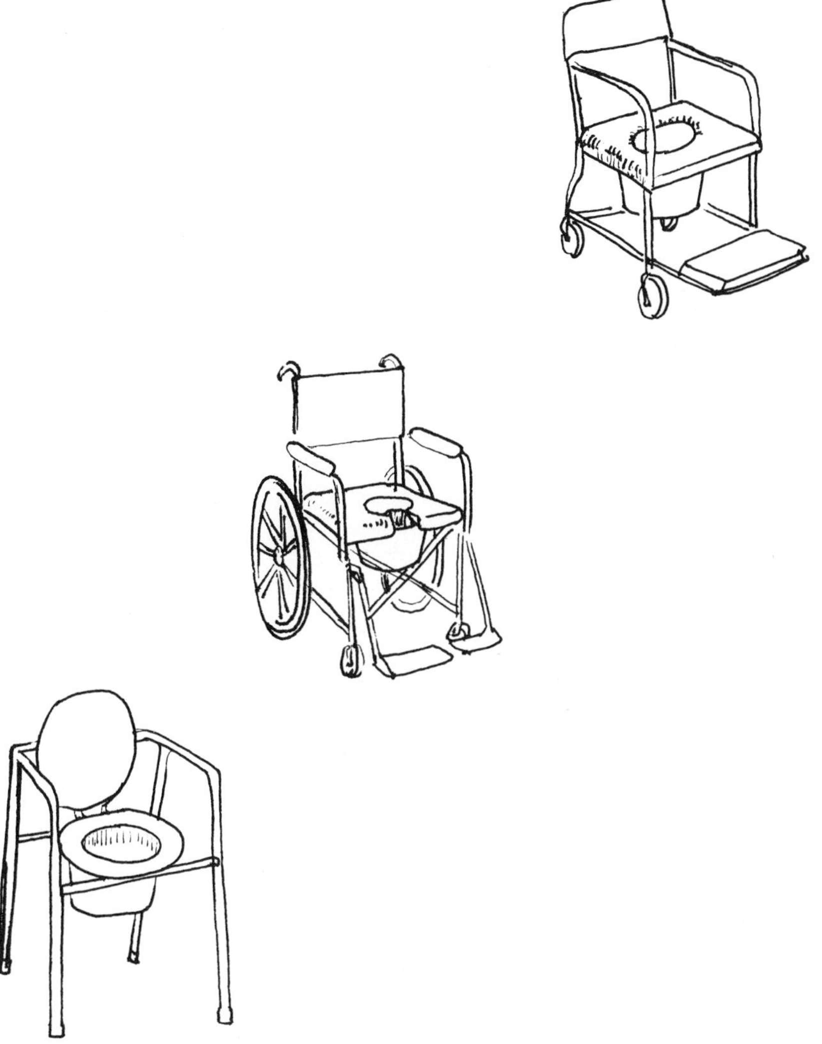

Figure 9–3. *Commodes.*

female urinal that can be used by those in wheelchairs (see Fig. 9–5*B*). Another option is the system consisting of a perineal funnel and tubing, which can drain directly into a toilet or a urine collector bag (see Fig. 9–5*C*).

Women in wheelchairs might find hand-held urinals easier to use with specially adapted wheelchair cushions. Cushions can be designed with a cutout that can be removed to accommodate a urinal. Split cushions can be designed to accommodate a long, narrow pan to catch urine without the woman having to change position in the wheelchair.

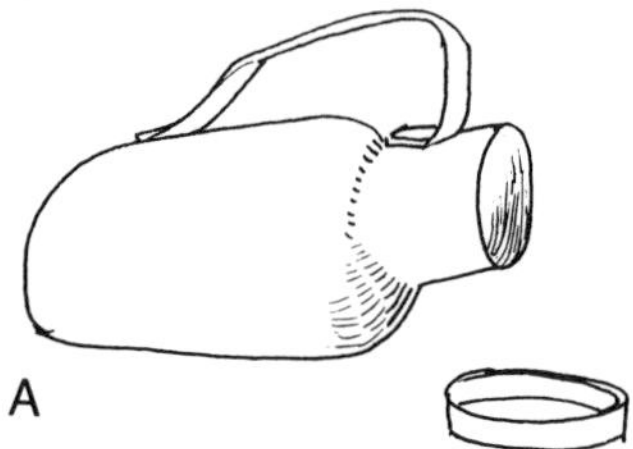

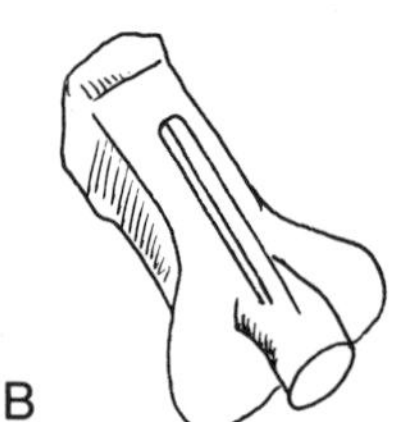

Figure 9–4. *Male hand-held urinals can be of a traditional design* (A) *or can be specifically designed for use in wheelchairs* (B).

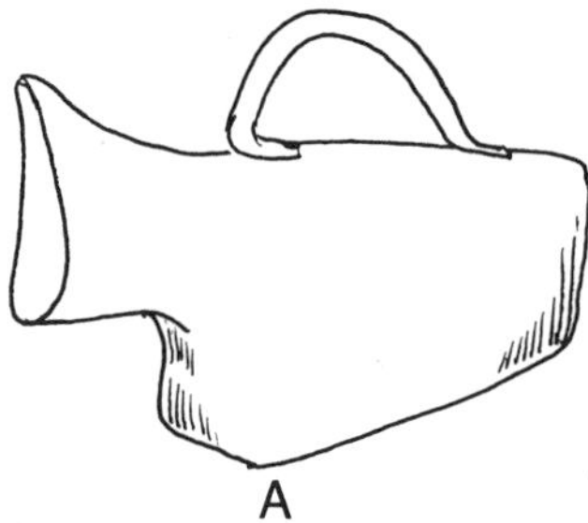

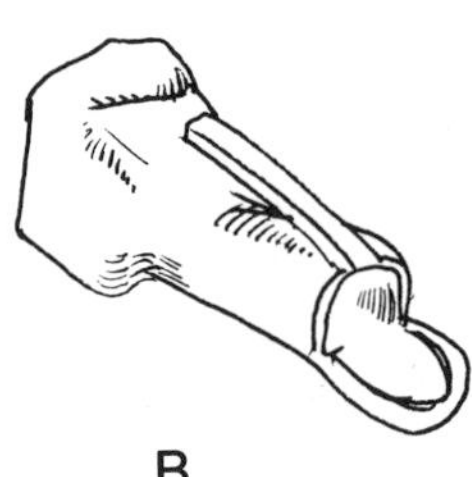

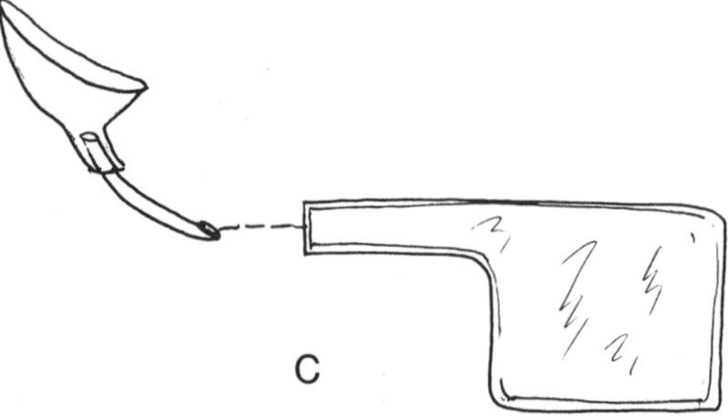

Figure 9–5. *Female hand-held urinals can be of a traditional design* (A), *can be specifically designed for use in a wheelchair* (B), *or can be of a funnel design* (C).

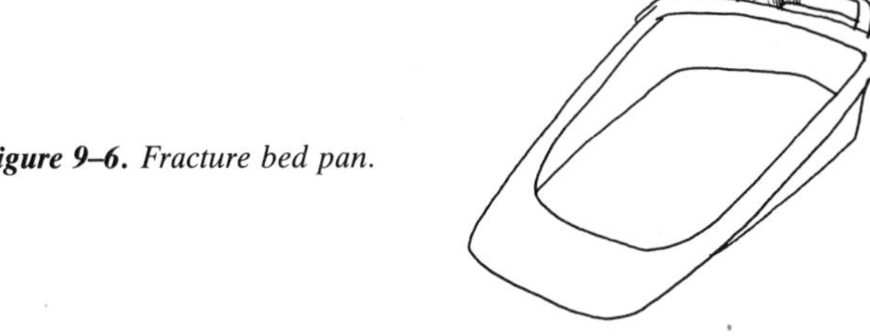

Figure 9–6. *Fracture bed pan.*

An incontinence device that is secured in the vagina was marketed in 1988 (Chap. 13). To date not enough women have used it to determine its efficacy.

CLOTHING

Persons with impaired physical mobility can be helped to maintain continence by wearing suitable clothing.

Men with limited dexterity might find Velcro fly closures easier and quicker to open than zippers. Extending the fly opening down to the crotch seam makes using a hand-held urinal easier. Generally, loose-fitting boxer shorts allow quicker access than bikini-type or fitted briefs. When dexterity is severely limited, men might choose not to wear underpants at all.

Women with limited dexterity will probably not be able to wear slacks, because it requires considerable agility to get them out of the way for urination. Tight skirts and layers of underclothes such as slips, corsets, and pants also require time and agility to maneuver out of the way.

Loose-fitting clothes with minimal undergarments are most functional. A wrap-around skirt provides the easiest access when using a hand-held urinal and is most functional for clearing clothing out of the way during toilet transfers. Although open-crotch or loose-fitting underwear facilitates the use of hand-held urinals, not wearing underpants is probably most functional (as it is for men).

References

Mumma, C.M. (ed.): Rehabilitation Nursing: Concepts and Practice. A Core Curriculum. Evanston, IL, Rehabilitation Nursing Foundation, 1987, pp. 8–9.

Paralyzed Veterans of America: Design Guidelines Qualifying for the Tax Advantages of Section 190. Washington, D.C., Paralyzed Veterans of America, 1986, p. 4.

Leslie Oliver, RN

10 The Neurogenic Bladder

For many people with incontinence and other bladder problems, the underlying cause is damage to the delicate neurologic control mechanisms that regulate bladder function. Continence depends on long nerve pathways, which are vulnerable to disease or trauma affecting the nervous system (Chap. 2).

The problems of people with neurogenic bladder dysfunction are often exacerbated by the fact that bladder control is seldom the only impairment. Many of these individuals have varying degrees of physical or mental disability, or both. When poor bladder function and disability coexist, the problems of coping with micturition and incontinence are compounded. The specific problems associated with physical disabilities are discussed in Chapter 9.

Damage to nerve pathways at any point between the cortical bladder center and the bladder itself can impair continence. Dysfunction depends on the exact site and the extent of the lesion—there are five possible sites of damage (Fig. 10–1). Diffuse neurologic damage, such as that from multiple sclerosis or multiple injuries, can produce any combination of these problems.

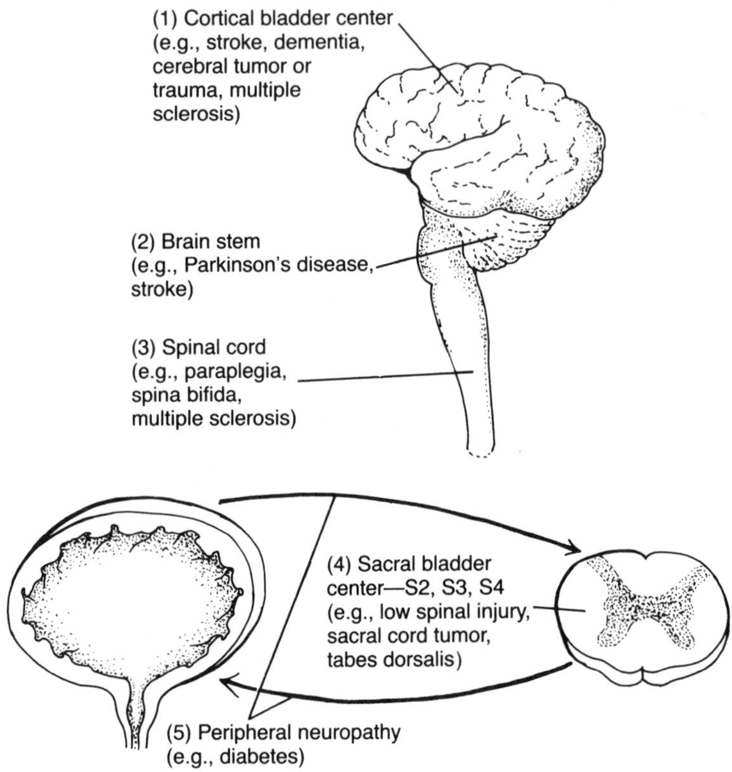

Figure 10–1. *Sites of neurologic damage leading to neurogenic bladder problems.*

SITES OF NEUROLOGIC DAMAGE

Cortical Bladder Center

The higher cortical centers that control micturition can be involved in processes such as a cerebrovascular accident, diffuse cortical failure, dementia, or multiple sclerosis, and can be damaged by a cerebral tumor or head injury. "Normal" age changes in the brain result in impairment of function in a high percentage of older people. Damage impairs the ability to inhibit the sacral reflex arc efficiently (see Fig. 2–2). Often bladder sensation is retained so that urgency is felt, but the important inhibiting signal is weak or absent, and urgency and urge incontinence can result. This condition is identical to detrusor instability (Chap. 2), and the term "unstable bladder" can be used to describe an uninhibited bladder of neurogenic or idiopathic origin.

Brain Stem

Centers in the brain stem are vital in coordinating the complex series of reflexes and feedback loops involved in the act of complete voluntary micturition. Damage (e.g., in Parkinson's disease, multiple sclerosis, other dementias) results in a poorly coordinated and often incomplete voiding sequence. During micturition the detrusor contracts and the urethra relaxes synergistically, functioning together to effect rapid and complete bladder emptying without interruption, straining, or residual urine. Brain stem damage can result in detrusor-sphincter dyssynergia—the sphincter does not relax adequately as the detrusor contracts, or the bladder contraction is unsustained. This can result in a total inability to void, in all voiding being by abdominal effort only, or in interrupted and incomplete emptying.

Spinal Cord

After the initial phase of spinal shock is over, complete transection of the spinal cord above the level of the sacral bladder center usually results in an "automatic" bladder that is decentralized from all cerebral control. Immediately after spinal injury most people experience a phase of silence, during which all spinal reflexes are disrupted or absent. The bladder is completely atonic, without any activity. Retention of urine results. Once this phase ends and the spinal reflexes return (which can take from a few days to several years), the bladder starts to "wake up" again. If the sacral bladder center is undamaged, the spinal reflex arc becomes re-established. The patient has no sensation of bladder activity nor any control over reflex contractions. Because the bladder is cut off from the coordinating center in the brain stem, these bladder contractions, although often powerful, are frequently not sustained, and incomplete emptying with residual urine results. The patient experiences sudden, uncontrollable incontinence, but this does not always leave an empty bladder. When transection is incomplete some conscious sensation and some voluntary control might be retained.

Sacral Bladder Center

If spinal cord damage involves the S2 to S4 segments, the spinal reflex arc is disrupted. There will be neither conscious sensation nor voluntary control of the bladder, and the detrusor contraction reflex will be absent. The bladder is atonic in response to filling, although local synapses in the bladder wall could cause minor ineffectual contractions. This atonic bladder becomes increasingly distended and overflow incontinence usually develops. Any bladder emptying will be by abdominal effort alone.

This type of bladder was once commonly seen in tabes dorsalis of tertiary syphilis. Nowadays those with low spinal injury or tumor and spina bifida are the most frequently affected.

Peripheral Nervous System

Disease of the peripheral nervous system can attack the local nerve supply to the bladder. This is especially common in those with diabetic peripheral neuropathy, which can affect both sensory and motor pathways. Because sensation is deficient, the bladder might become overdistended. Motor damage leads to inefficient bladder emptying and overflow incontinence can develop. Similarly, extensive pelvic surgery can disrupt peripheral nerves.

Neurogenic bladder problems fall into two broad categories of dysfunction: those resulting in an unstable or uninhibited bladder (e.g., cortical or spinal damage) and those causing voiding problems (e.g., brain stem, spinal, sacral, or peripheral damage). Even if these two coexist, they should usually be managed as two distinct entities and treated separately.

DIAGNOSIS

Neurogenic bladder problems should always be investigated fully prior to treatment. Urodynamic investigation is essential to accurate diagnosis. Cystometry (Chap. 3) should be done at a predetermined rate of filling, depending on the nature of the patient's symptoms. A fast rate of filling (300 ml/minute), however, can cause reflex detrusor contractions. Radiography is helpful if voiding difficulties are suspected, because the bladder neck and urethra can be visualized during attempted voiding (videocystourethrography). Electromyography can help to diagnose dyssynergic sphincter activity.

If the patient is disabled, a careful assessment of mobility, dexterity, and life-style is also vital in planning realistic goals (see Chaps. 3 and 9).

TREATMENT

The Unstable Neurogenic Bladder

Treatment of the unstable neurogenic bladder is similar to management of detrusor instability of non-neurogenic origin. Uninhibited contractions can often be reduced in magnitude and number, even eliminated, by drug therapy. Care must be taken in patients with neuropathy, because a few are hypersensitive to medication and can be put into retention or experience exaggerated side effects, especially from anticholinergic therapy. New treatments should therefore be introduced gradually and monitored closely.

Accurate charting reveals whether there is a pattern to the instability and incontinence. If the volume of bladder filling at which contractions occur is relatively constant, it is often possible to plan a toileting program designed to anticipate incontinence. This obviously varies with fluid intake and might need to take the patient's activities into account, because movement can provoke bladder contractions. The role of bladder training has not been well evaluated for those with an unstable neurogenic bladder, but it is likely to be effective for some patients (Chap. 4).

Many of those with an unstable neurogenic bladder have restricted mobility (e.g., after a stroke or spinal injury). This complicates the problems of managing a bladder that is unpredictable and provides little if any warning of impending micturition.

Neurogenic Voiding Difficulties

Incomplete bladder emptying can lead to various problems. Urinary tract infection is common, because the bladder is never completely emptied. It is extremely difficult to eradicate, even with antibiotics. Reinfection and a shifting spectrum of invading organisms are common. If the residual volume is large, in particular over 400 ml, there is risk of renal damage from back pressure through the ureters. If hydronephrosis is present, with or without ureteral reflux, renal infection usually follows bladder infection. This carries a high risk of morbidity and possibly of mortality.

Residual urine often leads to overflow incontinence and also reduces functional bladder capacity. If the bladder capacity is 500 ml, with a residual urine volume of 400 ml, the functional capacity (the capacity that can be used) is only 100 ml. This will obviously increase voiding frequency. Those with the double problem of a residual volume and instability (e.g., people with multiple sclerosis or spinal injury) often have a small margin between their residual volume, which is always in the bladder, and the volume at which uninhibited contractions develop. This can result in incontinence occurring soon after voiding. Indeed, some have almost continuous episodes of incontinence, because as soon as the volume in the bladder exceeds the residual volume, the bladder contracts and expels the excess.

Voiding Techniques

Some people with voiding dysfunction can find a technique to help stimulate complete emptying. If the elements of the sacral reflex are intact but merely uncoordinated (e.g., cut off from the brain stem), it is often possible to initiate a detrusor contraction by stimulating trigger areas. Alternatively, a direct increase in abdominal pressure, especially in women, can raise the intravesical pressure to the point where urethral resistance is overcome and voluntary voiding occurs (Valsalva or Credé maneuver; see below). If either of these can be done before overflow occurs, continence can be achieved.

Trigger Areas. Patients without sacral damage may find a "trigger" to initiate a bladder contraction. Tapping the abdominal wall suprapubically is a common method. The abdomen is firmly and repeatedly tapped, usually by the tips of the extended fingers of one hand, until voiding starts. Often the contraction generated is unsustained, so the tapping and voiding must be repeated several times until the bladder is empty. Abdominal tenderness or weak fingers can be a problem and using this method can become time-consuming and demoralizing. Because bladder contraction usually helps to open the urethra, however, the potential for damage is low. Using this method is preferable to straining or pushing.

Other trigger mechanisms include pulling pubic hairs, stroking the abdomen or interior aspect of the thighs, and digital anal stimulation and dilation (Johnson, 1980). Patients managing their voiding in this way should experiment to discover which technique works best and most easily for them.

Valsalva and Credé Maneuvers. The Valsalva and Credé methods are only suitable for those whose sphincter mechanism is not in complete spasm—usually patients with damage at the sacral bladder center level, where sphincteric resistance is often low and easily overcome.

The Valsalva maneuver (inhaling deeply and then exhaling forcefully against a closed glottis) greatly increases the intra-abdominal pressure and can enable the bladder to be emptied. In some people, this pressure increase can trigger a bladder contraction. This type of straining is inadvisable, however, certainly on a long-term basis. It raises intracranial pressure and impedes cardiac return and should definitely be avoided by anyone with cardiovascular or cerebrovascular disease. Straining can eventually weaken and damage the pelvic musculature and bladder neck, leading to sphincter incompetence (stress incontinence).

The Credé maneuver (manual bladder expression) involves applying considerable pressure suprapubically, usually with the ball of the hand or fist, directly over the bladder. As with the Valsalva maneuver, this can work to empty the bladder, either by raising bladder pressure directly or by triggering a contraction. Unfortunately, if no contraction occurs, the bladder neck remains closed, and a high pressure is needed to open it. Eventual sphincter damage is a risk. Some people find expression uncomfortable. If sensation is deficient, great care should be taken to avoid bruising. Obese people and those with weak hands or arms also have difficulty. Sometimes someone else can be taught to apply the pressure. If reflux from the bladder to the ureters is suspected, use of the Credé method should be avoided. Whether its repeated use can create reflux is unproven.

Intermittent Catheterization

The biggest single advance in the management of neurogenic voiding difficulties has been the introduction of intermittent catheterization. The method involves the regular introduction of a catheter to empty the bladder and then removal of the catheter, leaving the patient catheter-free in between.

Sterile intermittent catheterization was originally introduced for the immediate management of patients with spinal injury as an alternative to the use of an indwelling catheter in the phase of spinal shock, when the the bladder is areflexic. A strictly aseptic technique is used and the procedure is performed often enough to keep the urine volume below 400 ml.

The procedure involves considerably less risk of infection and complications than does the use of an indwelling catheter, and carries a better long-term prognosis in regard to catheter-free continence. In a hospital, or wherever catheterization is done by someone other than the patient, the risk of cross-infection is high and it is always best to maintain a strict aseptic policy.

In the past 10 or 15 years the technique of intermittent nonsterile ("clean") self-catheterization has become widely adopted for the long-term management of people with persistent large residual urine volumes. Most work has been done with children suffering from spina bifida (Kaye and Van Blerk, 1981) and spinal injury patients (Pearman, 1976). More recently it has been used for all categories of those with incomplete bladder emptying. Many people, with a wide range of physical abilities, can be taught self-catheterization. If this proves impossible, a relative or caregiver can be taught instead.

The clean technique was introduced by Lapides in the United States in the early 1970s (Lapides and associates, 1972). Much to the surprise of professionals indoctrinated in the importance of strict asepsis in catheterization, patients using a clean rather than a sterile technique did not tend to encounter frequent problematic urinary tract infections. In fact, many who previously had chronically infected residual urine found that infection decreased when intermittent catheterization was used, because the focus of infection (the residual urine) was removed. Complete, regular emptying of the bladder is probably an important factor in the prevention of infection in the urinary tract.

Many nurses are skeptical when first introduced to the use of this procedure and worry about infection risks and the dangers of trauma to the urethra from repeated catheter insertion. In practice the risks are slight, and certainly nothing approaches the problems associated with indwelling catheterization. Few patients have to abandon intermittent catheterization, provided that the procedure is taught correctly and the program closely supervised in the initial stages.

To be selected as a suitable candidate for intermittent catheterization, the patient usually must have a residual urine volume persistently greater than 100 ml and have problems of overflow incontinence, recurrent bladder infection, or both. If self-catheterization is to be successful, a reasonable degree of manual dexterity, intelligence, and motivation is necessary. Usually the parents of young children are taught to carry out the procedure until the children are old enough to be responsible for it themselves, usually by the age of 7 or 8 (Fay, 1978). A close relative or constant attendant might be able and willing to help a disabled adult. Before this option is considered, however, it must be ascertained whether it will be acceptable both to patient and caregiver, and that the relationship between them will not be unduly stressed by this additional dependence.

The technique of intermittent catheterization should be fully discussed with the patient prior to teaching the method. Many patients are fearful of using a catheter initially; they might want to discuss the possibility of hurting themselves and the long-term effects of the procedure. A few, especially women, are embarrassed at the idea of touching the genitals. Whoever teaches the patient should impart a feeling of optimism that the patient will be able to carry out the procedure and will benefit from it. The alternatives, including voiding techniques, the use of an indwelling catheter, surgery, or drugs, and continuing with the voiding difficulty and overflow incontinence should also be discussed, with the advantages and disadvantages of each. For many patients intermittent self-catheterization is the treatment of choice and should be strongly recommended by professionals.

People vary greatly in their aptitude for self-catheterization. Teaching should take place in a relaxed, private, and unhurried atmosphere. When several different staff members are involved it is prudent to have a written and consistent policy, so that the patient is told the same thing by everyone. A full and detailed explanation of the local anatomy should be given, usually with the aid of diagrams (Fig. 10–2). Few people have an accurate idea of the length of the urethra or of the interrelationship of the various genital organs. Some are afraid that the

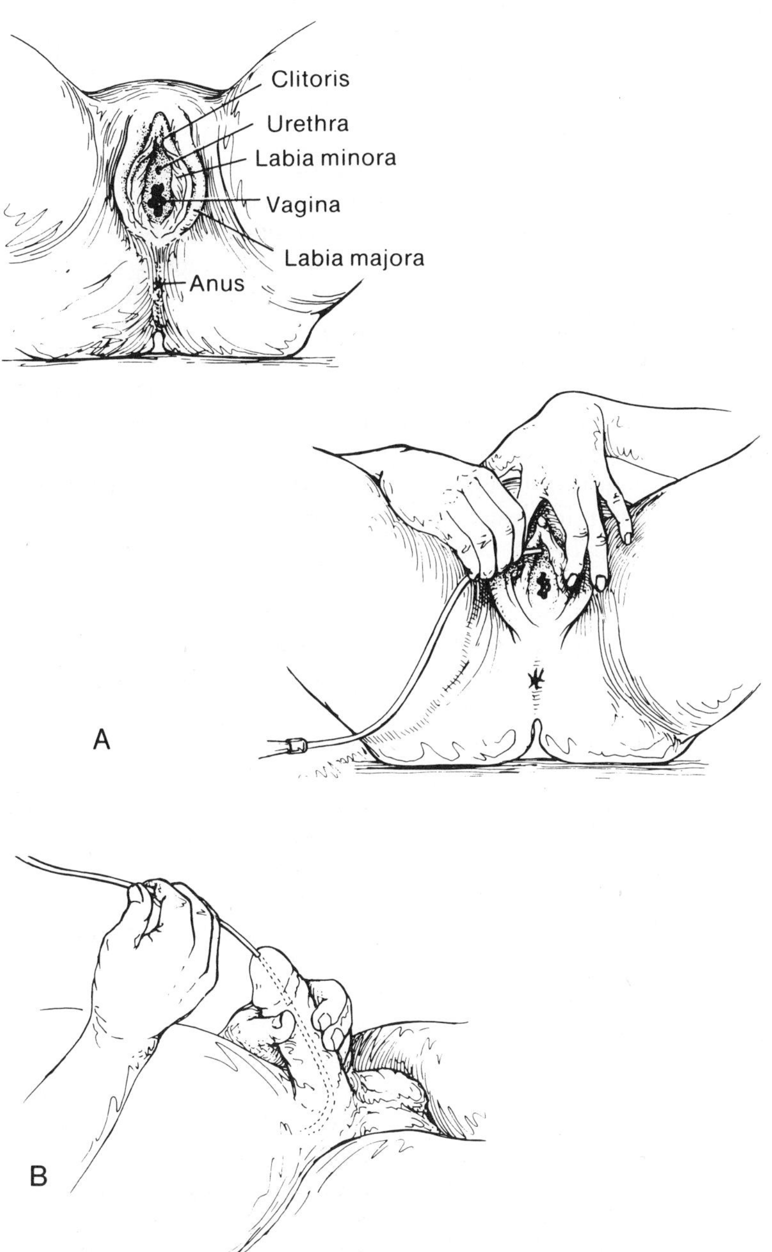

Figure 10–2. *Diagrams for teaching self-catheterization.* A, *Female patients.* B, *Male patients.*

catheter might get lost inside or that the bladder might be punctured if the catheter goes in too far. Patients can be catheterized in the semirecumbent position while a detailed commentary is given. Usually the teacher (physician or nurse) should be using aseptic technique (because of the risk of cross infection), and it must be explained to patients why a clean technique is safe for them to use outside the hospital. Most people understand the explanation that everyone has a certain resistance to their own bacteria and because the bladder will be completely and regularly emptied, any bacteria that are introduced will be drained out again and thus cannot take hold and cause an infection. Health professionals should wear gloves and take extra precautions to protect patients from the bacteria of other patients and to protect themselves from the patients.

Once the catheter is in position, women should be shown the position of the urethral meatus in a mirror and be taught to locate by touch how far it is from an easily identifiable landmark (e.g., the clitoris or labia). The woman should then withdraw the catheter herself and reintroduce it by separating the labia with the nondominant hand (Fig. 10–2*A*) and locating the meatus in a mirror. With practice most women can learn to self-catheterize by touch (indeed, some never manage to get a reasonable view in the mirror).

Having successfully introduced the catheter two or three times while lying down with the legs abducted, patients are then asked to catheterize sitting on a toilet, by touch if possible. If a mirror is needed, a shaving mirror can be adapted to hook over the front of the toilet seat or a suction pad can be attached to the seat or front of the bowl. Some women cannot manage this. There are various positions that should be considered and tried to suit individual preferences or disabilities. Squatting, standing with one foot on a stool or toilet, sitting on the edge of a chair or wheelchair (with a "U" cut-out cushion, if necessary), or using a posterior approach if the legs cannot be abducted—any of these might be suitable, depending on the patient's physical abilities and agility.

Male patients have far less difficulty than women in locating the urethral meatus and can self-catheterize lying, sitting, or standing (Fig. 10–2*B*). Men should use a water-soluble lubricating jelly on the catheter prior to inserting it into the urethra. Some women also prefer to use lubricating jelly on the catheter.

Many patients can learn to self-catheterize competently in a single outpatient session. People with multiple handicaps might take considerably longer to find a position and method that is reliable. Patients with limited movement in their hands and wrists might have to try a few different types of catheters to find the most suitable one.

The frequency of catheterization varies among individuals. Some people empty the bladder almost completely at micturition and have a residual urine that slowly accumulates over a few days. Others are in complete retention and need to catheterize five to six times a day. Self-catheterization should be done often enough to avoid incontinence whenever possible or as often as required to ensure that the volume of residual urine obtained is always below 400 ml. Once the technique has been mastered, the patient can be dismissed with an adequate supply of catheters and a simple instruction sheet and diagram (Tables 10–1 and 10–2; Fig. 10–2).

Further Considerations. Patients should be reminded that, although it is not necessary to wash themselves before each catheteriza-

Table 10–1. *SELF-CATHETERIZATION FOR WOMEN*

Directions for Patient

1. Perform the catheterization as often as your physician or nurse has suggested. To start with, this should be every ______ hours.
2. Get your catheter, a mirror, and lubricant gel, if you need it.
3. Wash your hands thoroughly and rinse the catheter with water.
4. Situate yourself in the most comfortable and convenient position. If you do not sit on the toilet, you will need a container for the urine.
5. Separate the labia with one hand and, holding the catheter 2 to 3 inches from the tip, gently insert it into the urethra until urine flows (Fig. 10–2*A*).
6. When urine stops flowing, slowly withdraw the catheter. If the flow restarts, stop withdrawing until the bladder is empty. The bladder should be emptied completely at each catheterization.
7. When the catheter is out, wash it with a mild soap, rinse it thoroughly, and shake it dry. Dry the outside with a clean paper towel or tissue and store it in a clean, dry place, ready for the next use. If you are keeping a chart, record the urine volume obtained.
8. Each catheter can be used for several weeks before a new one is needed. Most patients use each catheter for a month at a time. A supply of catheters is available by prescription from ________________.
9. You should drink 3 to 4 pints of liquid (any type) every 24 hours. Discuss the amount and types of liquid you should drink with your physician.

Questions Patients Frequently Ask

The following are questions that are frequently asked by women who are being taught to self-catheterize, along with suggested answers. Of course, patients should always be advised to contact their physician in an emergency.

1. "What should I do if I see blood in the urine or on the catheter?"
   Answer: "If it is a few specks, don't worry. If the bleeding persists or becomes heavy, contact your physician."
2. "What should I do if the urine becomes smelly or cloudy, or if burning or a fever develops?"
   Answer: "Bring a urine specimen to the laboratory or physician's office. You probably have a mild infection."
3. "What should I do if I cannot get the catheter in?"
   Answer: "Don't keep trying. You will irritate your urethra. Abandon the attempt and try again later. If the difficulty persists and you are unable to pass urine yourself, seek help within 12 hours."
4. "What should I do if I miss and put the catheter in my vagina by mistake?"
   Answer: "You will know because it will feel different and no urine will come out. Take the catheter out, wash it, and start again."

Table 10–2. *SELF-CATHETERIZATION FOR MEN*

Directions for Patient

1. Perform the catheterization as often as your physician or nurse has suggested. To start with, this should be every ______ hours.
2. Get your catheter and lubricant gel.
3. Wash your hands thoroughly and rinse the catheter with water.
4. Situate yourself in the most comfortable and convenient position. If you do not sit on the toilet, you will need a container for the urine.
5. Squeeze a small amount of lubricant gel along the catheter.
6. Holding the penis in a vertical position, gently insert the catheter until urine flows (Fig. 10–2*B*). You might find that coughing or deep breathing helps to overcome any resistance at the sphincter.
7. When urine stops flowing, slowly withdraw the catheter. If the flow restarts, stop withdrawing until the bladder is empty. The bladder should be emptied completely at each catheterization.
8. When the catheter is out, wash it with a mild soap, rinse it thoroughly, and shake it dry. Dry the outside with a clean paper towel or tissue and store in a clean, dry place, ready for the next use. If you are keeping a chart, record the urine volume obtained.
9. Each catheter can be used for several weeks before a new one is needed. Most patients use each catheter for a month at a time. A supply of catheters is available by prescription from ________________.
10. You should drink 3 to 4 pints of liquid (any type) every 24 hours. Discuss the amount and types of liquid you should drink with your physician.

Questions Patients Frequently Ask

The following are questions that are frequently asked by men who are being taught to self-catheterize, along with suggested answers. Of course, patients should always be advised to contact their physician in an emergency.

1. "What should I do if I see blood in the urine or on the catheter?"
   Answer: "If it is a few specks, don't worry. If the bleeding persists or becomes heavy, contact your physician."
2. "What should I do if the urine becomes smelly or cloudy, or if burning or a fever develops?"
   Answer: "Bring a urine specimen to the laboratory or physician's office. You probably have a mild infection."
3. "What should I do if I cannot get the catheter in?"
   Answer: "Don't keep trying. You will irritate your urethra. Abandon the attempt and try again later. If the difficulty persists and you are unable to pass urine yourself, seek help within 12 hours."

tion, routine personal hygiene should be maintained. A shower or daily bath, with good washing of the genital area, is sufficient.

Each catheter should be washed out after use (e.g., with a mild soap solution), rinsed in running water, and dried (by shaking it and wiping the outside with a paper towel). It is then stored in a clean, dry place until next use, when it should again be held under running water prior to insertion. Many people use a self-sealing plastic bag and keep the catheter in a handbag or pocket when not being used. Soaking the catheter in a strong antiseptic solution is unnecessary and is not recommended. This could be irritating to the sensitive urethral mucosa and could kill off normal flora, leaving the patient vulnerable to infection by more harmful micro-organisms. Similarly, swabbing of the urethral meatus is not encouraged unless a discharge or vaginal infection is present. Each catheter is used for approximately 1 month and then thrown away (except in hospitals, where a new catheter must be used each time to decrease the possibility of cross-infection).

The importance of hand washing should be stressed. Women are instructed just to wash their hands, part the labia, and insert the catheter until urine flows. Once the flow ceases the catheter is withdrawn slowly, stopping if the flow starts again. Men should do exactly the same and should also use lubricating jelly when inserting the catheter (see above).

Symptomatic infection is relatively uncommon. It results more commonly from catheterizing too infrequently than from too frequently (Champion, 1976). It usually occurs in one-quarter to one-third of patients at some time and generally responds to a single dose of trimethoprim (400 mg), because most infections are caused by Escherichia coli from bowel contamination. If there are recurrent episodes, it might be advisable to give the patient a small supply of trimethoprim to take when needed. A urine specimen should be cultured if symptoms fail to respond. Recurrent infections become a problem with a small minority of patients, and such patients should be observed for faulty techniques. The volume obtained should be measured to ensure that it is consistently below 400 ml. Occasionally it is necessary to advise sterilizing the catheters or changing them more frequently. Only rarely does self-catheterization have to be abandoned altogether.

Asymptomatic bacteriuria is common in people who are self-catheterizing (Lancet, 1979). Unless the patient has vesicoureteral reflux or is very young (under 5 years old), this can be left untreated. There is little point in obtaining routine urine samples; this is only indicated in the presence of symptoms.

If a patient has the dual problem of residual urine and unstable contractions, the aim of therapy should be paralysis of the bladder pharmacologically to abolish the contractions and drainage of the bladder by intermittent catheterization. This works well for many people with spina bifida, multiple sclerosis, or spinal cord injury.

Results with the use of intermittent catheterization are excellent. Up to 80% of patients with a large volume of residual urine of neurogenic origin can regain continence. Many have thereby avoided insertion of a permanent indwelling catheter, with all its attendant problems (Chap. 15), or a urinary diversion. Some people can gradually phase out catheterization as normal voiding is re-established. Others must continue to catheterize indefinitely. Some people with ileal conduits are now being "undiverted" back to using their own bladder with intermittent catheterization. The technique is also being increasingly used in elderly patients with voiding dysfunction (Chap. 8).

Drug Therapy

Various drugs can be used to assist voiding. Some decrease the contractions of an unstable bladder (e.g., oxybutynin). Others reduce outflow resistance (e.g., phenoxybenzamine or diazepam). All have significant side effects and should be used with great care.

Surgery

Formerly, many men with neurogenic voiding dysfunction had their urinary sphincters transected to preserve renal function, thereby creating total incontinence. Current surgical techniques are more selective. A careful bladder neck incision or resection or a urethrotomy can decrease outflow resistance to the point where a voiding technique can be effective without creating incontinence. Many quadriplegic and some paraplegic men do become incontinent after surgery to preserve renal function, however, and use condom drainage on a long-term basis.

A urinary diversion into a stoma should be a last resort in the management of neurogenic incontinence. This involves major surgery, and the long-term prognosis for renal function is uncertain. If all else fails to restore continence, especially if renal function is threatened by recurrent infections, urinary diversion might be considered as an alternative to the insertion of an indwelling catheter (Chap. 15). This is especially true for women, for whom there is not yet a satisfactory external collection device. Adjustment to surgery can be excellent with careful preoperative counseling, and certainly an incontinent stoma is easier to manage effectively than a totally incontinent female urethra. If there is little prospect of continence, a stoma can be offered to the female patient relatively early, rather than waiting until she has endured years of misery and incontinence. Continent urinary diversions are now being performed, and patients might wish to discuss this option with their physician. Counseling by an ET nurse, if available, can help patients and their families to reach an informed decision.

Bladder Management After Spinal Injury

It is crucial for the rehabilitation of paraplegic patients that effective bladder management be started immediately after injury. Initially the patients will be in spinal shock, with complete retention. If the bladder is allowed to become overdistended at this time permanent progressive damage to the local nerve supply can result. Intermittent sterile catheterization should be started immediately on admission and a careful record kept to ensure that the bladder is never allowed to hold more than 400 ml of urine.

Soon after injury patients should be encouraged to participate in their own bladder management. They are taught to self-catheterize as soon as they can and to keep their own charts.

After a variable length of time the bladder will begin to "wake up" as reflex contractions start to occur. At first these will be inefficient and a decision must be made on an individual basis as to whether the contractions should be augmented by drugs or by tapping to achieve voiding or to suppress them pharmacologically and continue intermittent catheterization.

The paraplegic, who has deficient or completely absent direct bladder sensation, can often learn to be sensitive to other stimuli that can help to monitor bladder fullness and activity. Some people have autonomic cues as to when the bladder is full (commonly tachycardia, but often other individual signs). Others can feel it by abdominal distention or by effects on the gut. It is important that these patients learn to interpret their internal signals correctly, because they are of great help in achieving continence. Nursing spinal cord injury patients requires extensive teaching from the onset of injury.

In men, an unstable bladder with dyssynergic voiding is often the outcome. This sphincteric resistance is useful in maintaining continence, but might need to be modified by drugs or surgery if voiding difficulty is significant. Alternatively, intermittent catheterization can be continued.

Women often fare less well than men. Serious incontinence often results, because the sphincter is less efficient once the reflexes have been re-established. Drug therapy can be helpful, but for some women incontinence is so severe that urinary diversion is considered.

References and Further Reading

Barry, K.: Neurogenic bladder incontinence: The consequences of mismanagement. Rehab. Nurs., *10:*12, 1981.

Blaivas, J.G.: Neurologic dysfunctions. *In* Yalla, S.V., et al. (eds.): Neurourology and Urodynamics: Principles and Practices. New York, Macmillan, 1988, pp. 343–357.

Champion, V.L.: Clean technique for intermittent self-catheterization. Nurs. Res., *25:*13, 1976.

Clean intermittent catheterization. Lancet, *2*:448, 1979.

Diokno, A.C.: Clean intermittent self-catheterization. *In* Yalla, S.V., et al. (eds.): Neurourology and Urodynamics: Principles and Practices. New York, Macmillan, 1988, pp. 410–416.

Fay, J.: Intermittent non-sterile catheterization of children. Nurs. Mirror, *146:*xiii, 1978.

Hartman, M.: Intermittent self-catheterization. Nursing, *78:*72, 1978.

Holland, N.J., Weisel-Levison, P., and Schwedelson, E.S.: Survey of neurogenic bladder in multiple sclerosis. J. Neurosurg. Nurs., *13:*337, 1981.

Johnson, J.H.: Rehabilitative aspects of neurologic bladder dysfunction. Nurs. Clin. North Am., *15:*293, 1980.

Kaye, K., and Van Blerk, P.J.: Urinary continence in children with neurogenic bladders. Br. J. Urology, *53:*241, 1981.

Khanna, O.P.: Cystometry: Water. *In* Barrett, D.M., and Wein, A.J. (eds.): Controversies in Neurology. New York, Churchill Livingstone, 1984, pp. 9–30.
Lapides, J., et al.: Clean intermittent self-catheterization in the treatment of urinary tract disease. J. Urol., *107:*458, 1972.
Pearman, J.W.: Urological follow-up of 99 spinal-cord injured patients initially managed by intermittent catheterization. Br. J. Urol., *48:*297, 1976.
Spiro, L.R.: Bladder training for the incontinent patient. J. Gerontol. Nurs., *4:*28, 1978.

Diane Krasner, RN, MS, ET

11 Incontinence in Varied Settings

The problems of incontinence vary from one setting to another. This is true in an acute or extended care facility, an institutional or residential setting, or the patient's or a relative's home. Location-related factors can cause or exacerbate incontinence or at least work against successful cure or management.

HOME CARE

Nurses who have worked exclusively in hospitals often fail to realize how different problems can be when experienced by patients at home. The vast majority of incontinent people live at home. Most cope with their incontinence, often remarkably well, and manage to control their problem so that it creates only minimal disruption to their lives. At best, there might be only a little extra laundry or more items for disposal. If incontinence is a major problem and poorly managed, however, it can become such a burden that it dominates home life, eventually leading to the inability to live independently or be maintained at home by caregivers. Success in managing heavy incontinence at home depends on who is available and willing to help, what washing and disposal facilities are available, and which services can be mobilized for assistance.

Assessment at Home

Assessment of incontinent people in their home environment provides the nurse with a clearer picture of the problem than could be obtained in a hospital or clinic setting. Assessment at home, however, is not without drawbacks. The nurse, as a guest in the home, is often less in control of the situation than in the hospital, and it might be difficult to keep some people, especially the lonely elderly, to the point of the discussion. The interview invariably takes longer at home, so it is important to allow plenty of time when planning an assessment visit. Some people deny their incontinence when visited at home. If the patient does not live alone, it could be difficult to ensure privacy and the patient might be unwilling to talk frankly in front of others.

Physical examination is often more difficult to carry out at home. The bedroom might be cold and poorly lit, and a physical examination could be almost impossible if done on a sagging mattress in dim light. Some people object to being examined at all. Any specimens obtained will be less fresh by the time they arrive at the laboratory than are specimens obtained in a clinic.

Unlike the assessment of patients in the hospital, the home assessment is based on a short observation period. A special effort may have been made to clean up, hiding the real effect that incontinence is having on the home. Sometimes several visits are necessary, both to gain the patient's full confidence and to establish a realistic picture of the problem.

Many people who are visited by a home health nurse are incontinent without the nurse's realizing it. The alert nurse, whether visiting to dress a leg ulcer or to do a developmental check on a child, will discover other health care problems, including incontinence, and take appropriate action. A mutual pretense that incontinence is not occurring—denial by the patient and failure to inquire by the nurse—only helps to reinforce the myth that incontinence is inevitable and untreatable.

Discharge from the Hospital

When an incontinent person is to be discharged from the hospital, successful transition to home depends on careful planning and liaison between hospital and community services. Rehabilitation in the hospital must be geared to the realities of the home circumstances. Because someone can cope with incontinence in the hospital, an environment with ready availability of products and assistance, this does not necessarily mean that the person can cope as well at home.

Unfortunately, there is often a lack of communication. Patients are frequently sent home with inadequate preparation and without their new caregiver(s) being fully informed about all their problems. Arrangements should be made in advance, particularly if home modifications are needed, and also for services such as nursing, laundry, or home help. Patients and families should be instructed in the hospital about how to use the products that will be needed in the home and where to purchase them in the community. The hospital nurse should teach patients and caregivers how to cope with problems like skin care and should give advice on practical management at home. To do this effectively, the hospital nurse must be fully aware of the difficulties that are likely to be encountered in the home.

Self-Care

Those with limited ability to carry out self-care are vulnerable at home. Many bowel problems are a result of constipation from a poor diet, which could be caused by the high cost of fresh foods, the inability to shop or cook, or the lack of motivation to prepare meals, especially for someone living alone. People who receive Meals on Wheels might find the food to be unpalatable or cold—for example, some meals are delivered too early, when the recipient does not feel like eating. Some people cannot even make themselves a drink, and they become dehydrated at home. This aggravates any bowel or bladder problems and can, in extreme cases, lead to a confusional state.

Personal hygiene can be a problem for some people at home. Incontinent persons need to be especially scrupulous in avoiding skin problems and odor. If they cannot manage effectively, they might depend on home caregivers for their personal hygiene.

Caregivers at Home

In a hopsital, however short of staff, there is always someone around 24 hours a day. This means that it should be possible to gear toileting times to an individual's requirements, which is crucial if help is needed in getting to or onto the toilet or in using a urinal. Someone who is not self-sufficient in toileting depends on others. The availability of help at the required time often determines whether incontinence occurs. Once wet, those with impaired physical or mental function may be unable to deal with the consequences independently and are forced to stay wet until help arrives. Dependence on others ranges from needing a verbal reminder that it is time to visit the toilet to help in rising from a chair to being transported to and lifted onto the toilet.

Some people with total incontinence might live alone or might live with someone who is just as (or even more) forgetful or frail. Many more are alone for at least part of the day. If dependence is total and the bladder unpredictable (as might be the case for someone with urge incontinence), continence is improbable without constant attendance. If incontinence does occur, the longer the interval between wetting and changing, the greater the likelihood of discomfort, skin problems, and odor. Some disabled people are incontinent, even if their bladder function is normal, simply because no one is available to help them. Many home care nurses come across people living alone who are almost helpless between visits by home care personnel. Few bladders can hold urine for 12 hours or longer, and sooner or later incontinence is inevitable. Sometimes it is possible, with forethought and planning, to organize a system to help the person use the toilet at intervals throughout the day (e.g., by spacing out the visits of such people as the visiting nurse, home help, and good neighbor). This is, however, unrealistic for many people. Men can manage with a hand-held urinal (Chap. 9), but many women cannot manage this alone. Every effort should be made to avoid the degrading situation in which an individual is forced to pass urine onto the bed or chair because no other help is available.

Even when someone is available, it is not always easy to transfer a disabled person onto the toilet. In the hospital, two nurses might manage easily, but a frail spouse might be unable to cope. Clear instructions can help a caregiver learn proper lifting techniques, and the nurse must ensure that faulty methods do not put the caregiver at risk for injury or disability. Often, co-ordinated equipment facilitates transfer—for example, a bed, commode, and wheelchair all at the same height, with detachable arms for sideways transfer, or an electric hoist, if appropriate. Strategically placed toilet substitutes, such as commodes, over-the-toilet commodes, or portable toilets, can be helpful if toilets are not close by. Urinals, bedpans, or external collection devices can be helpful for others (Brink and Wells, 1986).

Sometimes the help that is available is unacceptable, either to the patient or caregiver. Many elderly people are embarrassed if their spouse aids them with toileting, especially with assisting in the more intimate tasks of cleansing and washing. They might be ashamed of wet or soiled underwear being seen and prefer not to seek or accept help, even when needed. If children and aged parents are of the opposite sex, considerable reluctance is common, and many middle-aged people do not wish to see their parents naked. Never assume that, because a relative is willing to provide care, the relative will also be at ease with all the tasks this entails. An adult child who will readily feed, wash, and provide general care for an elderly parent might draw the line at cleaning up stool and urine.

It should never be forgotten just how disruptive incontinence can be in the home. A caregiver who will tolerate much inconvenience and hard work might find that incontinence is the "straw that breaks the camel's back."

Certain treatments for incontinence can be impossible to implement if no one is available to help. Bladder training can be particularly difficult. It is no use working out ideal toileting times for someone who is dependent and alone. No amount of medication or training can postpone micturition indefinitely. An alarm clock can be useful for the forgetful, but it must be responded to appropriately and then reset for the next interval after use. Many people who are forgetful about toilet visits cannot be expected to reset an alarm reliably. A 24-hour alarm system is needed that can be preset for variable intervals (e.g., by the nurse), with no need for the patient to reset it. Those who are hard of hearing might benefit from a vibrating or visual alarm system, but no such system is now available. This is not to suggest that bladder training is impossible for the disabled or forgetful at home (McCormick and Burgio, 1984). Many people have devised systems to help maintain continence, some involving neighbors or ingenious homemade devices.

The role of the family caring for a person with total incontinence in the home is crucial. For example, public assistance could be improved. Frequently those who appear to be coping well are left alone when they could actually use more help, both supportively and practically. Sometimes those in private voluntary organizations (e.g., National Multiple Sclerosis Society, National Spinal Cord Injury Association, or various locally run programs) can fill this need better than government agencies do. More could be done to ensure that home care continues, and possibly more people could be cared for at home. The development of support groups for caregivers, and more relief or holiday respite being provided, would do much to ease the burden.

The Home Environment

The home surroundings can present problems for two reasons: because incontinence is resulting in soiling the home or because the surroundings are not conducive to continence.

Most people are "house proud," at least to some extent. There can be little doubt that uncontrolled incontinence will ruin any home. Soiling of chairs, carpets, and beds, with the associated smell, can soon render a home unpleasant. Unlike institutions, few homes are planned with ease of cleaning in mind. Furniture and carpets are difficult or expensive to clean, and it might be impossible to eliminate a lingering odor. Waterproof covers for cushions and mattresses might help, but few people want to live on plastic chairs and linoleum. A visitor sitting on a wet chair inadvertently can create an embarrassing situation. Odor is often apparent and difficult to eradicate. It can be reduced by prompt cleaning after an episode of incontinence and by keeping soiled products and linens in airtight containers. Various deodorant products can help to reduce environmental odors.

Some homes make continence difficult for the elderly or disabled. The toilet might be inaccessible because of location or size. Ideally there should be a toilet on each level in a house, but this is seldom the case. Many modifications can be made, and public assistance funds might be available to help with the expense (Chap. 9).

Community Services

Community services might be available to help those who are incontinent at home. People are most likely to obtain these services if they have another disability or have been hospitalized at some point. Those who gradually become incontinent in their own homes, however, are less likely to seek or receive assistance.

The visiting nurse will be a key person in assessing individual needs, mobilizing resources, and making referrals for further help. The general practitioner should also be involved, but some are not motivated or interested and regard incontinence as a nursing problem. Some community services can provide skilled nursing care and nursing assistants for those with difficulties in personal hygiene, and, in some instances, can help provide attendant care. Home care nurses can advise patients and caregivers and teach methods of management or suggest sources of help. Visiting nurses can also be responsible for ordering incontinence products.

A social worker might also help provide advice on obtaining funds for home modification and other financial assistance. Physical therapists may help with mobility and advise on correct lifting and transferring techniques. Occupational therapists may assess self-care skills and improve these with instruction or equipment. The podiatrist or optician can help a person to cope independently by improving walking and vision. A co-ordinated effort by the home care team is often crucial in assisting the individual so that independence at home can be maintained.

Some day care centers provide assistance to incontinent individuals. This can be enhanced by training the staff about dealing with incontinence. Some centers, however, will not admit incontinent people. Keeping up the incontinent person's motivation and outside interests is vital in promoting continence. People need a reason to make the effort to be dry, and if they have have no outside contacts, apathy easily sets in.

Volunteers can provide practical help and emotional support. Many self-help organizations for those with a particular illness or disability act as powerful lobbying groups by demanding better services and providing help to their members.

Laundry and Disposal Problems

Laundry

Most incontinent people can, with a good appliance or absorbent product, minimize the amount of additional laundry. Some of those with severe incontinence who cannot afford good products suffer a considerable burden of extra washing. Nurses in the hospital, where soiled items disappear in a hamper or down a chute and reappear as if by magic on a linen cart, often give little thought to how a frail person with limited resources can manage at home. Even one change of clothing or sheets each day can be a problem. If incontinence is occurring often every day, the volume of laundry can be enormous.

Many incontinent people do not have adequate laundry facilities. Some do not even have a decent-sized sink, hot water, or access to a washing machine or clothes dryer. In some cases the home is literally taken over by the volume of soiled or drying linen. If only one sink is available, it is not hygienic to wash soiled laundry in the same place as food and dishes. Those with arthritic hands cannot wring out linens effectively, and the weak might not be able to wash efficiently and remove all trace of soiling, so that unpleasant odors could result.

Large quantities of clothes and sheets are needed if washing is not to become an almost continuous task. Repeated laundering shortens the life of linen. Replacement costs money and might be impossible for those with limited income. Hot water, detergent, electricity, and laundromat costs can also be a burden.

As the use of good-quality disposable products increases and as supply problems are overcome (Chap. 13), the chore of doing extra laundry will be lessened. This will enable more of those severely affected by incontinence to remain in their own homes rather than going into institutional care.

Disposal

If large numbers of briefs or pads are used, disposal can be a problem because of the sheer volume involved. Most people simply wrap used briefs or pads in newspapers or plastic bags and put them in the trash can, which can easily be filled within a week. Those who live in high-rise apartments with communal trash chutes or containers can experience difficulties. Bags can break open. Domestic animals scavenging in trash containers can distribute used incontinence products over public areas, leading to embarrassing questions as to where they came from.

Disposal is even more of a problem for incontinent people outside the home. Few male public rest rooms have disposal facilities, and even those for women, with sanitary napkin containers, seldom have a receptacle for larger products. When visiting friends or relatives it can be awkward to dispose of used products. If someone is staying away from home for several days it often becomes impossible to disguise the problem. Many incontinent people, whether out for the day or at work, have to wrap up their soiled products and take them home. This necessitates taking a large bag everywhere and worrying that an odor will be detected. Toilets for the disabled should have disposal bins for absorbent products available (although not all do). Able-bodied people might not be able to use these facilities without risking public disapproval.

With careful assessment of individual needs and proper planning of services and resources, most incontinent people can be cared for in the community. Indeed, some of those who are currently in institutional care might be enabled to live at home if services were improved. The nurse's aim must be to ensure that incontinent people do not have their lives dominated by their condition and do not lose their independence because of it.

ACUTE AND EXTENDED CARE

Institutions vary greatly in their approaches to incontinence, and it is difficult to make generalizations. Some offer excellent management and are geared to the promotion of continence, whereas other programs are less imaginative and allow patients or residents minimal opportunity to become or remain continent. A few common problems are presented in this section.

Acute Care

Much incontinence occurs in acute rather than in extended care settings. It often starts on an acute care unit and becomes the reason for transfer to an extended care facility rather than return to the community.

In acute care hospitals, priority is given to the care of life-threatening conditions. Dressings, intravenous infusions, and the administration of injections usually take precedence over toileting. With the increased use of the nursing process and individualized care plans, it is now easier to identify a patient's needs, but maintenance of continence needs to be given a much higher priority than it now receives. Most people would prefer to be taken to the toilet promptly when they ask and then have their bed made or lunch served on time. Nurses must learn to identify patients who are "at risk" of becoming incontinent in the hospital (e.g., those who are immobile, confused, or depressed and those on diuretics) and to take appropriate preventive action. If incontinence does occur, the nurse must find out the reason for it and plan care around treating the problem. Often the patient will be more disabled in the long run, not by the cause of the hospital admission (e.g., a fractured femur), but because incontinence was allowed to develop in the hospital.

There is a great temptation to use an indwelling catheter to manage incontinence in an acute setting—to protect a wound, minimize infection, or monitor urine output. This should be resisted unless there is a genuine need for a catheter (Chap. 15). Patients are often sent home with their catheter still in place when it has outlived its usefulness.

When a patient is in the hospital for rehabilitation, the success or failure of the rehabilitation program is often determined by whether incontinence can be brought under control, either by cure or appropriate containment. All members of the rehabilitation team should be involved in trying to restore the individual to continence: the nurse, by planning bladder training and creating a positive environment, possibly involving reality orientation or behavior modification (Chap. 8); the physical therapist, by mobilizing the patient; the occupational therapist, by improving dexterity and assessing which devices would be most helpful; the social worker, by arranging any necessary adaptations to the home; and the physician, by the appropriate use of diagnostic testing, medications, or both. Continence is everyone's responsibility, but it is usually the nurse who coordinates these efforts.

Extended Care

Individual Assessment

The importance of individual assessment of the patient or resident cannot be overemphasized. Many studies have found that multiple problems usually contribute to incontinence for each person, but that each has a unique combination of factors needing attention (Lepine and associates, 1979; King, 1979, 1980). Untreated medical conditions, drug side effects, constipation, urinary tract infection, immobility, depression, disorientation, and various other problems might be implicated (Chaps. 2 and 3 discuss the causes and assessment of incontinence). Until it has been established why each person is incontinent, any attempt at remedy is unlikely to be effective. Although this individual assessment is initially time-consuming, the long-term benefits are great, both in terms of the patient's dignity and more rewarding nursing management.

The Environment

Some extended care institutions are designed to meet the needs of the elderly or disabled. Suitably designed facilities can make continence easier, with plenty of accessible toilets within a short distance of beds and day rooms. Floors should be nonslip and easy to clean. Corridors need to be well lit. Signs and symbols should be legible and meaningful. Chairs and beds should be designed for ease of rising. The toilet area should be warm, clean, and private, with grab rails in reach.

Unfortunately, even some specially designed facilities do not meet all these criteria and many facilities are not specifically designed but are adapted from older buildings originally used for other purposes. Nurses are often "too good" at coping and "making do" in unsatisfactory environments. Wells and Brink (1980) have found that nurses tend to be uncritical of the toileting facilities provided, being more likely to adopt local routines rather than complaining or finding out how the situation might be improved. Residential homes may have been converted from large private houses with narrow corridors and many flights of stairs. This is not to say that these houses cannot be successfully modified, but a great deal of thought, planning, and money must be put into them if the renovation is to cater successfully to the needs of people with incontinence (Chap. 9).

It is possible for environmental factors to encourage incontinence, especially in those who are confused. It has been observed that if the institutional setting closely resembles a "normal" home environment, incontinence levels drop. Indeed, moving a group of patients from a hospital unit to an extended care facility, with more home comforts and an emphasis on reality orientation and personal responsibility, can dramatically reduce incontinence levels (Storrs, 1980).

Much can be done to transform an unsatisfactory environment. Nurses should become involved in planning, especially of new facilities, and should demand necessary alterations if conditions are poor. It is easy to put up with things and make do. In the long run this benefits no one.

The Staff

Institutions involved in the long-term care of incontinent people often have staffing problems. The work can be difficult and unpleasant and easily become a never-ending routine of changing, washing, and cleaning up, day after day. It can be difficult to attract staff, especially of a high caliber, and even more difficult to keep them. Staff turnover and sickness rates are often high and morale low. Staffing levels might fall below the numbers funded. In some hospitals it is regarded as a punishment or sign of disfavor to be sent to a unit where there are people with high levels of incontinence. In all facilities there tends to be a large percentage of untrained or unqualified staff members who, having had little training about incontinence, tend to accept it as inevitable.

Staff attitudes are an important factor in incontinence (Yu and Kaltreider, 1987). Even some trained staff have minimal knowledge about incontinence (Wells and Brink, 1980). It is easy, once working with incontinent people, to become so engrossed in the constant tasks of cleaning up that the reason for the basic problem is never questioned. It becomes accepted as inevitable, and once it is accepted, residents may never be given the opportunity to be continent. Routines become geared to mopping up rather than to promoting continence (Ramsbottom, 1980). It is common for management methods to make it impossible for the individual to be anything but incontinent. Once privacy and dignity have been lost, incontinence often becomes the norm.

Nobody likes cleaning up after incontinence. It is easy to see why staff members develop routines that attempt to make incontinence more tolerable. Making rounds with a cart of clean diapers and gowns and changing everyone in turn gets the job over with quickly and efficiently. To change people in a communal room, in public view while talking to them as if they were infants, must mean that those on staff are dissociated from the reality of another adult's dignity. The old, the demented, and the disabled are frequently dehumanized because of their incontinence. The nurse must always strive to devise methods of care that maximize the potential for continence. If this fails, incontinence must be managed with sensitivity. The first step toward achieving this humane approach should be to change the staff's attitudes about incontinence (e.g., with education and sensitivity training).

The Resident

Why do people who were continent at home start wetting soon after admission to an extended care facility? The reason might simply be the physical cause for admission, such as a stroke, immobility, or other disease. Sometimes the change of environment can be the cause—taken away from their usual surroundings and methods of coping, they may be too shy or embarrassed to ask for help or to mention that they always keep a commode by their bed at night. Disorientation or not knowing the proper words to use to ask for help can lead to incontinence. People might find the staff threatening or unhelpful and become unwilling to ask for assistance.

If the admission is for permanent care, it is not unusual for a person to become depressed. This can be mistaken for "settling down" and adapting to the routine. The resident who sits quietly in a chair and makes no demands can make life easy for staff, but depression as the reason for this behavior is often missed. Apathy can soon follow depression, and incontinence can result. Why bother, if everyone else is incontinent and it seems to be expected? With the loss of independence in all the tasks of daily life, some people regress to the point where everything has to be done for them; they cannot take responsibility for any aspect of life, including elimination.

Other factors can compound the problem. Lack of stimulus or motivation to keep active can lead to immobility. Arthritic joints stiffen and independent walking becomes impossible. It therefore takes longer to get to the toilet and help is needed. Immobility often leads to constipation, which in turn aggravates urinary or fecal incontinence. Immobility can also aggravate fluid stasis in the lower extremities, which might then be treated with diuretics.

Once incontinence has become established, people affected by it and those around them assume that nothing can be done, and accept it as inevitable.

Toileting Routines

It is common for extended care facilities to develop rigid toileting or changing routines. This usually involves toileting or changing (usually both) all residents at set times. This can be before or after meals and snacks or at a time that fits conveniently into the general routine. Such practices often go on year after year, regardless of whether they have any beneficial effect. Usually no record or chart is kept and the mindless routine is never changed.

This obviously does not fit with the concept of individualized patient care or a therapeutic regime. Although residents of institutions lead regular lives, with regular fluid intake and activities, and are likely to need toilet facilities at predictable times each day, these times are different for each person. One might always need to pass urine half an hour after a cup of tea, but another might need to go 2 hours later. Trying to toilet everyone at the same time means that some will not need to go and for others it will be too late. It can create problems if not enough toilets are available, placing pressure on staff. If task allocation persists, it is often the unfortunate newcomer who is assigned the job of toileting a large number of people in a short time and having them all ready for lunch. Under such circumstances, people are bound to feel hurried (and thus inhibited from bladder emptying). Privacy is difficult if there is a line outside the door.

In many institutions and extended care facilities, all incontinent people are treated identically by putting them on a toileting program. This involves taking them to the toilet at preset intervals (e.g., every 2 or 4 hours). It has the advantage of being easy to remember, so that staff members find compliance simple. It keeps a proportion of people dry by emptying their bladders before they really need to, but it does nothing to diagnose the cause of the incontinence or to retrain the bladder or patient. Rigid regimens such as these are best reserved for those people, usually only the very demented, for whom all efforts at retraining have failed and whose incontinence is intractable. It seldom applies to all patients in one location. If a rigid regimen is used, a chart should be kept to monitor the success (or failure) of the chosen interval.

For a retraining program to be successful, toileting times will have to suit individual needs. (Chapter 4 describes bladder training for the mentally alert; care of the elderly mentally impaired is discussed in Chapter 8.)

The success of bladder training depends on correct patient selection and diagnosis. It is pointless to try to "retrain" someone with stress or overflow incontinence; no amount of toileting can keep them totally dry. Bladder training is most suitable for those who are mentally alert, with urgency and frequency, and for those who are mildly to moderately confused who void wherever they are when they feel the urge. If the incontinence of a dependent patient has been caused by environmental factors, including a low staff level, it is more appropriate to retrain the staff to respond to the individual's needs and to recognize their most suitable toileting times than to train the patient's bladder. Offering toilet facilities when they are needed should be seen as part of basic nursing care and as a right for all patients. The term "training" should more properly be used in regard to efforts to change voiding intervals and increase independence.

Much of what has been said elsewhere in this book applies equally to people at home or in an institution, so this chapter should not be read in isolation. In practice, many settings are well designed, and those who care for incontinent people are doing all they can to promote continence and manage incontinence. There are many programs, services, and facilities available. Information and resources need to be more widely disseminated until standards of excellence exist in all settings.

References and Further Reading

Brink, C.A., and Wells, T.J.: Environmental support for geriatric incontinence: Toilets, toilet supplements and external equipment. Clin. Geriatr. Med., *2*:829, 1986.

Jirovec, M.M., Brink, C.A., and Wells, T.J.: Nursing assessments in the inpatient geriatric population. Nurs. Clin. North Am., *23*:219, 1988.

King, M.R.: A study on incontinence in a psychiatric hospital. Nurs. Times, *75*:1133, 1979.

King, M.R.: Treatment of incontinence. Nurs. Times, *76*:1006, 1980.

Lepine, A., Renault, R.K., and Stewart, I.D.: The incidence and management of incontinence in a home for the elderly. Health Social Serv. J., *89*:E9, 1979.

McCormick, K.A., and Burgio, K.L.: Incontinence: An update on nursing care measures. J. Gerontol. Nurs., *10*:16, 1984.

Mitteness, L.S.: The management of urinary incontinence by community-living elderly. Gerontologist, *27*:185, 1987.

Noelker, L.S.: Incontinence in elderly cared for by family. Gerontologist, *27*:194, 1987.

Ramsbottom, F.J.: Toileting and Changing Elderly Patients in Hospital. Birmingham, England, Department of Geriatric Medicine, University of Birmingham, 1980.

Storrs, A.: What is care? Br. J. Geriatr. Nurs., *4*:12, 1980.

Wells, T.J.: Problems in Geriatric Nursing Care. New York, Churchill Livingstone, 1980.

Wells, T.J., and Brink, C.A.: Promoting urine control in older adults. Helpful equipment (pictorial). Part 6. Geriatr. Nurs., Nov/Dec *1*:264, 1980.

Yu, L., and Kaltreider, D.: Stressed nurses dealing with incontinent patients. J. Gerontol. Nurs., *13*:27, 1987.

Nancy Faller, BSN, CETN

12 Toilet Training People with Mental Retardation

Most people with mental retardation, whatever their degree of impairment, have the potential to attain some degree of continence. Usually incontinence represents a failure to learn the skills necessary for continence. With some it might be related to performance (behavior) problems. In both cases it should never be accepted as inevitable until a serious attempt at toilet training has been made.

Some people suffer a coexistent physical handicap with mental retardation and might also have a neurologic problem. For such people it is always advisable to investigate bladder-sphincter function prior to initiation of a program. Training will not be effective if there is severe underlying voiding dysfunction. Similarly, any program for an individual who is so physically disabled that independence and self-help are precluded will have to be modified accordingly. Particular problems of the physically disabled and neurogenic voiding difficulties are discussed in Chapters 9 and 10.

Incontinence can be one of the most socially restricting aspects for people with mental retardation. It can rule out participation in otherwise feasible activities. If the person lives with relatives, incontinence is often a major burden of care. Furniture or carpets can become stained or the home can become impregnated with the smell of urine. Family members might have to restrict their social activities. In addition, the burden of laundry, especially for an older child or adult, can be overwhelming. The economic impact of incontinence has been outlined by Hu (1986). For people with mental retardation, this includes the expense of laundry, containment products, new furniture and carpets, and clothing and bedding worn out by excessive washing. As the individual grows, so can the problem, until it might become the reason for breakdown of family care (or breakdown of the parents' relationship). Additionally, it can precipitate requests for temporary or permanent placement away from home.

If the person with mental retardation requires a home away from the family, incontinence can be the deciding factor in placement. Many foster homes and community-based residential facilities will not accept a person with severe incontinence. Those with self-help skills, who are capable of some degree of independent living in all other respects, might be forced to live in an institution because of incontinence. Institutions that provide long-term care for people with mental retardation often have the highest levels of incontinence encountered in any setting. Current policy aims at a considerable reduction in the number of institutional beds for those with mental retardation and at placing as many as possible in a community setting. This means that attaining continence has become one of the most important aims in rehabilitation. Some people with mental retardation, who were incontinent of both urine and stool while in an institution, become continent when moved to a more homelike environment in a community setting (e.g., a group home).

Wherever people with mental retardation live, incontinence is likely to cause considerable problems. Thankfully, this is not inevitable, and it is increasingly being realized how much can be done in all settings. In the community, mental health agencies or school districts have or are setting up treatment teams to support clients, either in their own homes or in residential facilities. In institutions, attitudes are changing from a focus of providing custodial care to one of instituting more positive therapeutic interventions. These are aimed at maximizing each individual's potential, whether to enable eventual community placement or to improve their quality of life in the institution.

As with most skills, teaching the person with mental retardation to be continent is more likely to be successful if it can be started early. The ideal time to start training is probably around the second birthday, the age at which most children are toilet trained. (Some training can start as early as 15 to 18 months—for example, getting the child used to sitting on the potty.) This is usually part of a larger program aimed at achieving independence in activities of daily living. If training has not been started early, however, this by no means indicates that the chance has been lost. A high degree of success can be achieved with older children, adolescents, and adults who have either missed out on or failed with training earlier in life.

Toilet training people with mental retardation is not simple or easy. It should never be started lightly, without consideration of the full implications. All those connected with the individual's care must be enthusiastic and willing to cooperate and work together as a team. Ideally the program should be supervised by a professional, trained in working with this population and experienced in using behavior modification and operant conditioning techniques, (e.g., nurse, psychologist). Many behavioral consultants and special education teachers have extensive instruction in such techniques. Without such support, whether in an institution or the community, any toilet-training program will be difficult to implement and will stand less chance of success. It is probably best if those inexperienced in these methods request support and supervision when starting a program. The additional work and effort involved can rapidly lead to frustration and disillusionment.

TRAINING METHODS

The ideal aim of toilet training is independent toileting and continence, but this might not be realistic for all individuals. Certainly there are so many factors involved that it is usually best to break down the skills required into a series of intermediate target steps or behaviors, which can be worked on separately or in combination. One method of dividing the steps has been devised by Tierney (1973) (Table 12–1). The ultimate goal is to achieve the top final target behavior in all four columns. Progress is indicated by ascending any of the columns from the base target behavior, through intermediate targets, toward the final target. An end point might have to be accepted that is short of the top in one or more of the goals, depending on a realistic assessment of the individual's mental and physical abilities.

Most programs are based on theories of behavior modification. The underlying principle is that behaviors that result in pleasant consequences are reinforced, tend to continue, and become an established element of the individual's behavioral repertoire. Behaviors that result in neutral or adverse consequences are not reinforced and tend to be discontinued, or extinguished. By close observation and careful planning, a program can be worked out to shape the desired behavior gradually by using appropriate reinforcers until a carefully defined target behavior has been attained.

Table 12–1. MODEL FOR SHAPING TOILETING BEHAVIOR

Final target behavior	Patient goes to toilet independently	Patient removes clothing independently	Patient sits down on toilet independently	Patient eliminates only in toilet and is otherwise continent
Intermediate target behavior	Patient asks to go to toilet	Patient removes or actively attempts to remove some clothing	Patient is helped to sit down on toilet and sits unrestrained	Patient eliminates in toilet regularly and has only infrequent episodes of incontinence
	Patient indicates need to use toilet	Patient actively assists when clothing is removed by nurse	Patient is placed on toilet and sits unrestrained	Patient has established some regularity and uses toilet more frequently than is incontinent
Base target	Patient is taken to toilet by nurse	Patient cooperates passively when clothing is removed by nurse	Patient is placed on toilet and is restrained to sit	Patient uses toilet when placed on it, but is incontinent at all other times

From Tierney, A. J.: Toilet training. Nurs. Times, *69*:1740, 1973.

Many different training methods have been used for people with mental retardation, and most achieve a reasonable degree of success. The program must be acceptable to and understood by all those who will carry it out, whether family, staff, or other caregivers. The main differences between approaches are in the timing of toileting and the use of reinforcers. In residential settings there is also the issue of whether people should be trained individually or in groups. Probably the most successful method is individualized, intensive training using regular-interval timed toileting and mild correction for incontinence (Smith, 1979). Whichever method is chosen, the most crucial factor in success is a consistent approach to training—that is, having everyone involved with the person approach the training in an identical manner throughout the training period.

Intensive training involves a great commitment on the part of the trainer and initially can be time-consuming. A method found to be successful in the hospital has been outlined by Smith (1979) (Table 12–2). It uses regular-interval timed toileting (rather than using scheduled times, when incontinence has been found to occur). This regular-interval training has usually been found to be simpler to carry out than toilet training based on the individual's own natural bladder functioning.

The use of punishment in training is controversial. Many early studies used punishment or "restitutional overcorrection" to eliminate undesired behaviors. Today this is usually seen as unethical, especially the use of physical punishment. It has also been found to be largely unnecessary and can be counterproductive if it produces a high level of anxiety, because this impedes learning. A reprimand or "time out"

Table 12–2. *GENERAL GUIDELINES FOR REGULAR-INTERVAL INTENSIVE TRAINING*

Training	Procedure
Bladder	Seat person close to toilet Prompt to toilet every half-hour Reinforce (i.e., reward) for using toilet Reinforce every 5 minutes for dry pants
Accident	Reprimand immediately and sharply when wet Feel wet pants for discrimination learning Do *not* change wet pants immediately Do *not* prompt to toilet "Time out from reinforcement" for 10 minutes
Independence	Fade prompts to toilet, physical → verbal → gestural (in this order) Stop prompts when self-initiated toiletings established Move gradually away from toilet

From Smith, P.: A comparison of different methods of training the mentally handicapped. Behav. Res. Ther., *17*:33, 1979.

from reinforcement or attention for a specified time interval, however, is commonly used in response to avoidable mistakes. This is most helpful if given consistently and promptly. Some training methods also require the individual to participate in rectifying the consequences of incontinence (e.g., changing the bed or clothes), and this has sometimes been found to facilitate learning (Barker, 1979).

Individual training is naturally used in the home. In residential settings a choice must be made between individual and group training. The former is much costlier in terms of staff time than the latter, in which one staff member might deal with a small group of patients, but individual training on a one-to-one basis usually requires less time to achieve continence and also tends to yield better results. Thus it could be more cost effective overall. If staffing levels are such that it is impossible to contemplate individual training, then training a small group (five or six) less intensively is a reasonable substitute.

BASELINE OBSERVATION

All toilet-training programs should start with a baseline observation period. This involves regular checks at predetermined intervals to ascertain whether the individual is wet or dry and careful recording of results. Close observation should be made of episodes of incontinence and of the preceding and consequent behaviors of both the person and caregiver.

Families or staff can develop styles of coping with and reacting to incontinence that could actually be eliciting the behavior. The most common mistake is to give a lot of attention and create a lot of activity when incontinence occurs and to almost ignore the person when dry or toileting. It is easy to see how this situation can arise. Incontinence is experienced as a nuisance, because if not dealt with promptly it can soil the environment and lead to odor. It is a natural reaction to hurry the incontinent person to the bathroom to clean up the mess. While washing and changing the person, most caregivers give at least some attention and contact, both physical and verbal. Even if the content of the verbal exchange is a rebuke, it constitutes attention. Some people with mental retardation tend to respond to any form of attention as if to a reward. In this case, it is the incontinence that is being rewarded. Conversely, dryness is seldom rewarded as consistently. When observing such a behavior pattern in caregivers it is important not to blame the parents or staff, who are probably very caring, but to point out tactfully that this kindness might be counterproductive and to suggest how the attention might be reversed to reinforce continence rather than incontinence.

Observation of the person can be helpful. Is any warning given of imminent voiding? Many people who are mentally retarded have no verbal skills, so that communication will usually be nonverbal, such as general agitation, getting up, or repetitive actions. Can the person discriminate between dryness and wetness? Again, this might be expressed by exhibiting agitation, wandering, pulling at clothing, or crying. Is the individual ever toileted, and, if so, is urine passed appropriately? How many other "paratoilet" skills does the individual already have? The abilities to walk, put on and remove clothing, sit upright unaided, wash hands, communicate simple needs verbally or nonverbally, and follow simple commands are all useful, although not essential. Sometimes specially adapted clothing can improve the potential for self-care.

During this baseline period it is also important to establish what constitutes reinforcement for each individual. Most people with mental retardation cannot conceptualize a distant (albeit worthwhile) reward once the goal has been achieved. Something must be found that acts as a reinforcer to behavior and that can be delivered immediately, simply, reliably, and frequently. This can be verbal (e.g., saying "well done" or giving a cheer). More often, nonverbal reinforcement can be better understood and appreciated. This can be anything from a smile, to a funny face, clap, pat, hug, or kiss. The reinforcer might be edible (e.g., a drink, sweet, or other food). Care should be taken with oral reinforcers, because the calories involved can lead to a weight problem and increased tooth decay. Similarly fluid intake might already be excessive (which will exacerbate incontinence). It has been found by caregivers that drinks act as pacifiers. This will not be harmful during training, because the greater the fluid intake, the more training opportunities will occur. Excessive frequency, however, once the person is trained, will be undesirable. Also, if drinks are used as reinforcers during training, they should be strictly reserved for the relevant purpose and not also given at indiscriminate times. Sometimes the reinforcer can be linked to the toilet itself (e.g., using a musical potty chair or setting up an apparatus that makes a noise when urine is passed onto it).

It should never be assumed that something will act as a reinforcer unless it has been proved that the individual will respond to it in some way. If the reinforcer selected is actually disliked or seen as neutral, it will not reinforce the desired behavior. A noise might be found frightening or a selected food disliked. Often a small reinforcement, such as a sweet, which can be easily kept in the trainer's pocket and delivered immediately, is the best choice. The effectiveness of reinforcers should be reviewed regularly, because the desire for a given reinforcer can reach the saturation point, so that it becomes ineffective. If this occurs, new reinforcers should be introduced.

To be selected as suitable for toilet training, the individual should be able to hold urine for at least 1 hour on some occasions and to respond to simple reinforcers. In addition, there should be someone, either a relative or professional, who is prepared to help carry out the program.

THE TRAINING PROGRAM

Most training programs take several weeks and sometimes several months to be effective. It is essential to keep accurate records throughout so that progress can be monitored and any necessary adjustments made (Woods and Guest, 1980). Records also provide feedback to help keep up the morale of all involved. This is probably the most crucial requisite for success—that the program be rigidly and consistently adhered to and not abandoned too soon. The community treatment team has an important supportive role in the home. Although the team members are not always able to carry out the training, they should be available to provide advice and encouragement and to help maintain caregiver motivation.

Once any target behavior has been achieved, prompts should gradually be withdrawn (e.g., from actually escorting the person to the lavatory to verbal and gestural prompts), so that the behavior becomes increasingly spontaneous and independent. This process is called fading. Reinforcers should also change from being continuous (one for every correct achievement) to intermittent, with a gradually decreasing frequency of delivery (termed "changes in reinforcement schedule").

Eventually the comfort and independence afforded by continence become rewarding enough in themselves to maintain the behavior for some individuals. Others need intermittent reinforcement and reminders to maintain continence after the program has ended. Some never achieve total continence and always need some help and reminders.

The introduction of toilet training in an institutional setting, if it has never been used before, often involves a considerable change in attitudes, particularly in the rethinking of nursing roles. This cannot be imposed from above or outside, because the staff must want to participate actively. At first it is often seen as a lot of extra work and pessimism about the outcome is common. It is usually best to introduce the idea through staff training. Sessions such as study days and seminars can be helpful. Toilet training should be started in those areas in which staff members express an interest or request a program. It is also a good idea to select those patients for training who the staff feel are appropriate and have a chance of attaining continence quickly. Pointing out the potential long-term benefits of reducing the proportion of time spent on toilet-related activities and a lighter workload can help generate enthusiasm for the project. All staff must understand the training procedures so that consistent responses are given by all members of the care team.

Some people with mental retardation exhibit other behavioral problems in addition to incontinence. It has been found that these often improve during a toilet-training program. As an additional benefit, levels of self-help skills and independence can increase. This is probably a result of the increased attention and stimulation offered within the learning environment afforded by toilet training.

Sometimes using a pants alarm (see Fig. 5–2) or toilet bowl alarm (Fig. 12–1) helps during the training. These devices enable caregivers to know immediately when incontinence or voiding has occurred and to take appropriate action promptly. The more closely the consequence is paired with the act, the stronger is the conditioning effect. Care

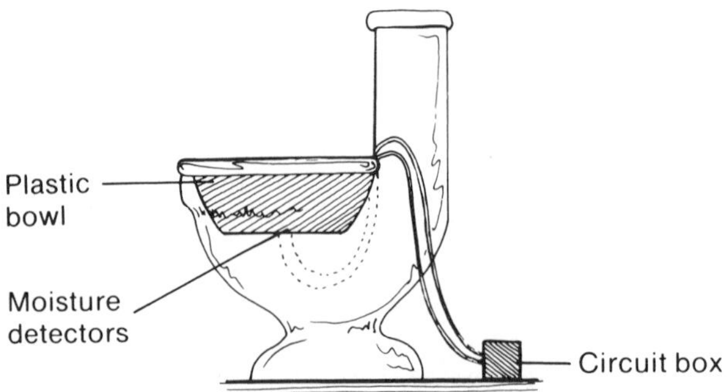

Figure 12–1. *Toilet bowl alarm.*

should be taken, however, that the individual does not respond paradoxically to alarms—that is, a few might enjoy hearing the pants alarm and wet intentionally to create the noise or, alternatively, might be frightened by the toilet alarm and withhold urine when on the toilet.

Nocturnal enuresis can be corrected by similar but obviously less intensive behavior modification programs. Dry beds should be rewarded and regular toileting encouraged at predetermined intervals. Participation in changing wet beds aids learning. An enuresis alarm can be effective if *well supervised* (Chap. 5) and used as part of a broader program.

CONTAINMENT

A minority of people with mental retardation are unresponsive to toilet training. Others live in situations, either at home or in an institution, in which training is not feasible. For such people an efficient method of containment is of paramount importance but often presents difficulties. Some might not tolerate appliances, and even pads and pants tend to be pulled at or removed. The problem of containment is even greater when the person with incontinence is an adult, who can empty a full bladder with considerable force.

Disposable or reusable absorbent products (Chap. 13) might be the best management for a mentally retarded adult who is totally incontinent and not amenable to training, but these tend to be expensive and could be out of reach financially. A good case of special need and priority often has to be made to procure supplies, but there can be little doubt that, if the provision of an expensive pad enables the individual to be cared for at home, it is a good use of resources on both humanitarian and financial grounds.

References and Further Reading

Barker, P.: Nocturnal enuresis: An experimental study involving two behavioral approaches. Int. J. Nurs. Stud., *16:*319, 1979.

Foxx, N.H., and Azrin, R.M.: Toilet Training the Retarded. Champaign, IL, Research Press, 1973.

Hu, T.: The economic impact of urinary incontinence: Clin. Geriatr. Med., *2:*673, 1986.

Sines, D.: Incontinence: Helping people with mental handicap. Nurs. Times, *79:*52, 1983.

Smith, P.S.: A comparison of different methods of toilet-training the mentally handicapped. Behav. Res. Ther., *17:*33, 1979.

Smith, P.S., and Smith, L.J.: Continence and Incontinence: Psychological Approaches to Development and Treatment. London, Croom Helm, 1987.

Tierney, A.J.: Toilet training. Nurs. Times, *69:*1740, 1973.

Tierney, A.J.: Toilet-training the mentally handicapped. Nursing, *1:*795, 1980.

Woods, P.A., and Guest, E.M.: Toilet-training the severely retarded: The importance of evaluation. Nurs. Times [Occas. Papers], *76:*53, 1980.

Katherine F. Jeter, EdD, ET

13 The Use of Incontinence Products

Even with the best nursing and medical care available, not all incontinent people can be cured completely. There will always be a minority whose problem persists despite all efforts. There will also be those who are too ill for therapy or who make an informed decision not to undergo recommended treatment. Some might be improved considerably, but still wish to use a product to give them confidence in public, and many need a temporary supply while awaiting or undergoing treatment.

A wide range of absorbent products and devices is available for incontinent people (App. I). These products make it possible to conceal and manage incontinence. By containing urine or stool they should enable the person to feel confident and socially acceptable.

SELECTION AND ASSESSMENT OF INCONTINENCE PRODUCTS

Criteria for Selection

People require and expect many different things from absorbent pads, garments, or collection devices. The ideal product should meet the following criteria:

1. It contains urine and stool completely and prevents leakage onto clothing, bedding, and furniture.
2. It is comfortable to wear and protects vulnerable skin from maceration, chafing, and pressure sores.
3. It is easy for the incontinent person to use. If this is not feasible because of physical or mental disability, it should be easy for a caregiver to use.
4. It disguises or contains odor.
5. It is inconspicuous under clothing, without bulk or noise.
6. It is easy to dispose of or clean, as required.
7. It is reasonably priced and readily available.

People have particular requirements depending on their age, sex, and lifestyle. Some like disposable products, whereas others prefer ones they can wash and reuse.

Formerly, many items were produced for incontinent people that were poorly designed, with little consideration given to the needs of the user. Pads were conceived merely as larger versions of babies' diapers or modifications of sanitary napkins. Today, considerably more thought is going into product design. Many companies realize that there is a vast market for adult incontinence products, particularly if those who now hide their problem can be persuaded to seek help.

Only recently has substantial investment been devoted to new product development, and the benefits of this are yet to come. Many items described in this chapter and depicted in Appendix I represent the results of the first wave of interest, and are likely to become outdated over the next few years.

There are many reasons why companies have taken so long to recognize the potential market represented by incontinence products. Incontinent people are difficult to identify for advertising and promotional purposes. There is little incentive to develop high-quality products if they do not sell. With increased professional interest and public discussion about incontinence, companies now foresee a profitable future for quality products.

A persistent problem has been the lack of clinical trials and technical quality control tests for almost all absorbent products and devices. It is impossible to tell how a product will perform without trying it. Some items that look and feel like they will be effective and comfortable might turn out to be hot, bulky, and of insufficient capacity. Other unlikely looking products might be the perfect solution for someone. It is imperative for nurses to become involved with clinical evaluations to familiarize themselves with the many excellent products appearing on the market.

Assessment

The key to the success or failure of a product lies in an accurate initial assessment of the patient's needs. No one product will suit everyone. Nurses must make their assessment with the person and range of available products in mind. It should never be forgotten that a patient's needs can change with time, so the assessment of suitability must be a continuing process and supply systems should be flexible enough to accommodate changes.

When assessing for an appropriate product, a number of factors are important in the decision-making process:

1. Patient considerations: sex; type of urine or fecal incontinence; ambulatory, bedfast, chairbound; physical limitations (e.g., arthritis, parkinsonism); financial status; living arrangements; proximity to retail outlet.

2. Product considerations: reliability; capacity; ease of application; disposability; affordability; comfort; safe to use; toll-free (800) telephone number provided?

The remainder of this chapter outlines broad categories of products. A more complete listing and illustrations of products and manufacturers are given in Appendix I.

ABSORBENT PRODUCTS

Adult Disposable Diapers

At least 30 manufacturers now produce disposable adult diapers, euphemistically termed "adult briefs" or "adult underpants" to lessen the stigma attached to their use. These terms were devised by the manufacturers, who have learned that most adults perceive wearing diapers to be embarrassing and degrading. Adult diapers might be necessary for a senile person who is totally incontinent of urine and stool. People who cannot be close to bathroom facilities for long periods of time, and who are completely incontinent, might prefer diapers. Disposable garments should fit snugly, be absorbent enough to contain a full void or continuous leakage for several hours, and have elastic gathers at the leg to prevent urine and loose stool from leaking onto outerwear and bed linens (Fig. 13–1). Several types are made with a superabsorbent polymer that gels fluid to prevent squeeze-out and buffers odor. "Superabsorbent" does not refer to more pulp or fluff material, but to an additive that absorbs many times its own weight.

Reusable diapers are made by several companies. Some are fitted or are of hourglass-shaped cotton. Others are simply rectangular. Some have a waterproof panel that eliminates the need for a waterproof pant.

When laundry facilities are convenient, extended care facilities and some individuals prefer reusable diapers and underpads, because they are less expensive than using disposable products and there is not the problem of where and how to dispose of pounds of wet and soiled disposable briefs. When making the choice between disposable and reusable products, laundry costs must be considered.

Reusable and disposable incontinence briefs are invaluable for selected patients, but are not without their disadvantages. Vigilant skin care must be practiced to avoid fungal infection and skin damage that predispose patients to pressure sores. According to Willington (1975) and Allman (1986), patients who are incontinent and immobile are at great risk for developing pressure sores.

Adult disposable diapers can cost as much as 85¢ each. Rarely is this reimbursed. A daily cost of $3.00 to $5.00 is prohibitive for many families. Often adult diapers are packaged in large cases of 50, which might be cumbersome for a frail elderly spouse or for someone without a car. Although they are termed "disposable," getting rid of adult diapers can be a real problem for those in certain living situations. Recently, several governmental and environmental agencies have turned their attention to the problems of waste management for medical supplies, including adult diapers.

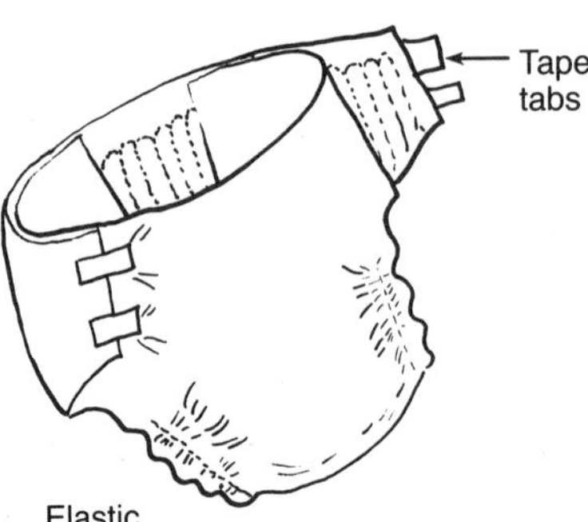

Figure 13–1. *Adult brief with elastic gathers at the leg.*

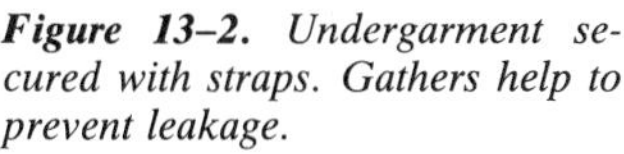

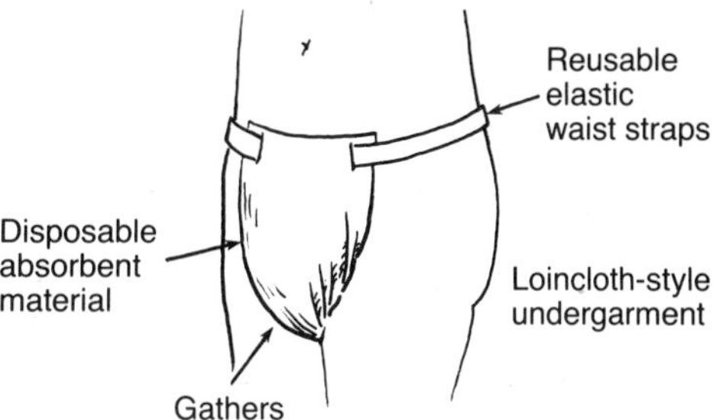

Figure 13–2. Undergarment secured with straps. Gathers help to prevent leakage.

Adult Undergarments

The term "adult undergarment" may have been coined by Kimberly-Clark to describe a loincloth-type absorbent product, called Depend, that is held in place by elastic straps. No outer pant or additional securement is required (Fig. 13–2). Several companies now make similar-style undergarments. Products of this design are particularly appealing to active people with moderate leakage. Patients and families should be told that this type of garment is rarely satisfactory for a heavy wetter and is usually ineffective for bedridden patients. Leakage usually occurs when the wearer is recumbent, because the garment does not fit snugly to the body.

Pants With Absorbent Inserts

Most people who need absorbent protection prefer a garment similar to their usual underwear. There are many pant-and-pad systems available. Some new pants are even made like men's fitted briefs and women's underpants to heighten their appeal (Fig. 13–3).

When the pant is waterproof, it is not necessary to have plastic

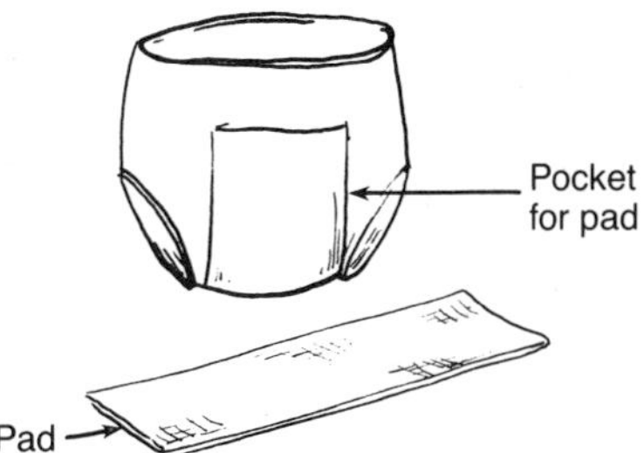

Figure 13–3. Pad and pant system. The pant is reusable; the pads can be disposable or reusable.

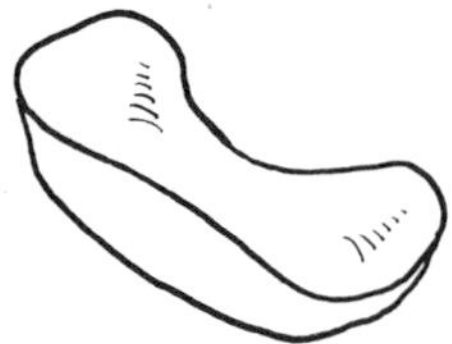

Figure 13–4. Contoured foam shell lined with superabsorbent (specifically for females).

backing on the absorbent pad. When the pad has a waterproof backing, a jersey, cotton, or mesh brief can be safely worn to hold the pad in place. Many new pads are made with superabsorbents.

Sanitary napkins have long been used by men and women to contain urine. In fact, some manufacturers believe that up to 10% of the sale of sanitary napkins is for urinary incontinence. This is unfortunate because they are only somewhat absorbent and do not help to control odor. There are a number of pads now on the market, specifically for urinary incontinence, that promise comfort and security against leakage and odor. One has been designed specifically for women and incorporates superabsorbents to prevent squeeze-out (Fig. 13–4). Some pads are contoured to fit the perineal area and buttocks and are particularly suitable for patients with large-volume urine loss and fecal incontinence (Fig. 13–5). These pads can be worn with regular underpants or stretch mesh briefs (Fig. 13–6).

Male Drip Collectors

Male drip collectors are handy for men with a small amount of urine leakage, but they require the penis to be long enough to fit into the pocket configuration (Fig. 13–7). Replacement drip collectors can

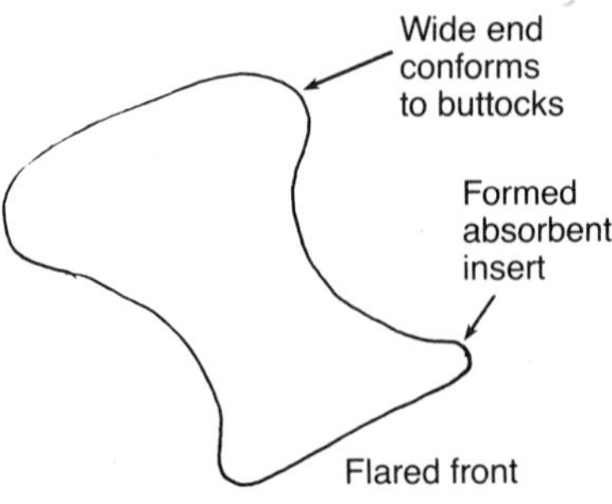

Figure 13–5. Contoured disposable pad ideal for patients with urinary and fecal incontinence. The flared front prevents the pad from slipping.

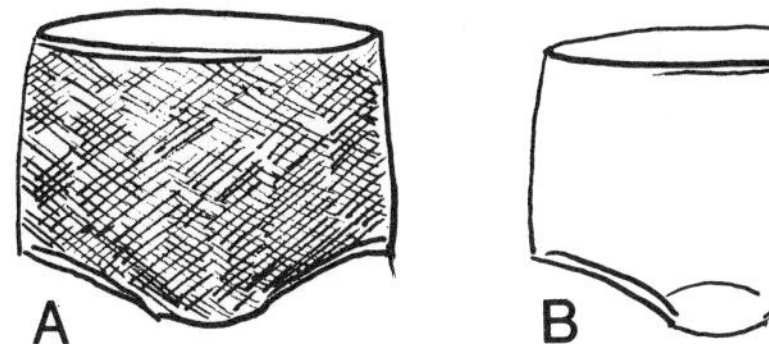

Figure 13–6. Stretch mesh briefs come in several sizes and are reusable. They are used to hold absorbent products snugly against the body. A, *Washable brief.* B, *Cotton or terry elastic (reusable).*

easily be tucked into a man's inside coat pocket or briefcase. Many men stain their underwear for a few days or weeks after a prostatectomy. A drip collector worn during this period can help spare them embarrassment. Some men have become conscious of a postvoid drip now that more men's briefs are constructed of nonabsorbent, single-layer fabrics. New styles in underwear, coupled with the fashion shift toward pastel and light-colored trousers, have increased the popularity of drip collectors. They are manufactured with superabsorbents and a waterproof backing. They are held in place with regular fitted undershorts, athletic supporters, or comfortable stretch mesh briefs.

Other pad-and-pant combinations are not male- or female-specific. Each manufacturer has incorporated certain desirable features: Gore-Tex pants for waterproof comfort, Velcro closures, adjustable legs and waist, and pads of varying lengths and absorbency. Patients need guidance in selecting these products, because they are expensive and rarely covered by insurance.

Few nurses realize how many excellent products are available. If nurses don't know, it is safe to assume that patients and the public are similarly uninformed. Furthermore, patients are reluctant to experiment with products that might look attractive and be effective because of their cost. When patients and families are helped to make a choice, the right absorbent product, regardless of price, will be cost-effective.

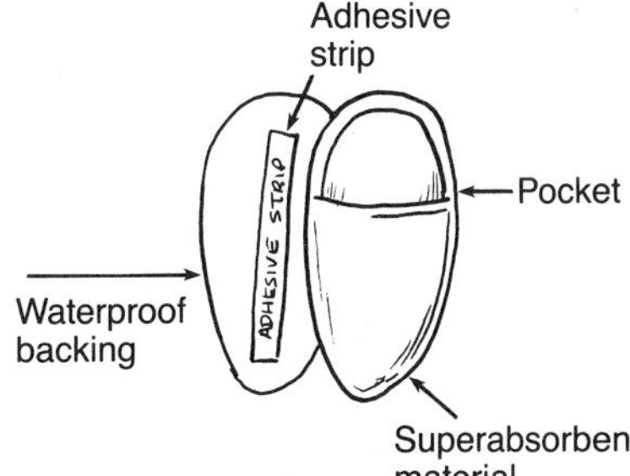

Figure 13–7. Drip collector fits over the penis. An adhesive strip holds the pad in a Jockey-style brief; the penis is inserted into the pocket. The pad is made of a superabsorbent material that gels fluid.

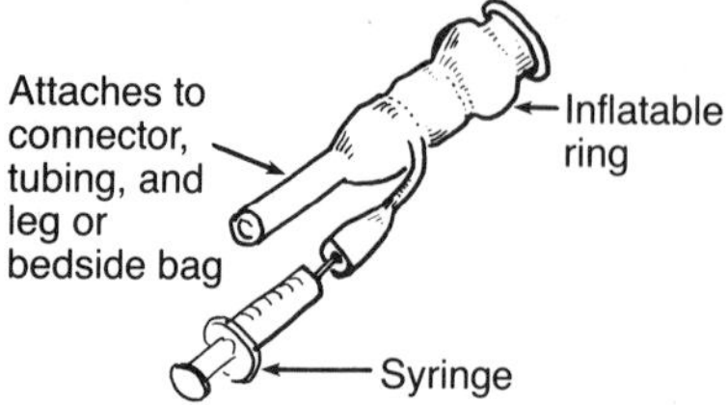

Figure 13–8. *Condom collector (for males). The syringe inserts air into the inflatable ring, which holds the condom catheter in place. The collector is made of latex, comes in various sizes, and can be reused, because it is held in place by the inflatable ring.*

COLLECTION DEVICES AND OTHER PRODUCTS

Condom Catheters for Men

Condom catheters might be the best solution for incontinent men who are not candidates for an artificial sphincter or other surgical procedure. The original "Texas catheter," which relied on an adhesive strap to hold it on, has been replaced by self-adhesive condom catheters, the sheath-and-liner concept, and one condom-style catheter that is held in place with an inflatable ring (Fig. 13–8). The most recent innovation for further versatility of a condom catheter is a removable tip that enables the wearer to perform intermittent catheterization without removing the entire sheath (Fig. 13–9).

The sizing of a condom catheter is extremely important. Most manufacturers furnish a sizing template to assist with the fitting. Institutions that try to make one size fit all are being penny-wise and pound foolish. There is much wastage with ill-fitting devices that do not remain in place.

Many elderly men have a retracted penis that cannot accommodate a condom catheter. A pouching system, much like an ostomy appliance, has been designed for men with a retracted penis (Fig. 13–10).

When external catheters are the product of choice, patients do best if they are "fitted" by a specialist in the hospital, clinic, urologist's office, or a home health store. Once the initial fitting and instruction have been accomplished, patients can order from the distributor that offers the best price and service. External catheters are covered by Medicare and Medicaid with a physician's prescription.

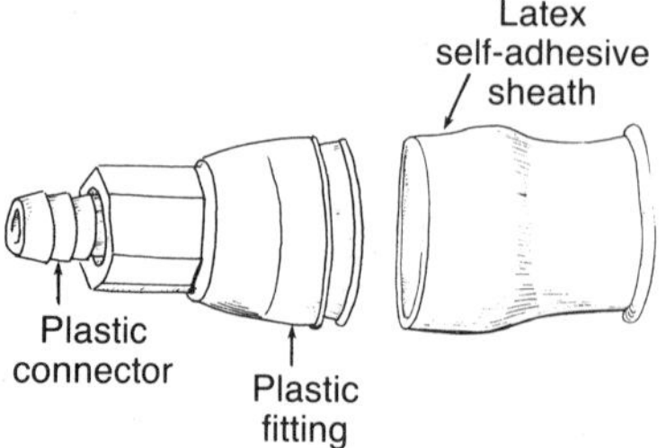

Figure 13–9. *Two-piece condom collector. It is designed for males to facilitate intermittent catheterization, but who leak in between, or it can be used for spontaneous voiding. The plastic secures the two pieces together with an easy twist.*

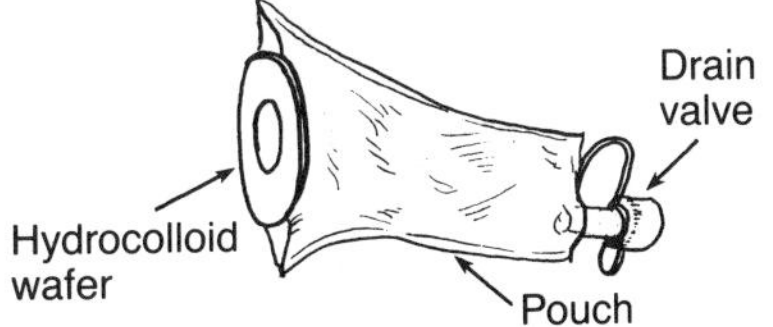

Figure 13–10. *Retracted penis pouch. The hydrocolloid wafer adheres to the skin, the pouch holds the urine, and the drain valve empties the urine into the toilet, or it can be connected to the leg or a bedside bag.*

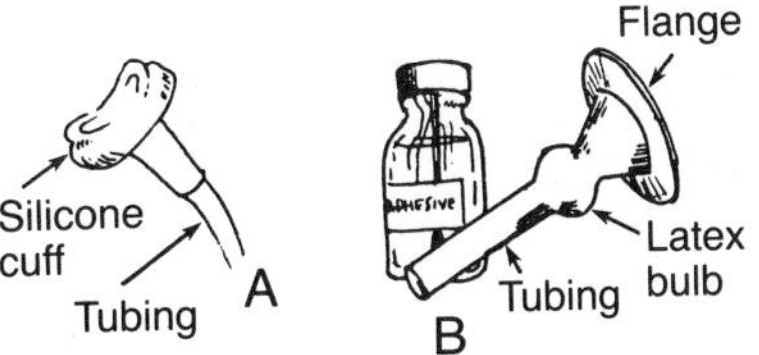

Figure 13–11. *Early external devices for females.* A, *Silicone cuff. This fits around the meatus by suction and glue; it is attached to the leg or a bedside bag by the tubing.* B, *Flange, with latex bulb and tubing. The flange adheres around the meatus with silicone adhesive, and is attached to the leg or a bedside bag by the tubing.*

Attitudes toward condom catheters differ. Many older men complain that the external catheter rolls off their penis or they cannot get it on in the first place. Some boys and young men prefer condom catheters, whereas others view them as a repugnant encumbrance on their genitals.

Collection Devices for Women

The quest for a satisfactory external collection device for women has been arduous and the solution elusive. Female astronauts are still launched and participate in extravehicular activity wearing a pad and a pant despite NASA's efforts to produce a satisfactory collecting system.

The earliest products for women were glue-on external devices (Fig. 13–11). Both have received mixed reviews, but they are satisfactory in selected cases.

Recently, an external device was designed that fits into the vagina and channels the urine from the urethra through a small hose into a leg bag (Fig. 13–12). Careful fitting and attention to detail in patient selection and application procedures are necessary for this device to be effective.

Accessories for External Collection Devices

Patients who use external collection devices should be provided with at least two leg bags and a bedside drainage receptacle that can

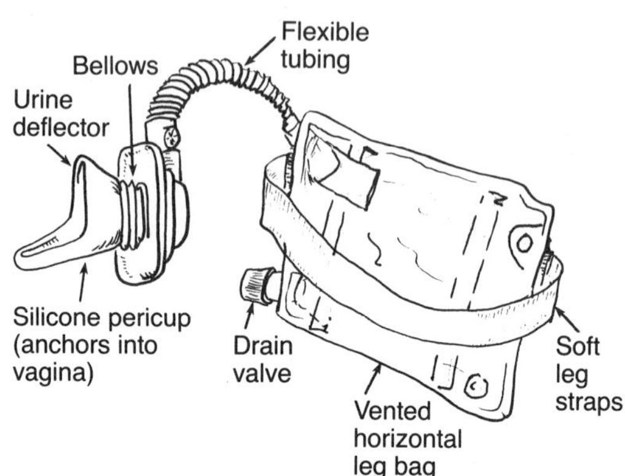

Figure 13–12. *External collection device for females. It is secured in the vagina and held in place by snug-fitting underpants. Urine drains into the vented leg bag. The bellows are available in two sizes to accommodate the distance between the distal labia and the periurethral floor.*

be washed and reused. The leg bag should be changed every 24 hours. The used bag should be cleaned with a solution of equal parts white vinegar and water or with a commercial decrystallizer. After soaking for 10 to 15 minutes, the decrystallizing solution should be drained and the leg bag hung to dry. The bedside drainage receptacle should be emptied each morning and cleaned in a similar manner. Hospital-style bedside bags are not easily cleaned and should not be given to patients for long-term use.

Wide soft straps should always replace the narrow rubber straps furnished with most leg bags. Some patients prefer their leg bag to be strapped around the ankle with an extender tube that allows them to empty the bag over a floor drain or onto the ground. This eliminates the need to take off outer clothing and can be helpful for people in braces or a wheelchair. Rehabilitation nurses and occupational therapists are particularly helpful in designing systems that provide maximum independence to persons with limited dexterity and mobility.

Skin Care Products

Skin care products are available that are formulated specifically for incontinent patients. They usually involve a three-step regime—a cleanser, moisturizing cream, and barrier. Incontinence cleansers allow for frequent washing of the skin without dehydrating it. The preferred creams vanish when rubbed in and do not accumulate to trap urine and stool. A cleanser and cream are usually sufficient to protect skin integrity, even when incontinence is continuous. When skin damage has already occurred, a barrier cream or film might also be needed to promote healing. Fungal rashes respond promptly to a prescription antifungal cream applied after the skin has been washed with an incontinence cleanser. Over-the-counter antifungal creams can be used to discourage fungal growth, but they are not the most effective products for treating these rashes when they occur.

Nursing homes often explain their lack of protective products as cost containment, labelling them "luxury items." One study in an acute care facility showed that total charges for treating patients with pressure sores were as high as $86,000, with a mean of $37,000 (Allman, 1986). A few hundred dollars spent in preventing skin breakdown can hardly be considered "frills." It is possible to maintain most frail elderly incontinent patients in diapers, without irritation or pressure sores, with meticulous skin care using the proper products. Specialty incontinence products can also mean the difference between a pleasant atmosphere and the offensive odor of urine and feces.

Deodorizers

There are deodorizers available for the environment and also chlorophyllin copper complex capsules and tablets that can be taken orally to deodorize urine and stool. When using room deodorizers it is important to select one that eliminates rather than masks the odor. Most nurses are familiar with the pungent scent of eucalyptus, orange, or lavender that pervades some facilities or homes. Deodorizers made especially for incontinence have little odor of their own and leave no lingering offensive scent.

Chlorophyllin copper complex is effective for some patients when taken orally. Products containing this ingredient do not require a prescription, and the effective dosage must be determined by the individual or caregiver.

Some families say that their elderly relatives are not as careful about personal hygiene as they were when they were younger, or that their olfactory senses have decreased with age. Some older people are not aware of or concerned by malodorous furnishings or clothing. It might fall on the visiting nurse or clinic nurse to investigate causes of and remedies for soiled clothing and personal odor.

SERVICES AND SOURCES OF SUPPLY

Adult diaper services are available in a few large cities. In other locales, existing baby diaper services have added large diapers and bed linens to accommodate adult invalids. Reusable products and laundry services might be more convenient and economical for some people than disposable products.

Sears publishes a specialty Home Health Catalog and the American Association of Retired Persons puts out the AARP Pharmacy Service Catalog, both of which feature various incontinence products. A number of major distributors have an extensive inventory of incontinence products and accessories. They usually have toll-free numbers and someone available who is knowledgeable enough about products to make recommendations to the caller. They will ship directly to the home.

One of the most noticeable changes in the past 5 or 10 years is the availability of adult absorbent products in grocery stores and pharmacies. Although the assortment in these retail outlets might be limited, good products are now available in almost every neighborhood.

Ouslander and colleagues (1985) have expressed concern that the manufacturers and distributors of incontinence products are lax in advising purchasers that most incontinence can be cured or palliated, and provide no warnings that products should not be substituted for diagnosis and treatment. Manufacturers and distributors have been criticized for having inadequate information on their packages regarding sizing, capacity, and skin care. Until these problems are remedied, nurses are responsible for telling consumers that incontinence is treatable and for referring patients to physicians or nurse specialists for diagnosis and treatment of voiding dysfunction.

SUPPORT GROUPS AND CONTINENCE CLINICS

Support Groups

HIP (Help for Incontinent People) is a nonprofit organization that was chartered in 1983. It is a patient advocacy organization founded to inform the public that incontinence is a symptom, not a disease, and to provide information to the public and health professionals about proper diagnoses and treatments for voiding dysfunction. HIP publishes a quarterly newsletter to supplement physicians' teaching. A small pamphlet explaining incontinence, and one-page leaflets on such topics as Questions To Ask Your Doctor and Pelvic Muscle Exercises, are available for a nominal cost. Other groups such as the Simon Foundation and Continence Restored have similar charters with varying foci (App. II).

As the movement toward public education by nurses, physicians, and support groups gathers momentum, there is concern that this information is outstripping professional education. People who have heeded warnings to consult a physician might have been told the following: (1) the condition is not bad enough to fix; (2) the problem is part of old age; and (3) people don't die of incontinence, but they have died from operations to cure it. Nurse specialists should be ready for the new patient population that is now forming as a result of increased media attention to the problems of incontinence.

Continence Clinics

Continence clinics and centers are being established in hospitals and in urologist's, gynecologist's, and geriatrician's offices. Nurse specialists, physicians, and hospitals are beginning to regard continence clinics as a lucrative marketing scheme. A continence clinic, however, must be more than a physician's office with facilities for urodynamic testing. Ideally, it should be a place where full diagnostic services are available, complemented by support personnel, educational materials, a biofeedback laboratory, and product displays. From the initial history to the final determination of the most appropriate management, caring for incontinent patients and their families requires time, space, and an interdisciplinary approach.

A support group can be part of continence clinic activity. This might appear to be another drain on the nurse's fragmented time, but it has the potential to find patients who would otherwise go untreated or be treated elsewhere.

For too long, incontinence has been viewed by nurses as a problem rather than a challenge. Nurses have an opportunity to provide information about the causes of voiding dysfunction and its many treatments. This requires further study and continuing education on the subject as our understanding of the various dysfunctional states of the lower urinary system evolves.

Millions of Americans reportedly endure the expensive and embarrassing discomfort of urinary incontinence. Nurses should be informed about the many procedures, products, accessories, and services that can help promote a cure and provide comfort for the large majority of incontinent people.

References

Allman, R.M., et al.: Pressure sores among hospitalized patients. Ann. Intern. Med. *105*:337, 1986.

Burgio, K.L., Whitehead, W.E., and Engle, B.T.: Behavioral treatment of urinary incontinence in the elderly: Bladder, sphincter, biofeedback and toileting skills training. Ann. Intern. Med., *104*:507–515, 1985.

Dugan, J.S.: Winning the battle against incontinence. Nursing 84, *14*:59, 1984.

Fowler E., and Goupil, D.: Managing an incontinence problem: Assessment, plan and products. J. Urol. Nurs., *4*:327, 1985.

Harrison, N.W., and Paterson, P.J.: Urinary incontinence in women treated by an electronic pessary. Br. J. Urol., *42*:481, 1970.

Kegel, A.H.: Physiologic therapy for urinary stress incontinence. J.A.M.A., *146*:915, 1951.

Linder, R.M., and Upton, J.: Prevention of pressure sores. Surg. Rounds, *6*:42–49, 1983.

Mahoney, D.T.: Bed-Wetting and Urinary Incontinence in Children. Stoughton, MA, Enuresis Institute, D.T. Mahoney, 1982.

National Institutes of Health: Urinary Incontinence in Adults. Program and Abstracts. National Institutes of Health, Rockville, MD, 1988.

Ouslander, J., et al.: Technologies for Managing Urinary Incontinence. Washington, DC, Office of Technology and Assessment, 1985, Health Technology Case Study 33.

Rudinger, E.A.: Bionic therapy for sexual dysfunction and stress urinary incontinence. Presented at the Armed Forces District Meeting, American College of Obstetrics and Gynecology, Las Vegas, September 20, 1976.

Turner, R.K.: A behavioral approach to the management of incontinence in the elderly. *In* Mandelstam, D. (ed.): Incontinence and its Management. London, Croom Helm, 1980, pp. 175–190.

Willington, F.L.: Management of urinary incontinence. *In* Urinary Incontinence. Caldwell, K.P.S. (ed.): New York, Grune & Stratton, 1975, pp. 129–167.

Linda L. Jensen, RN

14 Fecal Incontinence

If any problem is more embarrassing and less socially acceptable than urinary incontinence, it is incontinence of feces. Whether in the home or hospital, coping with fecal incontinence is a considerable burden and unpleasant for both the person and the caregivers.

As with urinary incontinence, fecal incontinence is a symptom that must have a cause. Accurate diagnosis of the underlying problem can lead to a high cure rate. With proper management persistent, uncontrolled fecal incontinence should be rare.

About 0.5% of adults (1 in 200) living in the community probably suffer regular fecal incontinence. It tends to be an underreported symptom that many elderly or disabled people and those with anorectal disorders or diseases of the colon accept and disguise without seeking medical help (Leigh and Turnberg, 1982). The highest incidence of fecal incontinence, however, is found in the elderly in extended care facilities. Many surveys of patients in geriatric or psychogeriatric hospitals have reported fecal incontinence in up to 50% of patients, and certainly a rate of 10 to 20% is common. On general hospital floors, 2 to 3% of patients are likely to be incontinent of feces (Egan and colleagues, 1983). In most cases, however, it is a reversible or avoidable situation.

PHYSIOLOGIC AND ANATOMIC CONSIDERATIONS

Most people maintain fecal continence by a delicate coordination of the neurologic and muscular activity of the colon, rectum, and anus. The main function of the large intestine is to receive chyme from the small bowel, to absorb water from the chyme and form feces, to correct some electrolyte imbalances, and to store and propel feces. About 600 ml of chyme are received daily, and this is eventually reduced to 150 to 200 ml of fecal matter.

Movement of feces or gas along the colon can be stimulated by physical activity, neurologic activity, emotions, or eating. Both eating and the sight or smell of appetizing food cause the cecum to empty into the colon (the so-called gastrocolic response, which is probably mediated hormonally), and this often stimulates a "mass movement" of feces over a great distance through the colon.

When feces enter the rectum there is an immediate sensation of rectal fullness and impending defecation. The sensory nerve endings responsible for this are probably located in the muscle around the rectum, rather than in the rectal wall itself. When the rectum is distended by about 150 ml of feces the internal anal sphincter, which is a smooth muscle (autonomic) sphincter, relaxes completely, allowing feces to pass into the anal canal. The external sphincter, however, which is a striated muscle, is under both autonomic and voluntary control (Fig. 14–1). If defecation is not convenient the external sphincter contracts and the full defecation reflex is inhibited from continuing to completion. The external sphincter maintains a continuous tonic

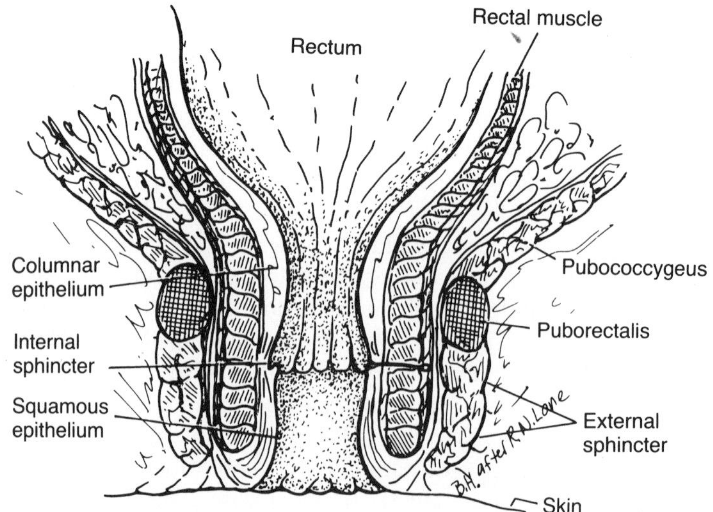

Figure 14–1. *Diagrammatic representation of coronal section through the pelvic floor.*

contraction, even at rest, and this can be greatly augmented for short periods by voluntary contraction. If the defecation reflex is voluntarily inhibited, the stool will be returned to the rectum until a more convenient time. The anal canal is lined with sensitive squamous epithelium, which can distinguish accurately between gas, fluid, and solid matter that enters the anal canal, even during sleep. This is an important consideration, because flatus can be passed without fecal incontinence occurring, and even fluid diarrhea can be retained by most people.

If the defecation reflex is not inhibited—that is, if it is convenient to defecate—the external sphincter relaxes completely and, with minimal abdominal effort, rectal contractions expel the stool, aided by gravity.

The muscular supports of the pelvic floor, especially the puborectalis muscle, help to maintain a double right angle between the anus and rectum, which acts as a flap valve (Fig. 14–2). This aids continence during physical activity. If abdominal pressure is raised, the pressure merely closes the valve more effectively, which is important in preventing stress incontinence of feces. There is also a reflex contraction of the pelvic floor in immediate response to effort.

"Normal" bowel habits vary greatly among individuals. Probably 99% of adults have bowel movements ranging from three times daily to once every 3 days (Connell and associates, 1965). It should be remembered, however, that what is regarded as "normal" for those on a highly refined Western diet is often far from optimal, as the high incidence of bowel disorders in the West testifies. One good-volume, formed, soft, and easily passed stool each day, without excessive urgency, flatus, or abdominal distention, is probably the best objective for most people to try to attain. Variations on one per day are seldom cause for concern unless the other criteria also fail to be achieved.

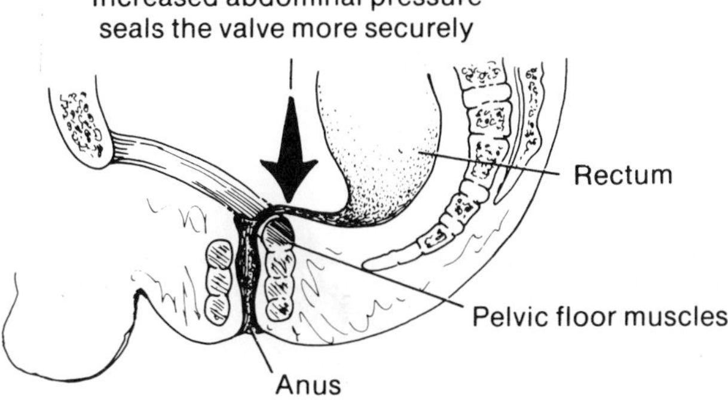

Figure 14–2. *The anatomic arrangement at the anorectal junction results in the formation of a flap valve. The anterior wall of the lower rectum impinges on the closed anal canal and any increase in abdominal pressure seals the valve more securely.*

CAUSES

Fecal incontinence is generally caused by underlying disorders of the colon, rectum, or anus, neurogenic disorders or fecal impaction.

Underlying Disorders

Severe Diarrhea

Severe diarrhea increases the likelihood of having fecal incontinence. The following are some of the more common disorders that can cause diarrhea: ulcerative colitis; Crohn's disease; villous papilloma of the rectum; carcinoma (can also cause constipation); infection; radiation therapy; effect of drugs (e.g., broad-spectrum antibiotics, laxative abuse, iron). Fecal incontinence tends to be a common, if seldom reported, accompaniment.

Those with impaired mobility, diminished sensation or awareness, or already impaired sphincter function are more at risk of diarrhea causing incontinence than otherwise healthy individuals. Lower bowel carcinoma is the most common malignancy of old age, and any recent change in bowel habit should be thoroughly investigated in those in all age groups. Remedying this incontinence involves treating or bringing under control the underlying disease process.

Muscle Ring Deficiency

The pelvic floor muscles support the anal sphincter, and any weakness will cause a tendency to fecal stress incontinence. The vital flap valve formed by the anorectal angle can be lost if these muscles are weak (Fig. 14–3). An increase in abdominal pressure would therefore tend to force the rectal contents down and out of the anal canal. This might be the result of congenital abnormalities or of later trauma (e.g., obstetric, after anal surgery, or direct trauma, such as in

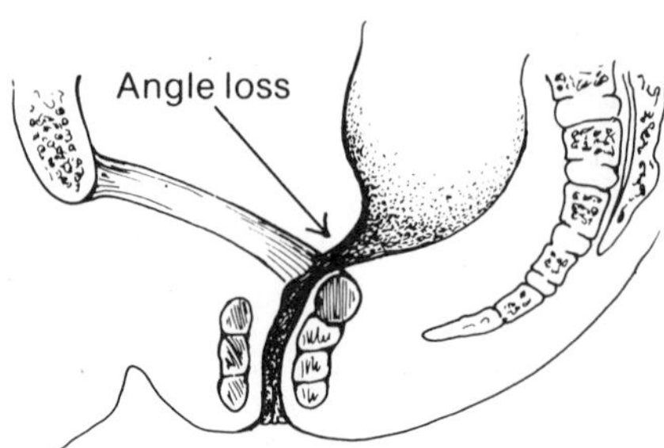

Figure 14–3. With muscle weakness the flap valve formed by the anorectal angle is lost.

a motor vehicle accident). A lifelong habit of straining at stool might also cause muscle weakness.

Mild weakness can respond to pelvic muscle exercises. These should be taught much as exercises for urinary stress incontinence (Chap. 6), but with concentration on the posterior rather than anterior portion of the pelvic muscles. Rectal tone should be assessed by digital examination and the patient instructed to squeeze. Regular contractions of the posterior portion of the pelvic muscles should then be practiced often (usually in sets of 25, 3 times a day), for at least 2 months.

The person must also be firmly instructed to desist from all straining during defecation. Most people with muscle weakness severe enough to cause incontinence of solid stool require surgical repair to restore continence. The most successful surgery involves restoration of the anorectal angle and flap valve mechanism (Parks, 1980).

Some evidence has shown that straining or obstetric trauma causes direct muscle damage and injures the nerve supply of the pelvic floor by prolonged stretching of the nerve fibers (Parks, 1980). If the straining has also induced rectal prolapse, it will require repair at the same time.

Neurogenic Disorders

The medulla and higher cortical centers of the brain have a role in coordinating and controlling the defecation reflex. Therefore, any neurologic disorder that impairs the ability to appreciate or inhibit impending defecation will probably result in a tendency to incontinence, similar in causation to the uninhibited or unstable bladder. For example, the paraplegic can lose all direct sensation of and voluntary control over bowel activity. Neurologic disorders such as multiple sclerosis, cerebrovascular accident, and diffuse dementia can affect sensation or inhibition, or a combination of both. Incontinence occurring in the demented person sometimes occurs because of a physical inability to inhibit defecation. With others it occurs because the awareness that behavior is inappropriate has been lost.

The Paraplegic Patient

Often the paraplegic patient can receive an indirect indication of when the rectum is full and defecation imminent. Various autonomic indicators, such as tachycardia, sweating, or flushing, are often present, and it is important for paraplegics to learn to become sensitive to their own internal indicators if continence is to be achieved. If the lesion is above the cauda equina, it is usually possible to stimulate a defecation reflex voluntarily once the period of spinal shock is past. This is only useful if the rectum is full, so each person must learn to diagnose a full rectum correctly and to act on it before an involuntary reflex causes incontinence. For many paraplegics the reflex can be initiated by dilating the anus, either with a finger or an anal dilator.

Cauda Equina Lesions

If the defecation reflex is disturbed because of damage to the S2 and S3 nerve roots, defecation is often extremely difficult to manage and total uncontrollable incontinence is common. The sphincters, devoid of nerve supply, are usually lax and patulous and simply allow the feces entering the rectum to pass straight out.

If a person with neurogenic fecal incontinence fails to achieve adequate voluntary control, the problem is best managed by inducing constipation artificially and planning controlled bowel evacuations. Some authors recommend the use of a constipating agent in the morning (such as codeine) and a laxative in the evening (e.g., a senna preparation). A more reliable method might involve constipating the patient over several days and then emptying the bowel every 3 to 5 days with the aid of an enema or suppository. Up to 7 days does little harm as long as no discomfort is experienced. A regimen should be worked out to suit the needs, diet, and lifestyle of each patient (Avery Jones and Godding, 1972).

Fecal Impaction

Severe constipation with impaction of feces is probably the most common cause of fecal incontinence, and it certainly predominates as a cause among the elderly and those living in extended care facilities. Chronic constipation leads to impaction when the fluid content of the feces is progressively absorbed by the colon, leaving hard, rounded rocks in the bowel. This hard matter promotes mucus production and bacterial activity, which causes a foul-smelling brown fluid to accumulate. If the rectum is overdistended for any length of time the internal and external anal sphincters become relaxed, giving a completely patulous sphincter that freely allows passing of this mucus as "spurious diarrhea." The patient's symptoms usually include fairly continuous leakage of fluid stool without any awareness of control. Obviously, if the true diagnosis is missed and the patient is treated for diarrhea with constipating agents, the condition is aggravated. Some of the hard stool can also be passed occasionally by gravity or pressure from the formation of more feces above. Most patients with an impaction have hard feces in the rectum but, in a few, the impaction is higher up and cannot be detected by digital examination.

Causes of Constipation

Constipation, the underlying cause of fecal impaction with consequent fecal incontinence, can have many possible causes (Table 14–1).

Constipation means different things to different people, and is difficult to define. In practice, frequency of defecation matters little, as long as the feces are of a soft consistency and easy to pass without undue effort or straining. Constipation refers to feces that are hard and difficult to pass, and that are usually passed at irregular or infrequent time intervals.

Simple Constipation. Simple constipation (i.e., with no underlying bowel pathology) is often self-induced. It can be caused by low food or fluid intake (low fluid intake often being caused by fear of urinary incontinence), poor diet, especially one low in fiber or residue (in the elderly this might be for financial reasons or because of absence of teeth to tackle fiber), lack of exercise, or a combination of these. Physical activity is an important stimulus to colonic activity, and large bowel movements are rare in those who are immobile. A person with diminished awareness might ignore the call to stool.

Environmental factors can be important in causing constipation. Many toilets are too high to allow the feet to rest comfortably on the floor, so additional help from the abdominal muscles cannot be employed during defecation. This can be especially important in the elderly, whose muscle tone might already be decreased. Bathrooms that are cold, uncomfortable, or inconveniently situated can encourage both the ignoring of rectal sensations and not allowing enough time for a bowel movement to be completed. Privacy is also important for complete defecation; if privacy is lacking defecation might be delayed or only partial. This could be true of a child at school, who might be inhibited by bathroom regulations or by the presence of other children. It could be the person who shares accommodations and fears that others are waiting. Or, it could be the hospital patient who hears the

Table 14–1. *COMMON CAUSES OF CONSTIPATION*

Cause	Example
Simple constipation	Low-residue (low-fiber) diet Dehydration Environmental factors
Motility disorders	Irritable bowel syndrome Idiopathic megacolon
Psychiatric disorders	Depression Confusion Anorexia nervosa
Local pathology	Anal fissure Hemorrhoids
General pathology	Endocrine disorders (e.g., diabetes, hypothyroidism); carcinoma
Iatrogenic factor	Drug therapy; immobility; nursing management

nurse hovering outside the door and "waits until next time" in the hope of less haste and greater privacy. Many people can delay defecation almost indefinitely, and impaction can result.

Motility Disorders. The normal transit time of food through the gastrointestinal tract has been measured by radiopaque markers and found to be between 3 and 7 days from mouth to anus for most people. Disorders such as irritable bowel syndrome, or diverticular disease (itself probably caused by the constipating effect of the Western low-residue, low-fiber, high-carbohydrate diet) can lead to constipation, sometimes alternating with diarrhea. Some people have an idiopathic slow transit time or megacolon, and transit time probably increases with advancing age.

Slow transit time (8 to 15 days is not uncommon) through the colon allows increased water absorption and encourages the formation of an impaction. In the elderly this can lead to the "terminal reservoir syndrome," in which a largely distended lower colon is never emptied completely.

Psychiatric Disorders. Depression can be a primary factor, and is an often neglected cause of constipation. Confusion and dementia also predispose an individual to constipation. Conversely, constipation can be the underlying cause of confusion. Anorexia nervosa, self-purgation, and some psychoses can underlie apparent constipation.

Problems Secondary to Local or General Pathology. A large bowel carcinoma can present as constipation. Hemorrhoids, anal stricture, or any painful anorectal disorder tends to cause inhibition of defecation and thereby result in constipation. Endocrine disorders, notably hypothyroidism and diabetes, can be underlying pathologic factors.

Iatrogenic Factors. Constipation can be drug-induced (e.g., analgesics, especially opiates, anticholinergics, and antiparkinsonian drugs), or can develop because of a period of enforced immobility (e.g., postoperatively). It can also be induced by nursing management—for example, requiring a patient to defecate while perched on a bedpan in bed, a most unnatural act because of the inappropriate position adopted and the lack of privacy. The straining and effort involved in attempting defecation on a bedpan, not to mention stress, are often considerably greater than the effort of getting up to use the commode or toilet. In cardiac patients straining at stool is a known precursor of cardiac arrest and sudden death.

Constipation in the Elderly

An older person can have a combination of many of the above-mentioned problems causing constipation. Wilkins (1968) has described a vicious circle of constipation in the elderly, which shows how factors combine to maintain constipation (Fig. 14–4).

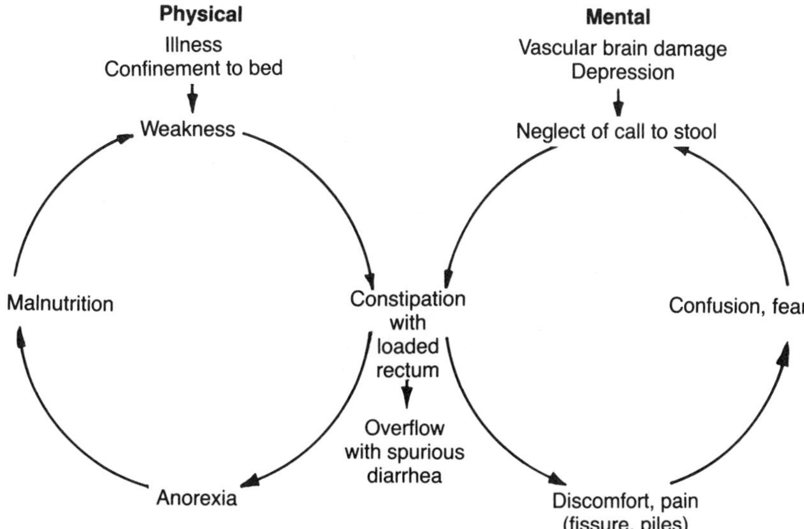

Figure 14–4. *Combination of factors that helps to maintain constipation in the elderly. From Wilkins, E.G.: Vicious circles of constipation in the elderly. Postgrad. Med. J., 44:728, 1968.*

Many elderly people are obsessed with their bowels, often resulting from a lifelong habit of weekly purgation and persistent beliefs that a bowel that is not completely cleared regularly can become toxic. Elderly people often attribute any feeling of malaise or ill health to infrequent bowel actions. Many are chronic laxative abusers (Connell and coworkers, 1965). This practice in itself can cause problems and eventually damage colonic activity, leading to nerve impairment and a "cathartic" colon. No evidence has shown that healthy, active old people are more likely to be constipated than younger people, and prophylactic laxative taking is best avoided unless constipation is a known problem that cannot be resolved by other means. Because of some atrophy of bowel mucosa and muscle with age, transit times do rise somewhat. Elderly patients should be reassured that decreased frequency of defecation is normal with age and taught not to equate this with constipation unless the feces also become hard and difficult to pass.

Investigation of Constipation and Fecal Impaction

Given the large number of possible causes, constipation with fecal impaction and incontinence should always be investigated and the underlying causes remedied, if possible. A rectal digital examination can reveal most impactions, although occasionally only soft feces are present and the rectum might even be empty. A plain abdominal film will reveal higher impaction if this is suspected. Many causes are easily treated, such as changing a drug or diet regimen, treating hypothyroidism or anorectal disorders, or acquiring a new set of dentures so that solid food can be chewed.

Further investigation depends on the clinical picture. Barium studies are useful if malignancy or diverticular disease is suspected. Defecography is a useful tool in diagnosing evacuation disorders. Endoscopy of the anal canal, rectum, and sigmoid colon can be useful. Blood and stool tests might be indicated. A few specialist clinics have facilities for sophisticated measurement of anal and rectal pressures, which are becoming essential diagnostic tools.

Nursing assessment of the patient with suspected impaction should include eliciting a careful history of the problem (with consideration of the patient's probable reluctance to discuss it because of embarrassment, and with as much privacy as possible). Diet, mobility, fluid intake, the environment and reactions to it should all be closely observed and their relevance determined. A checklist to help in the assessment of defecation can be useful (Fig. 14–5).

As well as causing incontinence, impaction can lead to intestinal obstruction, mental disturbances (including apathy and possibly agitation or confusion), rectal bleeding, and urinary retention (with possible overflow incontinence).

Treatment

Clearing the Impaction. The first necessity is clearing the fecal impaction. Manual evacuation of the feces is rarely necessary. Usually a course of disposable phosphate enemas, one or two daily for 7 to 10 days, or until no further return is obtained, is the treatment of choice for clearing impaction. A single enema is seldom efficient, even if an apparently good result is obtained, because impaction is often extensive and the first enema merely clears the lowest portion of the bowel. Fear of enemas stems from the days of large-volume soap-and-water enemas, which are both extremely uncomfortable and usually messy. These should no longer be used. The modern low-volume (100 to 150 ml) disposable phosphate enema causes minimal discomfort and, if administered with careful prior explanation and attention to privacy and dignity, does not generally cause much distress. The newer "microenemas" (5 to 10 ml) are even more acceptable.

If fecal incontinence persists once the bowel has been totally cleared (a plain abdominal radiograph can be helpful in confirming this), it can usually be assumed to be neurogenic in origin rather than caused by the impaction.

Prevention of Recurrence. Once the impaction has been cleared, every effort must be made to prevent recurrence. Attention to diet, fluid intake, mobility, bathroom facilities, and drug regimens can be sufficient. Some people also need to use agents to keep their bowel

Name: Assessment date:

Patient's usual term for defecation:
Usual frequency of bowel action: Range:
Usual time of day:
Any associated habits or events:

Does patient complain of constipation?
If so, what is understood by this?

Does patient get sensation of the need to defecate?
Does patient have to strain?
Average time taken for bowel movement:
Is defecation associated with pain?
Any bleeding? Fresh or altered blood:
Mucus:
Problematic flatus: Continent of flatus:
Hard stools: Ribbon stools:
Usual consistency of feces:
Usual amount of feces:
Does patient experience urgency? Time of warning:
Sensation of incomplete evacuation?
Diet: Any food taken for bowels?
Any food avoided for bowels?
Average daily fluid intake:
Laxative use: Present:
Past history of use:
Any constipating drugs taken?
History of perianal problems?

Fecal incontinence?
If yes: Nature of soiling:
Sensation of incontinence:
Frequency of incontinence:

Results of rectal examination, if done:
Any recent change in bowel habits:
Bathroom facilities:
Problems with using bathroom:
If bedpan or commode used, patient's reaction to this:

Ability to cleanse after defecation:
Mobility impaired:

Are any bowel problems anticipated with current illness or condition?

Figure 14–5. *Sample checklist for assessment of defecation.*

regular. A large variety of laxatives is available. They are of four general types—bulking agents, stool softeners, chemicals, and rectally administered evacuants (Table 14–2).

The bulking laxatives work by hydrophilic action (i.e., they attract water into the stool). Usually feces are 60 to 70% water, so a 10% increase in water content will soften the stool considerably. Natural unprocessed bran is probably the most satisfactory bulking agent, but proprietary brands (e.g., Metamucil, Citrucel, Unifiber) are available. Because bran is mixed with food and chewed, it is less likely to form a bolus and therefore has a low risk of leading to intestinal obstruction. Bulking agents eaten as granules carry a slight risk of adhering together

Table 14–2. *COMMONLY USED LAXATIVES*

Category	Examples	Comments and Contraindications
Bulking agent	Natural bran; Metamucil, Citrucel, Unifiber	Introduce gradually, only after impaction has cleared; avoid if patient has loss of rectal sensation or terminal reservoir syndrome
Stool softener	Liquid paraffin; castor oil	Avoid general use
Irritant or chemical	Senna; bisacodyl	Use minimal effective dose
Combined softener and irritant	Pericolace, Doxidan	Use mimimal effective dose
Rectally administered	Suppository (e.g., glycerin, bisacodyl); enema (e.g., phosphate, microenema)	Some patients might need assistance or find use unpleasant
Miscellaneous	Lactulose	Flatus can be problematic

as a bolus. It must be remembered that bulking agents take several days to reach the colon and any impaction should be cleared before starting use. If not, the additional bulk merely accumulates above the impaction and adds to the amount of feces that needs to be cleared. Bulking agents increase the water content and size of stool and decrease gut transit time, thereby increasing the frequency of defecation. They should be used with care for patients with diminished rectal sensation, those who ignore the call to stool, and those with known terminal reservoir syndrome. The gradual introduction of bulking agents can help to minimize problems.

Stool softeners act to alter stool consistency. The most common softener was once liquid paraffin. The use of liquid paraffin has been discontinued because so many harmful effects were noted, including interference with digestion, binding of fat-soluble vitamins, possible deposits in the lungs from inhalation, leading to lipoid pneumonia, paraffinomas (deposits in the tissues), and fecal incontinence. Similarly, castor oil should not be regularly used because it works by stimulating the small bowel to massive activity and usually leads to complete bowel clearance within 2 hours. It is therefore suitable for complete bowel preparation (e.g., prior to radiographic examination), but the water, electrolyte, and nutrient loss involved makes it unsuitable for repeated use, especially in the elderly.

Chemical (or irritant) laxatives work by stimulating colonic peristalsis. The most commonly used are senna (Senokot) and bisacodyl (Dulcolox). They are selective to the colon, so they do not upset the whole gut and have a minimal effect on fluid and electrolyte balance and on gut flora. For prolonged administration the smallest effective dose should always be used.

Pericolace and Doxidan are combinations of a softener and chemical laxative. They have been found to be effective in the long-term regulation of bowel function. Lactulose, a sugar, does not really fit into any category. Taken orally, it is not absorbed but attracts water and thus softens the stool. Some patients find it causes a bloated feeling and excessive flatus.

Of the rectally administered laxatives, the disposable small-volume enemas are probably the most convenient and effective, but their use usually requires assistance. For lesser problems, glycerin or bisacodyl suppositories can be effective and can be used independently by many people.

Often the best regimen for each individual is found by trial and error. It is most important to prevent recurrence of impaction or incontinence will usually return. When dealing with patients in an extended care facility or hospital this often involves close observation of each patient's bowel habits. The traditional nursing practice of merely asking patients if they have had a bowel movement and marking "yes" or "no" on the TPR chart or in the Kardex is not good enough. Extra vigilance is needed to avert the preventable condition of incontinence caused by impaction. Patients must be asked in more detail about their bowel movements (e.g., consistency, amount, ease of passage), and about any feelings of discomfort, bloating, or incomplete evacuation. The nurse must respect the patient's dignity and be sensitive to likely embarrassment, and should request this information in private. Questions asked in front of visitors or other patients are less likely to be fully answered and spontaneous comments might be discouraged. If the patient cannot be relied on for an accurate account, it is the nurse's responsibility to observe the stool and note its characteristics. The difficult passage of one small hard pellet each day, which often is recorded as a bowel movement and assumed to be evidence that all is well, is usually the exact opposite—an indication of impending impaction. If this is suspected, the nurse must perform a rectal examination to ensure that impaction is not developing. The momentary discomfort caused by a digital rectal examination is minimal compared to the distress and inconvenience caused by fecal impaction and incontinence.

Meticulous observation, coupled with optimism and a belief that impaction is avoidable, can greatly reduce the prevalence of fecal incontinence in the hospital or extended care facility.

PREVENTION

Fecal incontinence can generally be prevented. Alterations in lifelong dietary habits can help to prevent many disorders that later cause incontinence, such as diverticular disease and possibly carcinoma. Regular laxative use or abuse should be avoided, because it can cause colonic and nerve damage. Avoidance of straining at stool can help to preserve pelvic-muscle integrity, as will better obstetric care, with a shortened second stage of labor. Public education about fluid intake, diet, the importance of establishing a regular bowel habit, and avoiding laxatives and straining might prevent many future problems.

For those who come under the nurse's care, greater thought should go into their need for privacy, comfort, and adequate time for defecation. Again, the importance of diet, fluids, exercise, and relevant drug regimens must be stressed. Nurses who create an environment geared to the promotion of continence, who have an attitude that this is a preventable or reversible condition, and who prepare to make strenuous efforts to monitor the bowel function of all their patients closely can do much to prevent the misery of fecal incontinence.

INTRACTABLE FECAL INCONTINENCE

Protection

If fecal incontinence proves to be intractable for any reason, as it may for a small minority of people, protection will be needed to preserve the person's dignity and protect the environment. Many of the products and devices used for urinary incontinence are also suitable for fecal incontinence (Chap. 13), especially those with a disposable pad worn directly against the perineum. If fecal incontinence alone is present, high absorbency is usually not necessary and relatively thin pads can be used. If large formed stools are passed, some people find a "wing-folded" pad to be most helpful for containing the stool until it can be disposed of. Marsupial pants and washable underpads are not suitable for fecal incontinence.

Smell

The odor of feces is a particularly difficult problem. Obviously, prompt disposal of the feces and scrupulous personal hygiene (with regular baths, if possible) is the best management, but even this does not always prevent smell. Proprietary deodorants, such as Ostozyme or Hex-On, can help if used on a pad or clothing, or in the air. Each person might find that certain foods aggravate the smell of their feces and are best avoided. Unpleasant odor is still one of the unsolved problems associated with fecal incontinence.

Colostomy

A person with severe, persistent fecal incontinence might wish to be considered for surgical diversion of the bowel in a colostomy. The feces can then be collected in a discreet, odor-free collection device or appliance and the person can regain social acceptability. This obviously represents a last resort, but it should not be forgotten as an alternative if the incontinence is severely limiting a person's lifestyle and activities. It can, with good advice and support, be a positive choice for someone whose life is otherwise ruled by the incontinence.

FECAL INCONTINENCE IN CHILDREN

Most children are continent of feces by the age of 4 years, but 1% still have problems at 7 years. More boys than girls are incontinent, suggesting that developmental factors can be relevant, because boys mature more slowly. Fecal incontinence or soiling in childhood (sometimes referred to as encopresis) has, like nocturnal enuresis, long been regarded as evidence of a psychiatric or psychologic disorder in the child. Psychologic factors are certainly important, but it is not true that most fecally incontinent children are disturbed (Morgan, 1981).

Usually it is easy to see how the incontinence arises. Such a child usually has fastidious, overanxious parents who are intent on toilet-training. The child is punished for soiling, so defecation tends to be inhibited, both in the underwear and in the toilet. Often when attempting toilet training the child is repeatedly seated on the toilet in the absence of a full rectum and simply cannot perform. The situation becomes fraught with anxiety and bowel movements become associated with unpleasantness in the child's mind. The child therefore retains feces and becomes constipated. Defecation then becomes difficult and painful as well.

The tension created while the child is on the toilet is often relieved later. "Respite defecation" occurs when the child relaxes—a formed stool is passed into the underwear. This might seem like deliberate naughtiness to the parent, who has just spent time encouraging the passage of stool in the correct place.

Once this pattern has been established, the child might even become impacted and suffer paradoxic incontinence or spurious diarrhea. Tension at home or lack of privacy at school can both lead to deliberate retention. Such children are made to feel guilty about the incontinence, although they have no control over it, and can try to conceal it by hiding the feces or clothing. This could be misinterpreted as intentional, but in fact, it is rare for a child to use deliberate smearing or soiling as a weapon against parents.

Both parents and incontinent child should be assessed for their attitudes to the problem. A rectal examination will reveal impaction, idiopathic megacolon, or a painful fissure. Rarely, a congenital abnormality of the rectum or anus is present. Most children can be treated by disimpaction of the bowel, simple explanation and reassurance, and the use by parents of simple rewards for appropriate defecation. Punishment for soiling should not be used, because this merely aggravates the child's anxiety over defecation. Also, clean underwear should not be rewarded, because this might reinforce retention of feces.

Regular laxatives and sensitive counseling and support remedy most problems. Sometimes advice includes practical measures, such as using a footstool to support dangling legs to aid defecation, lowering the lock so that the child can reach it and ensure privacy, or allowing more time before school to have a bowel movement. If the child does prove to be disturbed, however, as a few do, psychotherapy might be indicated.

The child with mental retardation might be in exactly the same position as the normal child—retaining feces because of the unfavorable response they produce in others. Conversely, incontinence can produce much commotion and attention and thus become reinforcing. Behavior modification programs using appropriate, prompt reinforcers and gradually withdrawn prompts can cure many children with mental retardation of incontinence (Chap. 12). If the incontinence is of neurogenic origin (e.g., spina bifida), the same constipating and planned evacuation program as that for adults can be followed.

The caregiver has an important role in educating parents to avoid many problems of fecal incontinence that arise in children. Clear practical advice on toilet training, and support for those experiencing problems, can often help to prevent incontinence at an early stage.

FECAL INCONTINENCE IN DEMENTIA

Severe dementia or confusional states can result in fecal incontinence caused by the loss of awareness of what is socially appropriate behavior. The person who has no conception that defecation should only be in a clearly defined receptacle has no reason to delay defecation voluntarily, so the stool is usually passed as soon as it enters the anal canal. Sometimes the knowledge that certain receptacles are designated for the purpose is retained but the ability to identify them is lost, and the demented person might use a totally inappropriate receptacle in which to pass feces, such as a wastepaper basket or a sink. Others remember to remove clothing and to sit or squat, but do so wherever they happen to be at the time. Some lose all apparent awareness and pass stool into their underwear or the bed. Some demented people lose all appropriate toilet behavior, but retain an appreciation that something is wrong and become agitated or start wandering, apparently aimlessly, just prior to becoming incontinent.

It should never be assumed that dementia alone is sufficient reason to explain fecal incontinence without the investigation and exclusion of other causes. Continence is deeply ingrained in most of us, and it is often one of the last social skills to be lost. The demented person might be incontinent because of diarrhea from any cause, because the same neurologic damage that has caused dementia has also affected the ability to control the defecation reflex voluntarily or, most commonly, because of fecal impaction. Most demented people are not fecally incontinent. Unless the dementia is profound, incontinence is most often found to have other causes.

When an individual gives any signs of impending defecation, there will usually be enough time to prevent incontinence by getting the person to a bathroom. Of course this depends on all those looking after that person being aware of exactly what signs to look for and what they mean. Spotting this characteristic behavior for each individual is vital to the nursing assessment of fecal incontinence in the demented person.

It might be possible to retrain the demented person to more socially acceptable habits. Often a routine of defecation can be established—for example, half an hour after a hot meal or drink. The principles of behavior modification (Chaps. 8 and 12) are equally applicable to fecal as to urinary incontinence. Reinforcing continent behavior can restore continence in many demented people. If this is unsuccessful, the same regimen as that outlined for the neurogenic bowel (see above) can be used—artificial constipation alternating with planned evacuation. Such a program requires meticulous nursing care and record keeping to keep the patient's condition satisfactory.

References and Further Reading

Alteresue, V.: Theoretical foundations for an approach to fecal incontinence. J. Enterost. Ther. *13*:44, 1986.

Avery Jones, F., and Godding, E.W.: Management of Constipation. Oxford and London, Blackwell Scientific, 1972.

Bainton, D. and Edington, A: "D" is for dignity. Health Soc. Sci. J. *90*:50, 1983.

Bartolo, D.C.C.: Pelvic floor disorders: Incontinence, constipation, and obstructed defecation. *In* Schrock, T.R. (ed.): Perspectives in Colon and Rectal Surgery, Vol. 1. St. Louis, MO, Quality Medical Publishing, 1988, pp. 1–29.

Breckman, B.: Stoma Care. Beaconsfield, England, Beaconsfield Publishers, 1981.

Brocklehurst, J.C.: The large bowel. *In* Brocklehurst, J.C. (ed.): Textbook of Geriatric Medicine and Gerontology. 2nd ed. Edinburgh and London, Churchill Livingstone, 1978, pp. 368–384.

Brooks, S.: Disturbances of bowel function. Nursing '84, *30*:870, 1984.

Connell, A.M., et al.: Variation of bowel habits in two population samples. Br. Med. J., 2:1095, 1965.
Egan, M., et al.: Incontinence in patients in two district general hospitals. Nurs. Times, *79:*22, 1983.
Henry, M.: Fecal incontinence. Nurs. Times, *79:*61, 1983.
Johns, C.: Encopresis. Am. J. Nurs., *85:*153, 1985.
Leigh, R.J., and Turnberg, L.A.: Faecal incontinence: The unvoiced symptom. Lancet, *1:*1349, 1982.
Morgan, R.: Childhood Incontinence. London, William Heinemann, 1981.
Mowlan, V., North, K., and Myers, C.: Managing fecal incontinence. Nurs. Times, *82:*55, 1986.
Parks, A.G.: Faecal incontinence. *In* Mandelstam, D. (ed.): Incontinence and Its Management. Brookenham, Croom Helm, England, 1980, pp. 76–93.
Schiller, L.R.: Fecal incontinence. Clin. Gastroenterol., *15:*687, 1986.
Smith, L.E.: Trouble in the anorectal zone: Incontinence and constipation. Emerg. Med., *18*(6):134, 1986.
Wilkins, E.G.: Vicious circles of constipation in the elderly. Postgrad. Med. J. *44:*728, 1968.

Georgeann Constantino, RN

Catheterization 15

The use of a hollow tube, or catheter, for urine drainage has a long history. The ancient Egyptians used gold catheters and the Greeks had bronze tubes for the relief of urinary obstruction (Cule, 1980). Current technology has produced a wide variety of catheters suitable for use in different situations. This chapter outlines how proper catheter management can help in the successful control of voiding dysfunction. Two methods of catheterization are considered; one that uses the indwelling urethral (or Foley) catheter and one that uses the suprapubic catheter. (Chap. 10 discusses intermittent catheter regimes.)

INDWELLING URETHRAL (FOLEY) CATHETERS

It was not until the 1930s that Fredrick Foley perfected the technique of dipping and coagulating latex on metal forms to manufacture a one-piece catheter and balloon. The Foley catheter is now the most commonly used of all urinary catheters. In its usual form it has a double-lumen shaft (one lumen for urine drainage, the other for inflation and deflation of the retention balloon), a rounded tip, and two drainage eyes proximal to the balloon (Fig. 15–1).

There are many variations on this standard design, both in regard to materials and construction. Table 15–1 summarizes the most com-

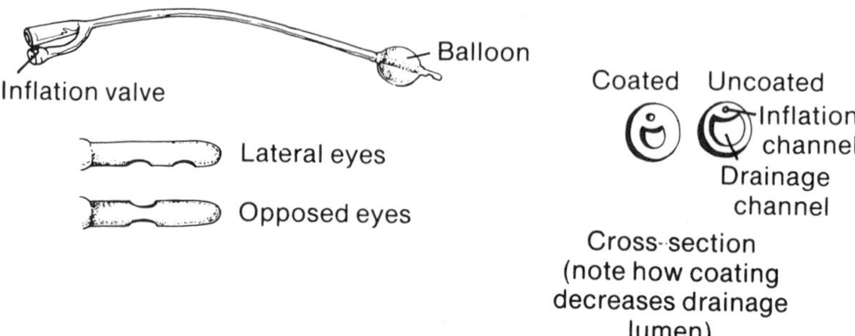

Figure 15–1. *Standard Foley catheter.*

monly used variants. The size of a catheter is measured on the Charrière (ch) or French gauge (F) scale. Actually these are identical systems that measure the external circumference of the catheter in millimeters, usually in 2-mm graduations. A 14-F catheter therefore has an external circumference of 14 mm.

Indications

There are many situations in which an indwelling urethral catheter can be used. The most common indications are post-operative drainage, particularly after urologic or gynecologic surgery, and acute illness, in which accurate monitoring of urine output is needed. Chronic or acute retention of urine is often managed by catheter, either on a short-term basis until the retention is treated or on a long-term basis if treatment is impossible or unsuccessful.

Table 15–1. *TYPES OF INDWELLING CATHETERS*

Type	Length (cm)	Sizes (F)	Balloon Sizes (ml)	Material	Comments
Standard Foley	40–45	8–30, in 2-mm graduation	3 (child), 5, 5–10, 30	Plastic	Short-term use
				Latex rubber	Short-term use
				Latex catheter with hydromer coating	Provides lubrication for insertion
				Siliconized	Provides lubrication for insertion
				Teflon-coated	Long-term use
				Silicone elastomer-coated latex	Long-term use
				100% silicone	Long-term use
Three-way	40–45	16–26	5–10, 30–50, 75–100	Plastic or latex rubber	Some are reinforced to prevent collapse with suction; used for continuous irrigation

Those who are terminally ill can benefit from the use of a catheter if frequent or painful urination, incontinence, severe skin problems, or pressure ulcers become a management problem. A catheter can make the difference between relatives being able to cope at home and the dying person needing institutional care.

Intractable urinary incontinence, from any cause, can also be managed by an indwelling catheter. It must be stressed that this should be a last resort. A catheter should never be the first line of management for incontinence. If people remain so incontinent after full investigation and trial of available treatments that the quality of their life is impaired and a normal lifestyle is impossible, a catheter can be a positive method of management. Patients who are too ill or frail to undergo therapy for incontinence can also obtain relief. Insertion of a catheter to control incontinence should only proceed after a full discussion of the implications between physician, patient, nurse and significant others (e.g., relatives), and after all agree and accept the decision. A catheter should never be inserted for the convenience of staff—it must always be a decision made for the well-being of the patient. For severely incontinent people a catheter might be the only way of being socially accepted. For some it can allow an independent life, free from the need for institutionalized care, or allow care by relatives who otherwise could not or would not cope with incontinence at home. For carefully selected patients, a well-managed catheter can restore social continence and a full range of normal activities.

Selection of the Catheter

Once the decision has been made to use an indwelling catheter, the choice of catheter type is crucial. It is not acceptable merely to use the first catheter that comes from central supply. Whoever is inserting the catheter should be aware of the selection available and their different intended functions.

Size

The primary consideration when selecting catheter size is to choose the smallest catheter that will drain adequately. For an adult this is normally a 12, 14, or 16 F. Size 8-F catheters are the smallest available for children. An infant feeding tube can be used to catheterize infants. Except where heavy hematuria is anticipated, sizes larger than 18 F should never be used for initial catheterization in adults and larger sizes are rarely indicated, even after prolonged catheterization.

A catheter is not intended to occlude the urethra completely, like a cork in a bottleneck. The folds of the urethra normally close on

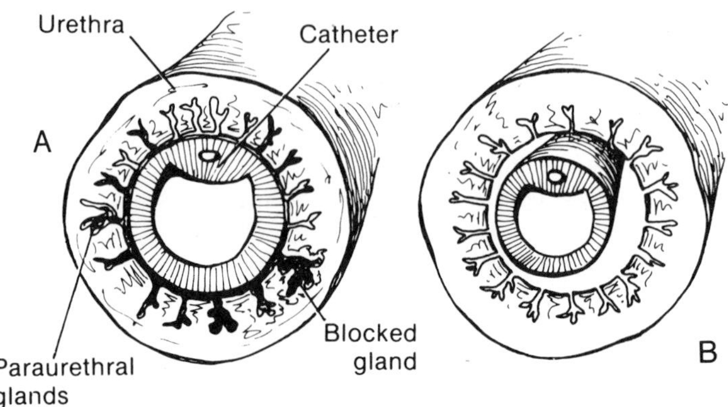

Figure 15–2. *The importance of catheter size.* A, *Too large a catheter blocks drainage from the paraurethral glands.* B, *A smaller catheter permits secretions to drain. (Blandy, 1981).*

themselves, and the smaller the catheter the more easily the urethral folds can close around it.

There should be adequate space around the catheter so that secretions from the paraurethral glands can drain. If these glands become occluded the secretions accumulate and the glands tend to become infected, which can lead to abscess or stricture formation (Fig. 15–2).

A catheter that is too large carries the risk of urethral erosion in men, either where it is gripped at the external sphincter or where it bends over the penoscrotal junction (Blandy, 1981). This can be followed by development of a sloughing granuloma and stricture formation (Fig. 15–3). This is occasionally seen after major non-

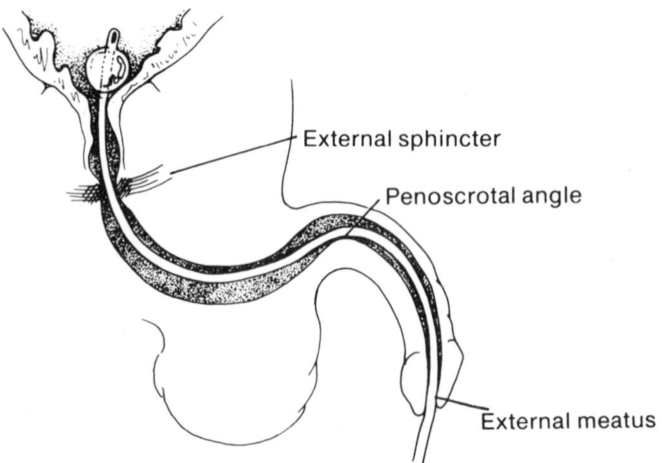

Figure 15–3. *Sites for catheter stricture. (Blandy, 1981.)*

urologic surgery (e.g., cardiac surgery), in which an inexperienced person has inserted a very large catheter to monitor postoperative urinary output. The patient might recover from the original complaint and be left with a urethral stricture.

Larger catheters do not necessarily have proportionately larger eyes. They will block just as easily as smaller ones. Coated catheters have an especially small eye and lumen size in proportion to their French size (see Fig. 15–1).

Balloon Size

Manufacturers indicate on the package the maximum amount of fluid that should be used to fill the catheter balloon, usually 5, 5 to 10, or 30 ml. Very large balloons (75 ml and larger) are specifically intended for controlling postoperative hematuria and should not be used for general purposes. The stated amount is commonly misinterpreted as the amount that must be used in that balloon rather than its maximum capacity. Inflating the balloon with 5 to 10 ml of sterile water is usually recommended as adequate to retain the catheter in the bladder and prevent it from being expelled (McGill, 1982). Occasionally a 30-ml balloon catheter, filled to capacity, is used to secure the catheter in place for routine drainage. If the only catheter available has a stated balloon capacity of 30 ml, as little as 15 ml can be used, although less than this will lead to uneven balloon inflation. Some experts (Kelly and Griffiths, 1983) believe that the recommended amount (30 ml) should be instilled into this size balloon. Anything less than this can result in difficulty deflating the balloon, thereby risking operative removal (Moisey and Williams, 1980), mucosal ulceration (Milles, 1965), and occasionally erosion leading to bladder perforation (Spees and colleagues, 1981).

The balloon is not designed to occlude the urethra or prevent leakage. (This is accomplished by the bladder neck and sphincters gripping the catheter lumen). The inflated balloon just retains the catheter in the bladder and prevents it from falling out. Few patients need more than 5 to 10 ml of fluid for this purpose.

A major problem caused by too large a balloon is the leakage of urine around the catheter. The drainage eyes are above the balloon. Use of a 5-ml balloon would cause a small amount of residual urine to be left around the balloon. If the balloon contains 30 ml of water, the residual urine volume is much larger (Fig. 15–4). Also, a larger balloon is more irritating to the bladder and can provoke contractions, especially in an unstable bladder. Contractions force the residual urine out around the catheter. A larger residual also has an increased likelihood of becoming infected.

Thirty milliliters of water is also heavy, especially when resting on

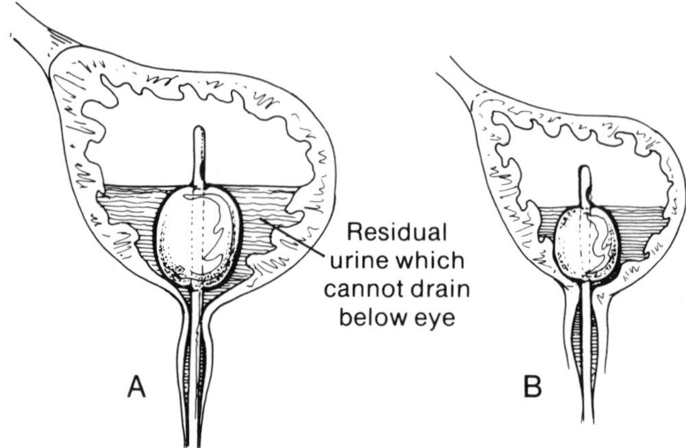

Figure 15–4. *Balloon catheters.* A, *30-ml balloon.* B, *5-ml balloon.*

the delicate and sensitive trigone of the bladder. This can lead to a feeling of discomfort or dragging from the catheter. If there is repeated traction or pulling on the catheter, this weight can damage the bladder neck. It is sometimes stated that a large balloon is necessary to prevent confused patients from pulling the catheter out, but these patients can and do pull out a fully inflated 30-ml balloon. If there is a chance that patients will pull the catheter out, it is infinitely preferable for them to pull out a smaller rather than a larger balloon. The additional discomfort from pulling out a larger balloon is seldom enough of a deterrent to a confused patient.

Actually, the weight and discomfort caused by a 30-ml balloon in the bladder could be why the catheter is being pulled out. Repeated traction on a smaller balloon is less likely to damage the bladder neck. Some nursing texts recommend restraining or using mittens on the confused catheterized patient. It is better to avoid the use of a catheter if a confused or uncooperative patient might pull at it.

Material

Until relatively recently most catheters were made either from plastic (polyvinylchloride or polyurethane) or latex rubber. Red rubber is used, but it tends to be irritating. Plastic is soft at body temperature but rigid at lower temperatures, and is often found by women to be uncomfortable, especially when sitting. Both plastic and latex rubber tend to develop cracks and encrustations with extended use (after about 2 weeks). Plastic might become less encrustated because its negative surface electrical charge discourages particle adhesion, although the clinical results of this are unproven. Both plastic and latex catheters are relatively inexpensive.

Many attempts have been made to improve the latex catheter—prolong its life, reduce encrustation and infection, and increase comfort. "Siliconizing" the surface of a latex catheter produces a lubricated surface, which is thought to ease insertion and provide some lubrication while the catheter is in place. Because lubricant is always used on insertion and the coating dissolves after insertion, the extra cost of siliconized catheters is of debatable value. Latex can be coated with Teflon or, most recently, a lubricating hydromer coating, which gives the catheter a smoother surface. This can reduce urethritis and stone formation, although it has not been proven that Teflon reduces encrustation.

Many extravagant claims have been made for catheters coated or dipped in silicone elastomer (silicone coated; this should be distinguished from the siliconized catheters described above). There seems to be less encrustation with silicone-coated than latex catheters in long-term use and some reduction in tissue reaction. Some manufacturers claim that they can be safely left in place for 3 to 6 months without changing. Latex has been found to be equally long-lasting if well managed (Blannin and Hobden, 1980). Encrustation itself might not be a major factor in catheter life span. Many are changed for other reasons, especially leakage, long before encrustation becomes a problem. If silicone-coated catheters are not used for their intended life spans, it must be questioned whether they are worth the extra cost (often twice that of a latex catheter). It has not been determined whether the reduced lumen from the coating actually impairs drainage, encourages blockage, and shortens the catheter's life.

Manufacturers are developing new urologic products in an attempt to reduce the risk of urinary tract infections and increase patient comfort. Recently 100% silicone catheters were introduced. Because they are not coated their internal lumen tends to be proportionately larger. Because silicone permits gas diffusion, however, they tend to allow balloon deflation over time. Without close supervision some patients find that the catheter falls out.

It may be best to choose an inexpensive catheter (latex) for initial or short-term use. If catheterization is well tolerated or indicated for long-term use, the additional cost of an all-silicone or silicone-coated catheter might be justified. If well managed, it could remain in place for up to 2 or 3 months. If patients experience repeated problems that necessitate frequent catheter changes, a latex catheter is more cost-effective. The more expensive catheters have no proven advantage for short-term use.

Design

Most catheters have a semirigid rounded tip. Variations include the Tiemann (olive-tip coudé), which is curved to aid insertion past an enlarged prostate, and whistle-tip, which is open-ended to facilitate drainage of sediment. Most catheters have two drainage eyes. These can be lateral (on the same side) or opposed (on opposite sides, which are less likely to block; see Fig. 15–1).

Insertion

The decision to institute drainage by indwelling catheter is a medical one and should always be made by the responsible physician. The actual insertion should be done by a nurse or physician who has received full instruction and who has had supervised practice in the technique. There is little reason for the tradition that male physicians or nurses catheterize men and female nurses catheterize women. As long as local hospital policies are followed, a competent professional should be able to catheterize any patient.

Prior to insertion, the balloon should be inflated and then deflated to detect any leakage or defects in the balloon or valve. Failure to perform this check may necessitate surgical removal.

Except for persons managed by clean intermittent catheterization, strict asepsis should be employed in the insertion of a catheter (Luckmann and Sorensen, 1987). When an indwelling catheter is indicated, a preconnected closed drainage system should be used to minimize or prevent infection from contamination through disconnection (Brunner and Suddarth, 1988). Ideally, the patient should have a bath prior to catheter insertion. If this is not possible, thorough cleansing of the genital area with soap and water is essential.

For women, the key to successful catheter insertion lies in visualizing the urethral meatus. The patient should lie semirecumbent with the knees bent and abducted to either side as far as possible. A gooseneck light directed at the vulva can be helpful. A cotton swab can be used to help locate the meatus if it is disguised among skin folds. If the opening is concealed it might be easier to find with the patient in the left lateral position and with her knees drawn up onto her chest, so that the anterior vaginal wall can be visualized from behind.

In men, the foreskin should be retracted and the glans penis thoroughly cleaned. A well-lubricated catheter is then inserted into the urethra. Some men find the procedure very uncomfortable. In such cases, it is appropriate and helpful to insert 10 ml of a local anesthetic gel (e.g., lidocaine, 1%) before re-attempting catheterization. After the anesthetic gel has been instilled into the penis, gentle pressure is applied for a few minutes to allow the anesthetic to take effect. The catheter is inserted while extending the penis vertically with a gentle but firm lateral grasp. If resistance is met at the external sphincter (5 or 6 inches), the patient is asked to relax and to pretend to pass urine. The catheter should never be forced in, but should be gently advanced. After urine begins to flow the catheter should be advanced 1 inch further to ensure proper placement in the bladder. Inflate the balloon and gently tug on the catheter to ensure proper placement. When the catheter is in place, reduce the foreskin. Tape the catheter to the patient's leg or abdomen to avoid penile necrosis resulting from excessive pressure.

If the catheter fails to pass, a different size, texture, or type (e.g., coudé, for men) of catheter can be tried. If this fails, urologic assistance should be sought.

Most facilities have their own detailed procedures for catheterization, and these should be consulted and followed accordingly.

Drainage Bags

If a closed catheter drainage system is not available, the catheter should immediately be connected to a drainage bag. The type of bag varies according to the needs of the individual patient. Most bags have a one-way valve at their inlet to prevent urine refluxing once it has entered the bag. Bags without this valve should not be used with an indwelling catheter (Fig. 15–5).

The patient who is bedridden or receiving continuous bladder irrigation will usually need the 2-liter capacity bag, which can be supported by a bed hanger or floor stand. These bags are also used for a short-term catheter and for overnight drainage with a long-term catheter.

Ambulatory patients, especially those whose catheters are to be in for more than a few days, will need a leg bag for daytime use (Fig. 15–6). This can have a capacity of 350, 500, or 750 ml. It is secured to the leg with straps that can be of latex, fabric, elastic, foam rubber, or Velcro. Leg straps can cause problems if they are too tight (a full bag can be heavy), and some people develop a sensitivity to latex. The inflow tubing can be short for thigh wearing or long for wearing over the knee or on the calf (under trousers). The calf bag is emptied by lifting up the bottom of the trousers. A thigh bag can be emptied more easily if a small Velcro-fastened opening is made in the inner trouser seam. Small leg bags can be concealed discreetly out of sight while wearing regular clothing.

It is important to select an outflow spigot that the patient can manage easily. Some bags have a removable rubber cap that could be easily dropped, and this is obviously unsuitable for those with poor manual dexterity. Some people find a push-pull valve easy, whereas others prefer a twist-and-pull type. Larger valves are often easier to

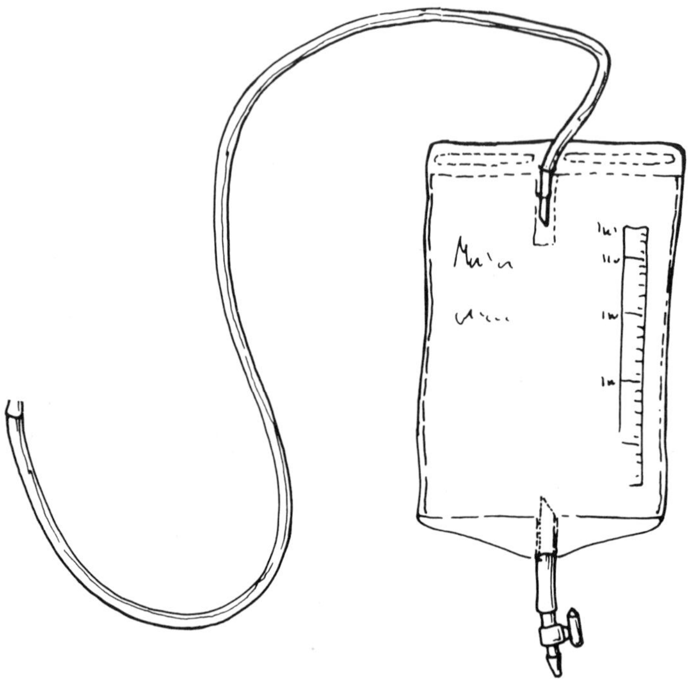

Figure 15–5. *Straight (night) drainage bag.*

manage, but can dig into the leg. Maintaining a closed sterile drainage system is the ideal but, for those patients who switch to a leg bag during the day, a larger drainage bag should be used at night. Prior to switching the drainage bags, proper hand washing should be carried out. Also, the catheter-tubing junction site should be cleaned with an antiseptic solution.

Some bags now incorporate baffles to spread the urine more evenly and allow the bag to conform to the contour of the leg.

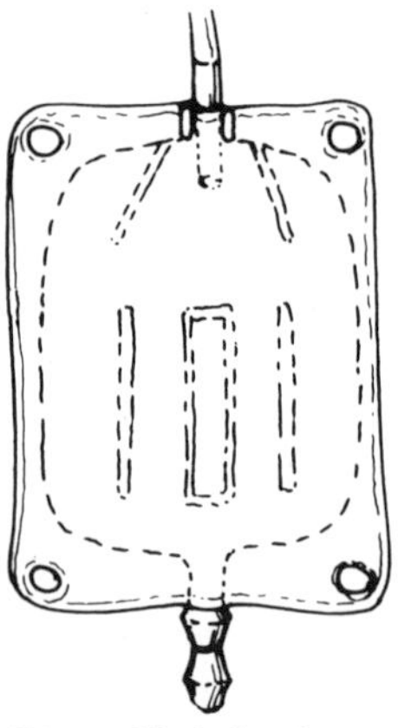

Figure 15–6. *Leg bag.*

Risk of Infection

The normal urinary tract has several defenses against infection. Complete bladder emptying, the regular scouring action of micturition, and a competent sphincter mechanism all help to prevent bacterial invasion and eradicate any microorganisms promptly and completely. The introduction of an indwelling catheter into this normally sterile system provides three potential entry portals for infection: on the catheter itself during insertion; along the catheter by way of the urethra; and on the path of ascent up the lumen of the catheter. The first can be largely discounted if strict aseptic technique is used for insertion. The second is more of a problem in the short female urethra, but defenses can be bolstered by ensuring that the catheter is small enough to allow free drainage of urethral secretions.

Ascending infection by way of the catheter lumen was the major source of infection in catheterized patients until the early 1960s. Prior to that time catheters were maintained on "open drainage," with the end of the catheter open and draining into a nonsterile vessel. With this system, almost all bladders were infected within 3 or 4 days of catheter insertion. Although this could be reduced to some extent by continuous antiseptic irrigation, infection rates remained high until the introduction of closed urinary drainage directly from the catheter into a sterile, sealed bag. Closed drainage lengthened the interval for development of infection from 4 to 30 days after catheter insertion. This has been the biggest single advance in catheter care.

Infection rates for catheters in place for less than 5 days can usually be kept below 10%, provided that the closed system is not interrupted (i.e., the catheter is never disconnected from the bag). After 5 days an increasing proportion of patients with catheters acquire a urinary tract infection. Despite precautions, nearly all are infected at 1 month. No method has been found that can significantly reduce this rising infection rate, except for keeping the system scrupulously uninterrupted. Routine bladder irrigations, systemic antibiotics, and antimicrobials in the drainage bag have all failed to alter the infection rate.

Catheters in place for an extended period inevitably become infected. The microorganisms are usually from the patients' own excretions (e.g., Escherichia coli), but almost any organism can invade the catheterized bladder, including more exotic bacteria, fungi, and yeast. A decision to use a catheter for long-term bladder management must be made with the awareness that infection will inevitably result.

Is there a consequence of this catheter-related infection? One in ten patients admitted to the hospital will have an indwelling catheter at some point during their admission. Of all nosocomial (hospital-acquired) infections, 40% are urinary tract infections and 70% of these are associated with the use of an indwelling catheter. There is evidence that patients catheterized during admission are likely to have a longer stay in the hospital, suffer more complications, and possibly have a higher mortality rate than patients with similar illness without a catheter (Platt and colleagues, 1982). The incidence of gram-negative bacteremias following catheterization is low but, when it does occur, it carries a 40% mortality rate. Patients catheterized because they are acutely ill or following urinary tract surgery are especially vulnerable to risks of serious complications.

If the catheter is likely to be in place short term, it is worth every effort to prevent or treat infection. Once the catheter is permanent, infection is unavoidable. Most studies regarding the effects of infection from long-term catheters have been done on patients with spinal injury. Many of these patients suffered renal impairment. Renal failure was the most common reason for death, apart from injury-related causes, and many patients were found to have scarred kidneys with pus on postmortem examination (Warren and associates, 1981).

Management

Short-Term Catheterization

For short-term catheterization (intended duration less than 1 week), the primary aim of management is prevention of urinary tract infection. The first question must always be "Is this catheter really necessary?" Surprisingly, the answer is often "no." If the catheter is suggested because the patient has failed to void (e.g., postoperatively), spontaneous voiding can be promoted by ensuring that the patient is not in pain and has adequate privacy and comfort to void, preferably on a toilet or commode. Running water, adequate time, and extra liquids work well for many patients. Catheters are frequently passed because the patient was uncomfortable or inhibited in voiding on a bedpan. If voiding is not achieved in the presence of a distended bladder or discomfort, intermittent catheterization should be used until spontaneous voiding returns. An external catheter is preferable to an indwelling catheter for male patients who must have their urinary output closely monitored, provided that the bladder is emptying completely.

After urologic surgery, a suprapubic catheter is often preferred because it can be clamped while the patient tries to void. If this fails, the catheter can be unclamped. This overcomes the problem of repeated catheter insertion in situations in which voiding problems are common. Some hospitals use catheters routinely in certain situations (e.g., orthopedic surgery) without consideration of individual needs and the risks involved.

If a urethral catheter is necessary for short-term use the duration of catheterization must be kept to an absolute minimum, preferably less than 5 days. If at all possible, a closed system between the catheter and drainage bag must be maintained. If a break is essential (e.g., to irrigate a blocked catheter), strict aseptic technique must be observed.

The drainage bag should be emptied at least once every 8 hours, using a "no-touch" technique and a clean container for each patient. Hand washing before and after handling the catheter or bag is important and helps to prevent cross contamination. For the same reason the bag should always be hung from the bed and never allowed to touch the floor. Some experts believe that catheterized patients should be separated from one another to prevent cross contamination. Going even further, others have suggested separation of infected and uninfected catheterized patients (Plantemoli, 1984). The CDC Guideline for Prevention of Catheter-Associated Urinary Tract Infections has weakly recommended adopting this practice (Wong, 1983). Although this might sound appropriate in theory, it could be difficult and costly to implement.

The value of routine meatal care is unclear. Some have suggested (Friedman, 1982; Engram, 1983) that catheter care, for both short-term and long-term catheters, should involve careful washing of the genital area with soap and water at least twice daily. On the other hand, a study conducted by Burke and associates (1983) suggested that twice-daily meatal care with a polyantibiotic ointment is not beneficial in the prevention of urinary tract infections and that daily bathing is sufficient. The CDC has not endorsed the practice of meatal care (Wong, 1983). Using antiseptic solutions for catheter care has no proven value and, in some cases (e.g., povidone iodine), has been found to increase infection rates. When possible a daily bath should be taken, using only soap and avoiding additives. In men, the foreskin should be retracted, the glans penis cleaned, and the foreskin replaced. The genital area should then be dried thoroughly with a clean soft towel. Talcum powder should be avoided because it can block the meatus around the catheter and irritate the perineum. Careful washing after each bowel movement should also be encouraged. Women should be instructed on correct perineal cleaning (e.g., wiping from front to back, away from the catheter). If the patient has a discharge of blood or mucus around the catheter, it should be carefully cleaned away using soap and water.

Bladder irrigations should not be used routinely in short-term catheter management. They do not prevent infection and they break the system, providing an opportunity for bacterial invasion. Similarly, systemic antibiotics have no place in the prevention of infection and can even provoke the emergence of antibiotic-resistant strains, but they should be used appropriately to treat symptomatic infection.

Drainage bags on short-term catheters are not changed routinely. If the bag becomes clogged with sediment it is replaced using aseptic technique; otherwise, most bags last 2 to 4 weeks.

If a urine specimen is to be collected from a catheter, the closed system should not be broken to take the sample. Most bags have a self-sealing sample port on the drainage tubing. The tubing should be clamped just below the port and left for several minutes for urine to accumulate above the clamp. (The nurse should stay with the patient whenever the catheter is clamped to prevent overdistention of the bladder.) The sample port should be cleaned with alcohol. The specimen is taken using a sterile needle and syringe. The needle is inserted at an angle (to avoid piercing the tubing and the nurse's finger). Urine should never be squirted into a specimen container with the needle attached to the syringe, because this can destroy any cells or casts present. The needle should always be removed.

Urine specimens should never be taken from the drainage bag. The specimen should be delivered to the laboratory within 1 hour of sampling. If this is not possible, it should be refrigerated under 40° F (4.5° C) until it can be delivered.

It has been reported (Nanninga, 1980) that routine urine cultures are of little value and should be avoided. On the other hand, if the patient is symptomatic (e.g., fever, chills, lower abdominal pain, cloudy urine, hematuria, burning around the catheter), a culture should be obtained and sensitivity testing done to determine the appropriate antibiotic for treatment.

If a patient is gravely ill and a septicemia from the urinary tract is suspected, a urine culture should be obtained. Septicemia is a life-threatening situation and merits immediate attention.

Long-Term Catheterization

As stated earlier, the use of a long-term catheter can be a positive decision for patient management, but it must always be made with the risks of infection in mind. The likely benefits and costs should be considered for each individual. For younger patients with prolonged management by catheter, renal problems become a major cause of morbidity and mortality (Warren and colleagues, 1981). Renal impairment caused by prolonged catheter use is less likely to occur if the patient is elderly or has a limited life expectancy. For younger patients, who might need a catheter for decades, every possible alternative should be seriously considered (e.g., suprapubic catheter, intermittent catheterization, or urinary diversion).

Hospital Care. The long-term catheter in a hospitalized patient should be managed in much the same way as the short-term catheter, but with the knowledge that infection probably cannot be prevented and will only be treated if the patient becomes symptomatic. Hospitals are prone to harbor multiresistant organisms and the aim must be to minimize cross contamination.

Home Management. Home management of the long-term catheter is inevitably different. It is often impossible to adhere to rigorous aseptic technique. Actually, it is usually unnecessary, because organisms are likely to be from the patient's own excretions. It is most important for the patient or caregiver to understand fully how to care for the catheter. A fearful patient, afraid to touch the catheter, will be far less successful than the confident patient. To this end, time must always be allotted for the newly catheterized patient to discuss any worries. Careful instructions and comprehension by the patient and caregiver are vital to successful home management.

The following explanation and instructions to the patient can be useful:

1. The catheter is a hollow tube that is draining urine from your bladder into a bag. You will not need to pass water yourself. These simple instructions will help you to look after your catheter properly.

2. When possible, a daily bath is recommended. Wash the area around your urethra and the catheter thoroughly. This should be done with plain (unscented) soap and warm water and the area should be dried thoroughly with a soft towel. Avoid use of talcum powder in the area. Also, wash this area thoroughly after a bowel movement.

3. Drink 8 to 10 large glasses of fluid every 24 hours. This means about 1 cupful of liquid every hour when you are awake.

4. Wear the leg bag when you are up and use the bedside drainage bag at night. Always wash your hands thoroughly before and after changing the bags. Prior to switching the drainage bags, clean all tubing junctions with alcohol. After switching the bag, rinse it thoroughly with water. Fill it with a vinegar-and-water solution (one part vinegar and three parts water) or a commercial decrystallizer. Let it soak for 30 minutes, empty, and hang to dry before the next use.

5. The bags will need to be changed if they leak, become odorous or malodorous, have sediment build-up, or if the catheter is changed. Each bag will last about 1 month.

6. When possible, exercise daily.

7. Avoid constipation, because this can prevent the catheter from draining properly. If constipation is a problem, consult your physician.

8. Avoid bending or kinking the catheter tubing. Always keep the bag below bladder level to ensure good drainage.

9. Tape the catheter to your abdomen or leg, and allow some slack to prevent undue pressure.

The patient should also be told that some common problems can arise with long-term catheter use.

1. Bladder spasms or cramps in the abdomen are common when a new catheter has been inserted. They are nothing to worry about, and usually pass within 1 day. If they persist, consult your physician.

2. If no urine drains for several hours:

Is the tubing bent or kinked?
Is the bag below the bladder level?
Is the leg bag connected with the correct end toward the top?
Have you been drinking enough?
Are you constipated?
Try moving or walking around.
Irrigate the catheter to try to unplug it.
If the catheter cannot be cleared with irrigation it will be necessary to have the catheter changed.

3. If your catheter leaks it is not serious, but should be reported. Medication (e.g., Pro-Banthine or Ditropan) might be necessary to stop bladder spasms or leakage of urine around the catheter (or both).

4. If the catheter falls out, another one will have to be inserted.

5. If you see blood in the urine do not worry, but increase your fluids. If the bleeding is heavy or persists, consult your physician.

6. If your catheter is causing you problems during sexual intercourse, do not hesitate to discuss this with your physician.

Your physician is:
Address:
Telephone no. during office hours (_____ AM–_____ PM):
Emergency no. for other times:

7. Please feel free to discuss any problems or questions you might have about your catheter.

The patient must be shown and given supervised practice in caring for the catheter. This includes instructions on daily bathing, as well as hanging, emptying, and cleaning the bags. It is not necessary to use sterile drainage bags in the home, provided that good hand washing is done. A leg bag is used in the daytime and a bedside bag is used at night. After each change the bag is rinsed with plain water. Daily cleaning should include the instillation of a vinegar-and-water solution (one part vinegar and three parts water) or a commercial decrystallizer. This reduces sedimentation and odor in the bag. The bag is then hung to dry. Each bag can be used for at least 1 month, often longer if there is little sediment.

The patient is told to drink plenty of fluid (at least 2 liters per day), to exercise to avoid sediment accumulation, and to avoid constipation. (Some people who have had an indwelling catheter for an extended period of time find that drinking distilled water markedly reduces the rate of sediment accumulation.)

Catheter-Associated Problems

Catheter Cramps

Most people experience cramps (often likened by women to menstrual pains) when a catheter is first inserted. A mild analgesic and simple reassurance that the cramps will settle down within 24 hours and that this is nothing to worry about will suffice for most patients. If cramps persist and are troublesome, the cause is usually unstable bladder contractions. Sometimes a smaller catheter or a smaller balloon will stop this. An anticholinergic or antispasmodic drug is usually the most effective remedy. In some people the cramps are severe enough to make catheterization inappropriate, and another form of management must be used.

Urethral Discomfort

Some urethral discomfort is common with an indwelling catheter, and this often has to be accepted. Silicone or silicone-coated or hydromer-coated catheters might be more comfortable than latex. The discomfort can be caused by a large catheter mechanically distending the urethra or occluding the paraurethral glands, leading to infection, urethritis, and an offensive discharge around the catheter. A smaller catheter should be tried if this occurs. In postmenopausal women, discomfort can be caused by atrophic urethritis, and a course of estrogen replacement therapy relieves the discomfort (Chap. 8).

Leaking Catheters

One of the most common reasons for catheter failure and premature change is leakage around the catheter. It is present in up to 40% of all patients with a catheter and is the reason for one-third of unplanned catheter changes (Kennedy and Brocklehurst, 1982; Kennedy and co-workers, 1983). This is particularly irksome if the catheter was placed to control incontinence, because not only is the patient still wet, but there is the additional problem of catheter care.

A leaking catheter is usually caused by an unstable bladder. The bladder is irritated by the presence of the catheter and contracts, squeezing urine out around the lumen of the catheter. Often, using a smaller catheter or less water in the balloon decreases the irritation and thus reduces the leakage. Also, with a smaller balloon, there is less residual urine available to leak. If a catheter leaks some fluid should be taken out of the balloon and, if that does not help, a smaller catheter can be tried. Anticholinergic or antispasmodic medication can help to stop the contractions (e.g., propantheline or oxybutynin).

The catheter might be leaking because it is plugged. Irrigating the catheter with 50 ml of sterile saline solution can help clear it of the obstruction. (In the hospital, this can be done aseptically through the sample port by clamping the tubing below the port.) It might also be plugged because of kinked tubing or because the bag has consistently been above the bladder level.

Hematuria

A small amount of blood in the urine of catheterized patients is common and is of no importance. It is usually caused by trauma, infection, or both. If hematuria becomes heavy and persistent, urologic advice should be sought.

Infection

In the patient with a long-term catheter, infection is both inevitable and usually asymptomatic. It is futile to treat these infections, because generally the urine is cleared only for a few days, if at all (Brocklehurst and Brocklehurst, 1978), and there is a danger of more pathogenic organisms invading the bladder or of resistance developing. Prophylactic antibiotics or antimicrobial irrigations have no place in catheter management.

If the patient becomes ill, however, the infection must be treated. Symptoms can include fever, chills, suprapubic pain, significant hematuria and, in the elderly, the unexplained sudden onset of confusion (Conti, 1987). The catheter might have to be removed for treatment to be successful.

Erosion of the Bladder Wall

If a catheter is on continuous drainage, the tip of the catheter is always in contact with the bladder wall and can cause ulcers in the mucosa. Some evidence has shown that prolonged use of a catheter predisposes to bladder malignancies, and chronic irritation might be the cause. The practice of intermittent catheter release to reduce irritation is not usually advocated by urologists. If the catheter is left clamped inadvertently it can cause overdistention and infection (Bates, 1981). Proper venting of the drainage bag or catheter prevents erosion of the bladder wall from occurring (Kunin, 1984).

Sediment, Encrustation, and Stones

Infection and secretions indicate that most patients with a long-term catheter have some sediment in their urine. This is a particular problem in the immobile patient, because sediment accumulates and can eventually block the drainage eyes. Patients are therefore encouraged to be as mobile as possible. If the patient cannot move, regular passive changes of position are recommended.

All indwelling catheters become encrusted to some extent. The use of silicone or silicone-coated catheters can lessen the amount of buildup but does not prevent encrustation. This can block the lumen and eyes of the catheter and can make the balloon difficult to deflate. Some bacteria, notably Proteus, produce the urea-splitting enzyme urease. When urease splits urea it releases ammonia and free hydrogen ions. This process encourages the precipitation of salts from urine—typically the three phosphates of ammonia, calcium, and magnesium. Stones can form around the nucleus of clumps of bacteria or encrustations can accumulate around the catheter. Once stones are present it is impossible to eradicate infection, and the stones can cause pain or bleeding or block the catheter. In immobile patients, re-uptake of calcium from the bones can make calcium available in the urine for stone formation.

Some patients seem to be more prone to sediment, encrustation, or stones than others. A few are inveterate catheter blockers and, for these people, it is worth increasing fluid intake to 3 liters daily, if tolerated. Routine bladder irrigations are suggested for those patients whose catheter frequently becomes obstructed (Brocklehurst and Brocklehurst, 1978). The practice of routine irrigation is controversial among physicians in the United States. The CDC has recommended irrigating catheters only when necessary to prevent or relieve obstruction (Wong, 1983), along with liberal fluid intake, if not contraindicated.

If a patient's catheter becomes blocked repeatedly, it is pointless to use expensive catheters. A latex catheter can be used when the catheter needs to be changed. Alternatively, another form of management might have to be considered.

No Drainage

Urine normally drains into the bladder continuously, so it should drain out continuously. If a catheter has failed to drain any urine, or only minimal amounts, over a period of several hours, the cause should be investigated. Sometimes the drainage tube has been inadvertently left clamped or connections are kinked. The bag might be overfull and will not admit more urine. Rectal examination can reveal that fecal impaction is interfering with catheter drainage.

The catheter might be blocked, thus preventing drainage. It can be gently rolled between two fingers and encrustation might be felt. Bladder irrigation can unblock the lumen or eyes. Fifty milliliters of sterile saline solution can be instilled and allowed to drain back. If nothing returns, 50-ml increments can be added (unless of course the patient is already experiencing discomfort or has an overdistended bladder). The saline solution should not be removed by the suction of a syringe, because the walls of the catheter can collapse and occlude the lumen completely and the bladder mucosa can be sucked into the drainage eyes. If irrigation fails to unplug the catheter, it should be removed and replaced. The removed catheter should be inspected for the site and type of blockage. If the second catheter fails to drain, the patient might be anuric. Provided that the patient is not dehydrated, this is a sign of renal failure that requires urgent medical attention.

Sexual Activity

It is possible for both men and women who have a urethral catheter in place to engage in sexual intercourse. Men can tape the catheter back along the shaft of the penis. This is not generally recommended, however, because discomfort is common for both partners and hemorrhage can occur. Considerable trauma to the urethra is inevitable, and repeated intercourse might eventually cause stricture formation. Intercourse will not be the pleasurable activity it should be if there is discomfort. Urethral catheters are probably best avoided for the sexually active person (this includes both the elderly and the young), and alternatives such as suprapubic catheters should be considered, especially for men. If a urethral catheter is necessary it might be feasible to teach patients or their partners to remove the catheter prior to intercourse and to insert a new one afterward. Women with a urethral catheter can find that a lateral position is more comfortable for intercourse. Because sexual activity is a difficult topic for many people to discuss, it is usually up to the nurse to introduce it and encourage the discussion of problems.

Catheter Changes

The interval between catheter changes should be geared to the individual patient's needs. Some people experience repeated catheter plugging and it is best to change it routinely every 2 to 4 weeks to preempt problems (Nanninga, 1980). Others can be safely left up to 3 months without problems (Blannin and Hobden, 1980). Usually the first catheter is changed after 2 to 4 weeks, with the interval being increased until the patient's limit of tolerance is found. Sometimes catheters are left in place until problems develop. This approach is recommended by the CDC (Wong, 1983). Many change the catheter at a fixed interval, however, to circumvent problems. In the community it is preferable to anticipate problems, because they often occur at night or over a weekend. It is a good idea to leave a complete catheter set in the home so that, if a nurse unfamiliar with the patient is called in, the correct replacement catheter is at hand and the patient does not have to be brought to the hospital for the catheter change.

Catheter Removal

To remove a Foley catheter, the water is drawn out of the balloon with a syringe. The widespread practice of intermittent catheter clamping and release prior to catheter withdrawal, often called "bladder training" and said to restore "bladder tone," has no proven value. The functional bladder usually resumes normal filling and emptying soon after the catheter is out, provided that fluid intake is adequate and the patient is allowed enough time, privacy, and comfort in which to void. Micturition might be uncomfortable at first, and the patient should be reassured that this is temporary.

If voiding has not been achieved within 6 hours of catheter removal, or if the bladder becomes distended or painful, intermittent catheterization is performed until normal function returns. If normal function does not return, intermittent catheterization might need to be continued indefinitely.

The Nondeflating Balloon

Occasionally a catheter balloon will not deflate with a syringe. It is important when inflating a balloon to use only sterile water and to be sure that no contaminants come into contact with the water (e.g., powder from sterile gloves). The inflation lumen is extremely narrow and easily blocked. If saline or another solution is used, the solutes can precipitate out to block the lumen.

Attempting to break a nondeflating balloon with extra water is not recommended. (It takes up to 100 ml of water to break a 5-ml balloon and up to 200 ml to break a 30-ml balloon). The trauma can damage the bladder mucosa, and there is a high risk of leaving small particles of the balloon behind. These particles will almost always form the nucleus for stone formation. The balloon should not be dissolved (e.g., with ether). Chemicals can cause an acute chemical cystitis, again with the risk of some particles of balloon remaining inside the bladder. The inflation arm should not be cut.

If any of these problems occur, the urologist should be notified. The urologist might break the balloon using a long stylet through the inflation lumen. The urologist might puncture the balloon under anesthesia, by way of the perineum in men or the vagina in women, or under radiographic control by the abdominal route. With all these methods the catheter and balloon must be examined carefully and, if there is any suspicion that pieces have been left behind, the particles must be removed cystoscopically. Any faulty catheters should be reported to the manufacturer for investigation.

Catheter Teams

Catheterization teams have been formed in some health care facilities. In addition, allied health personnel are being educated in the placement and care of patients with long-term indwelling Foley catheters. Patients and their families are instructed in the self-management of their catheters prior to hospital discharge (Newman and colleagues, 1986). Nurses who perform these functions often greatly improve patient management by introducing planned regimes of catheter care, anticipating problems, and being of assistance in the patient's own home. The proper care of patients managed with catheters by home health care professionals can greatly reduce the need for repeated hospital visits, and can provide continuity of care between hospital and community for patients being discharged home with a catheter for the first time. Further research is needed to evaluate the cost-effectiveness and improvements in patient care provided by such nurse specialists.

Conclusions

The decision to catheterize must never be made lightly, and should always be made with both the benefits and risks in mind. One of the most important factors in the successful use of a catheter is effective communication between all persons involved: patient, family (or other caregivers), nurse, and physician. Written records should always be kept of catheter size, type, changes, and problems. As with any other aspect of nursing care, planned management rather than crisis intervention is of greater benefit to the patient.

The more the patient is involved in catheter care, the better. If self-care is handled confidently and without fear, independence will be greatly enhanced (Blannin, 1982).

The catheter must always be placed for a reason. Professional attention is often focused on sorting out catheter problems rather than asking why it is necessary. If the catheter is causing more problems than it solves, take it out. Much can still be learned about ideal catheter management, and more research is needed before optimum management is available for all.

SUPRAPUBIC CATHETER

A suprapubic catheter is a catheter inserted directly into the bladder through the anterior abdominal wall. It is placed by a physician, under either general or local anesthetic.

Indications

The suprapubic catheter is especially useful after pelvic or urologic surgery, when the patient might have difficulty in resuming voiding. The catheter can be clamped for a trial of voiding. If unsuccessful, the catheter can merely be unclamped again, thus avoiding repeated urethral catheterizations (Hilton and Stanton, 1980). The suprapubic catheter is also useful for patients with acute retention, because voiding can be attempted without catheter removal.

The suprapubic catheter can be used for long-term drainage, especially in sexually active patients and in those experiencing problems with urethral catheters. In some women the urethra might have been

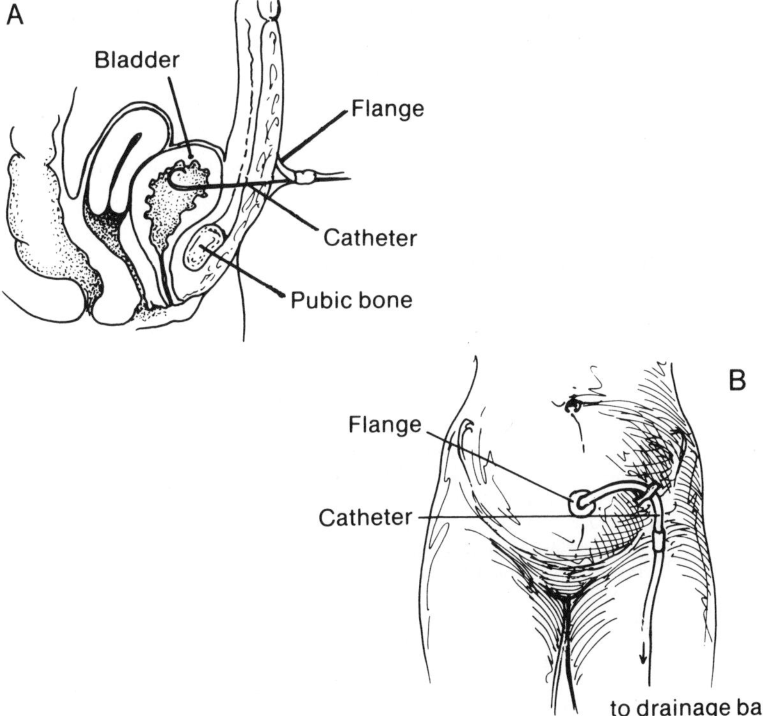

Figure 15–7. *Suprapubic catheter.* A, *Side view.* B, *Front view.*

closed surgically, thus necessitating the use of this type of catheter (Zimmern and colleagues, 1985).

The Catheters

There are several types of suprapubic catheter. Sizes range from 6 to 16 F. Some are secured to the abdominal wall by a retention disk, stitch, or tape; whereas others have a balloon for retaining the catheter (Fig. 15–7). Foley catheters can also be used.

Management

The use of suprapubic catheters is associated with lower infection rates than urethral catheters. The urethral defense mechanism is left intact and the entry site is relatively easy to keep clean. The entry site should be inspected daily, gently cleaned with a mild antiseptic, and covered with a dressing. Otherwise management is the same as for urethral catheters; the same bags can be used and the same instructions given to patients (see above). If the skin around the puncture site becomes infected, systemic antibiotics might be necessary.

Once the tract has been established, the catheter can usually be changed easily by medical or nursing staff through the original tract, without further anesthetic. When the suprapubic catheter is no longer needed it can be removed easily. The openings in the abdominal and bladder walls normally close spontaneously, without complication.

References and Further Reading

Bates, P.: A troubleshooter's guide to indwelling catheters. R.N., *44:*62, 1981.

Blandy, J.P.: How to catheterize the bladder. Br. J. Hosp. Med., *26:*58, 1981.

Blannin, J.P.: Catheter management. Nurs. Times, *78:*438, 1982.

Blannin, J.P., and Hobden, J.: The catheter of choice. Nurs. Times, *76:*2092, 1980.

Brunner, L.S., and Suddarth, D.S.: Textbook of Medical Surgical Nursing. 6th ed. Philadelphia, J.B. Lippincott, 1988.

Brocklehurst, J.C., and Brocklehurst, S.: The management of indwelling catheters. Br. J. Urol., *50:*102, 1978.

Burke, J.P., et al.: Evaluation of daily meatal care with poly-antibiotic ointment in prevention of urinary catheter-associated bacteriuria. J. Urol., *129:*331, 1983.

Conti, M.T., and Eurtopius, L.: Preventing UTI's: What works? Am. J. Nurs., *87:*307, 1987.

Cule, J.: Forerunners of Foley. Nurs. Mirror, *150:*1, 1980.

Engram, B.W.: Do's and don'ts of urologic nursing. Nursing '83, *13:*49, 1983.

Friedman, F.B. (ed.): Why not use a Foley? R.N., *45:*71, 1982.

Hilton, P., and Stanton, S.L.: Suprapubic catheterization. Br. Med. J., *281:*1261, 1980.

Kelly, T.W.J., and Griffiths, G.L.: Balloon problems with Foley catheters. Lancet, *2:*1310, 1983.

Kennedy, A.P., and Brocklehurst, J.C.: The nursing management of patients with long-term indwelling catheters. J. Adv. Nurs., *7:*411, 1982.

Kennedy, A.P., Brocklehurst, J.C., and Lye, M.D.W.: Factors related to the problems of long-term catheterization. J. Adv. Nurs., *8:*207, 1983.

Kunin, C.M.: Genitourinary infections in the patient at risk: Extrinsic risk factors. Am. J. Med., *76* (Suppl.):131, 1984.

Luckmann, J., and Sorensen, K.C.: Medical-Surgical Nursing: A psychophysiologic approach. 3rd ed. Philadelphia, W.B. Saunders, 1987.

McGill, S.: It's the size that's important. Nurs. Mirror, *154:*48, 1982.

Milles, G.: Catheter-induced hemorrhagic pseudopolyps of the urinary bladder. J.A.M.A., *193:*196, 1965.

Moisey, C.U., and Williams, L.A.: Self-retained balloon catheters: A safe method for removal. Br. J. Urol., *52:*67, 1980.

Nanninga, J.B.: Care of the catheter-dependent patient. Urol. Clin. North Am., *7:*41, 1980.

Newman, E., Price, M., and Magney, J.: Care of the Disabled Urinary Tract: Prevention of Renal Deterioration. Springfield, IL, Charles C Thomas, 1986.

Plantemoli, L.V.: When the patient has a Foley. R.N., *47:*42, 1984.

Platt, R., et al.: Mortality associated with nosocomial urinary tract infection. N. Engl. J. Med., *307:*637, 1982.

Spees, E.K., et al.: Unsuspected intraperitoneal perforation of the urinary bladder as an iatrogenic disorder. Surgery, *89:*224, 1981.

Stamm, W.E.: Guidelines for prevention of catheter-associated urinary tract infections. Ann. Intern. Med., *82:*386, 1975.

Warren, J.W., et al.: Sequelae and management of urinary infection in the patient requiring chronic catheterization. J. Urol., *125:*1, 1981.

Wilde, M.H.: Living with a Foley. Am. J. Nurs., *86:*1121, 1986.

Wong, E.S.: Guidelines for prevention of catheter-associated urinary tract infections. Am. J. Infect. Control, *11:*28, 1983.

Zimmern, P.E., et al.: Transvaginal closure of the bladder neck and placement of a suprapubic catheter for destroyed urethra after long-term indwelling catheterization. J. Urol., *134:*554, 1985.

Diane Smith, RN, MSN, CRNP
Diane K. Newman, RN, MSN, CRNP

16 The Role of Continence Nurse Specialists

Most of the suggested nursing interventions in this book do not require a specialist. Bladder retraining, pelvic muscle exercises, selection of products, intermittent catheterization, modification of the environment, and bowel management are well within the scope of the nurse's capabilities. Given adequate time and an understanding of necessary information, there is little difficulty in making a nursing assessment of the problem.

If incontinence is every nurse's business, is there a need for a continence nurse specialist? The answer is "yes." They need not be used for day-to-day management nor for the assessment and treatment of every incontinent person. They should serve as clinical support for nurses who have incontinent patients, as catalysts for improved care and coordination of services, and as educators and researchers.

DEVELOPMENT OF THE SPECIALTY

The United States currently lags behind Great Britain in nationwide promotion of continence through the development of nursing specialists or continence advisors. Many nurses now have great expertise in dealing with incontinence but there is no system comparable to that in England. Even in England the development of continence advisors (specialists) is a fairly recent phenomenon.

Almost all continence advisor positions in England started within the past decade. Different branches of the government fund these nursing specialists and assign them to a geographic area and scope of practice. Most of the original positions were created in the context of research-based urologic evaluation clinics. Often a nurse was hired on a research grant to assist with urodynamic investigations and to supervise patients during these procedures. From this limited role, many continence advisors became interested in the nursing aspects of incontinence and sought information on conservative and noninvasive methods for management. Such information was hard to obtain because little had been published. This prompted some nurses to conduct their own research and write nursing articles. A few obtained grants to conduct nursing research on incontinence. Most were asked to give talks and lectures to various groups of professional and lay people.

In the United States there has been no formal establishment of continence specialists. A number of nurses with advanced education see the importance of their work and achieve a high level of expertise.

Many of the present specialists saw the need for continence management and became involved in continence promotion because of the lack of medical support for incontinent patients. Many ET (enterostomal therapy) nurses have started to promote continence, as have other nurse specialists involved in research on incontinence. Some cities now have continence clinics that employ nurses with advanced education. These nurse specialists can be involved in the total assessment of the incontinent patient and in planning care. A few have continence clinics and private practices. It might be timely for these nurses to share their expertise and develop a recognized continence specialist role for nurses in the United States.

SCOPE OF A CONTINENCE NURSE SPECIALIST

The role of a continence nurse specialist should include patient assessment and management, teaching, involvement in urodynamic and continence clinics and outreach programs, providing advisory services, being familiar with continence products, engaging in research, and acting as links with manufacturers.

Patient Assessment and Management

Continence nurse specialists assess and manage incontinence. In some situations they may direct a self-referral clinic where they treat patients individually or suggest management techniques to caregivers. Nursing management of incontinent patients often involves noninvasive techniques, such as toileting programs and pelvic muscle exercises. These interventions are particularly helpful with elderly patients for whom surgery or pharmacologic treatment is not advised. The NIH Consensus Development Conference in 1988 suggested that these behavioral interventions be the front line of treatment for incontinence.

Involvement in Urodynamic and Continence Clinics

Many continence nurse specialists are part of the team in a continence clinic. They might direct the clinical aspects, including urodynamics, or they might have administrative responsibilities. Ideally, they provide consultation to acute and long-term care facilities. They might initiate the establishment and delivery of outpatient and home care services.

Teaching

Education should be the primary role of continence nurse specialists. This can include promotion of continence through community education and programs for professionals. Their time is best used to teach others how to assess and manage simple problems. Emphasis should be placed on the types of problems that should be referred to the specialist. Education also includes writing articles for publication.

Advisory Services

Continence specialists should act as resources. They should keep up to date with all current literature and trends in the field and should maintain a reference library. They should be available for consultation, by phone or in person, about all aspects of incontinence. This can include recommending a new product, references on catheter management, suggesting that a voiding diary for a specific condition be kept, and providing information about the latest research on urinary tract infections. Samples of continence products should be maintained so that patients and professionals can see what is available.

Familiarity with Continence Products

Continence nurse specialists should be familiar with products and local suppliers. A resource guide has been published by HIP (Help for Incontinent People, 1988). A list of current products is provided in Appendix I. When selecting products for patients, continence nurse specialists should consider functional and environmental constraints.

Research

Continence nurse specialists should be involved in research. If continence is to become recognized as a specialized area of nursing practice, it must become more research-based. This is true at every level, from small-scale descriptive studies to major research projects.

Links with Manufacturers

Continence nurse specialists must maintain liaison with industry to stay abreast of product research and development. Conversely, they can give manufacturers sensitive feedback on product performance and ideas for future development. Progressive companies are willing to invest heavily in education. They believe that increased awareness about incontinence will drive the market for improved quality.

Outreach Programs

There are many potential areas of interest for continence nurse specialists, but it is not possible to list them all here. Special areas of interest can include specialized mental health and geriatric programs, family planning or women's health clinics, nutrition sites for the elderly, and senior citizen clubs. Local circumstances and priorities dictate how far the continence nurse specialist can become involved in activities to promote continence.

THE DANGERS OF SPECIALIZATION

It has been argued that if every nurse were properly educated, specialists would be superfluous. This assumes that some future Utopia will exist, in which all nurses will have the basic education and desire to maintain current in every aspect of their practice, including continence promotion. This is unrealistic, especially in view of the current nursing shortage. Incontinence is a subject with so many factors involved that it is difficult to imagine how individual nurses could keep up with all new developments.

The various liaison functions outlined above merit a designated specialist to represent the interests of both patients and nurses.

Antipathy to the continence specialist in England has arisen because people feared fragmentation of patient care. It is not difficult to see how nurses might resent various specialists providing particular aspects of care, leaving the more "boring" routine work to the non-specialist.

The continence nurse specialist strengthens the validity of the role by freely sharing interventions with the purpose of enabling the general nurse to practice autonomously. When mutual suspicion gives way to mutual understanding and respect, specialists can make a significant contribution to nursing practice.

SUPPORT FOR THE CONTINENCE NURSE SPECIALIST

In England formal support is provided by the Association of Continence Advisors, which was founded in 1981 with the aim of opening up communication channels among interested professionals. Membership is multidisciplinary and is not confined to continence nurse specialists. The association holds one national conference annually, and a network of regional branches meets more frequently. Such an organization is needed in the United States to promote continence and the role of nurse continence specialists.

It seems safe at present to say that many nurses are not delivering the optimum possible care to their incontinent patients, and that they need advice on how to improve that care and support in implementing it. A large majority of incontinent people could regain continence if they were diagnosed accurately and treated correctly. Many of those with intractable problems could be helped to live fuller and more independent lives with appropriate management techniques. The continence nurse specialist must work with all nurses and other professionals, and with incontinent people and their caregivers, to help increase awareness, disseminate information, and provide facilities for tackling and alleviating this most distressing condition.

References

Badger, F.J., Drummond, M.F., and Isaacs, B.: Some issues in the clinical, social, and economic evaluation of new nursing services. J. Adv. Nurs., *8:*487, 1983.

Blannin, J.P.: Towards a better life. Nurs. Mirror, *150:*31, 1980.

Brink, C., Wells, T., and Diokno, A.: A continence clinic for the aged. J. Gerontol. Nurs., *9:*651, 1983.

Harris, J.: A positive step. Nurs. Mirror, *158:*16, 1984.

Incontinence Action Group: Action on Incontinence. London, Kings Fund Centre, 1983.

NIH Consensus Development Conference on Urinary Incontinence in Adults. Bethesda, MD, October 3–5, 1988.

Norton, C.S.: Challenging specialty. Nurs. Mirror, *159:*xiv, 1984.

Ramsbottom, F.: Advising the nurse. Nurs. Times, *78:*24, 1982.

Ramsbottom, F.: Is advice really cheap? J. Commun. Nurs., May:9, 1982.

Rooney, V.: A question of habit. Nurs. Mirror, *154:*ii, 1982.

Shepard, A.M., Blannin, J.P., and Feneley, R.C.L.: Changing attitudes in the management of urinary incontinence—the need for specialist nursing. Br. Med. J., *284:*645, 1982.

Wells, T.J., et al.: Urinary incontinence in elderly women—clinical findings. J. Am. Geriatr. Soc., *35:*933, 1987.

White, H.: Setting up an advisory service. J. Commun. Nurs., September:4, 1982.

Appendix I

PRODUCTS AND MANUFACTURERS

The product listings section in this appendix is divided into five subsections: (1) Disposable Products; (2) Reusable Products; (3) Devices; (4) Skin Care Products; and (5) Miscellaneous. The manufacturers' index section includes addresses, telephone numbers, and products. In addition, manufacturers are assigned an identification number. This number is given in the product section in parentheses and can be used to find manufacturers in the manufacturers' index.

To use this appendix, follow this example:

Title of subsection

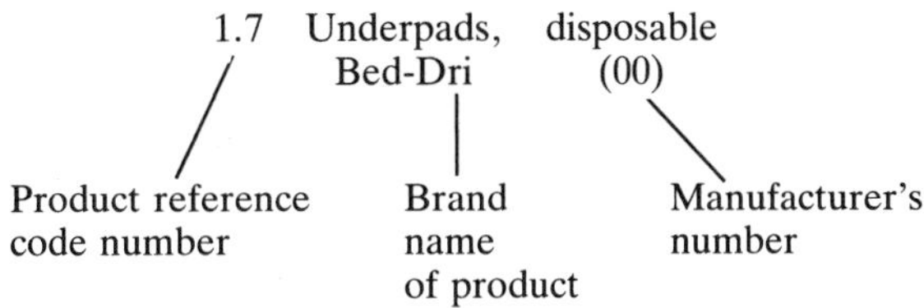

1. Look at the product reference code list (see below) and find the subtitle Underpads, Disposable. To the left of the title is its product code number, 1.7.
2. Now turn to the product section to find code 1.7. Here you will find a description of the item, a picture of the product, and a list of brands available.
3. The number in parentheses after the brand name is the manufacturer's number. The complete listing is given in the manufacturers' index (below). Note that national retail chain stores are not assigned a manufacturer's number.

From Resource Guide of Continence Products and Services, 3rd ed. HIP, Inc., Union, SC, 1988.

Product Listings

Throughout this product listing section the following symbols and codes are used:

* Asterisk indicates that the product has a superabsorbent layer to gel fluid.

*• Asterisk and circle indicate that the product is available with or without superabsorbents.

1.0 DISPOSABLE PRODUCTS

1.1 Absorbent brief with elastic legs
1.2 Absorbent brief without elastic legs
1.3 Pad-and-pant starter kit
1.4 Absorbent insert—flat
1.5 Absorbent insert—contoured
1.6 Undergarment
1.7 Underpads, disposable
1.8 Male envelope-style dribble collector

2.0 REUSABLE PRODUCTS

2.1 Diaper—flat
2.2 Diaper—contoured
2.3 Brief—reusable
2.4 Brief—mesh stretch
2.5 Drawsheet
2.6 Reusable liner—flat
2.7 Reusable liner—contoured
2.8 Underpads, reusable
2.9 Men's protective support
2.91 Men's protective brief
2.92 Men's drip collector
2.93 Men's protective boxer-style short

3.0 DEVICES

3.1 Condom catheter for men—self-adhesive
3.2 Condom catheter for men—with adhering strips
3.21 Condom catheter for men—with inflatable ring
3.3 Male urinal with supporter
3.3 Male urinal with supporter
3.4 Female external collecting device
3.5 Leg bag
3.6 Leg bag straps or holder
3.61 Catheter tube holder
3.7 Bedside drainage bag or bottle and covers

4.0 SKIN CARE PRODUCTS

4.1 Wet wipes
4.2 Cleanser
4.3 Deodorizer
4.4 Moisturizing cream, lotion, or salve
4.41 Antibacterial and antifungal cream
4.5 Barrier film, cream, or salve

5.0 MISCELLANEOUS

5.1 Catheters for intermittent catheterization
5.2 Enuresis alarm
5.3 Fecal incontinence collection system
5.4 On-the-go urinal for men and women
5.5 Oral deodorant tablets
5.6 Perineometer and pelvic muscle stimulator
5.7 Specialty leg bag emptiers, valves, drains, and clamps
5.8 Artificial urinary sphincter

DISPOSABLE PRODUCTS

1.1 Absorbent Brief With Elastic Legs

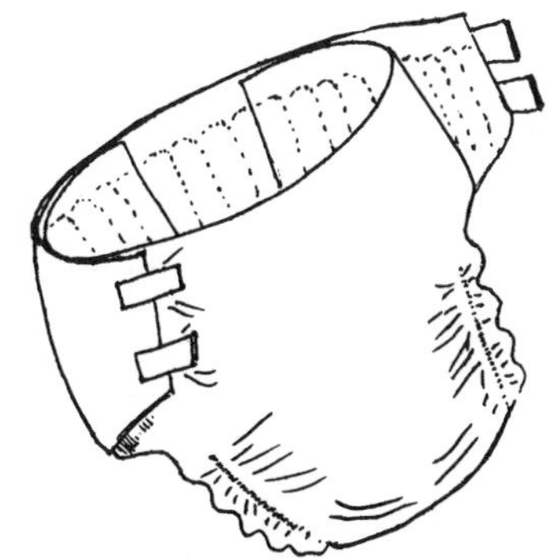

Diapers large enough to fit adolescents and adults. Outer plastic cover. Self-adhesive tape tabs. Elastic leg gathers to improve fit and prevent leakage.

Brand Name:

Attends	(86)	*PrimaCare II**	(92)
Assurance	(33)	*Provide*	(27)
Bard	(8)	*Sears*•*	
Curity	(51)	*Skin-Caring*	(94)
Curity	(52)	*Tranquility*	(85)
Depend	(53)	*Ultigard**	(87)
Dry Comfort•*	(42)	*UltraShield*	(112)
Kay Plus	(18)	*Wings**	(87)
*MaxiCare**	(66)		
PrimeTime	(66)		

1.2 Absorbent Brief Without Elastic Legs

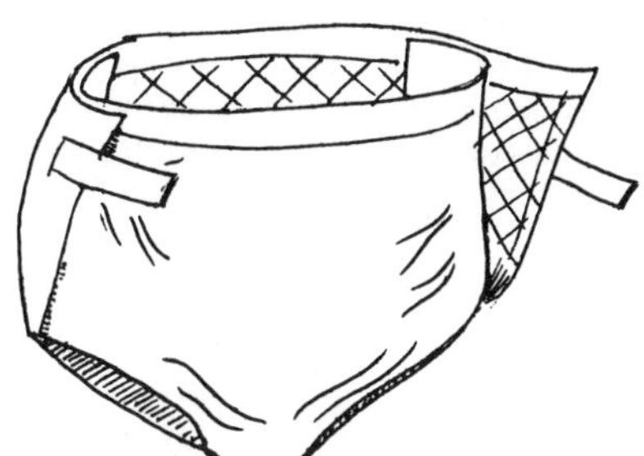

Diapers large enough to fit adolescents and adults. Outer plastic cover. Self-adhesive tape tabs.

Brand Name:

*Ables**	(66)	*Mark-Clark*	(58)
Ambeze	(112)	*Montgomery Ward*	
Bard	(8)	*Paper-Pak*	(80)
Bell-Horn	(10)	*Passport*•*	(59)
Curity	(52)	*Polysorb**	
Diaperbriefs	(36)	*PrimaCare I*•*	(92)
Go-Ahead	(36)	*Sears**	
JC Penney		*Unigard II**	(87)

1.3 Pad-and-Pant Starter Kit

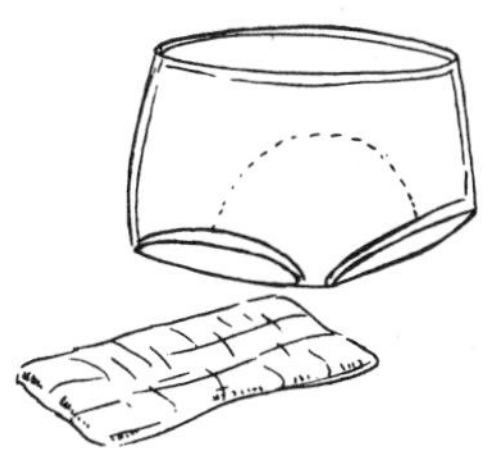

Some starter kits have a disposable pad and a reusable pant of cotton or a blend of nylon and polyester; some have a waterproof crotch.

Brand Name:

Bell-Horn	(10)	*Mark-Clark*	(58)
Brief Encounter		*Revco*	
Dignity	(45)	*Safe and Dry**	(55)
DRIpride	(27)	*Salk-Knit**	(92)
Geri-Care	(37)	*Tranquility*	(85)

1.4 Absorbent Inserts—Flat

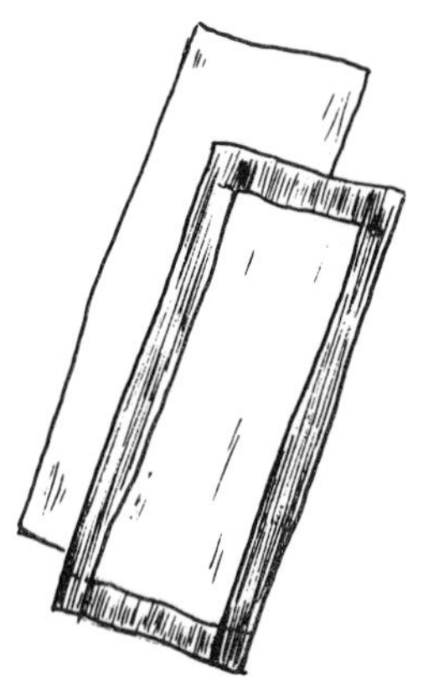

Also called "liners." Rectangular and have a waterproof cover. Held in place by incontinence pants, close-fitting underwear or both. Available with or without adhesive strips to hold pad in pant.

Brand Name:			
*Aquagel**	(92)	*Mark-Clark**•	(58)
Assurance	(33)	*Mark One**	(59)
Bell-Horn	(10)	*MaxiShield*	(112)
Content I and II	(27)	*MiniGard*	(112)
Curity	(51)	*Montgomery Ward*	
Curity	(52)	*Prefer**	(92)
Dignity	(45)	*Promise*	(94)
DRIpride	(27)	*Safe and Dry**	(55)
Dry Comfort	(42)	*Salk-Knit**	(92)
*Free & Active**	(45)	*Sears**•	
*HandiCare**•	(66)	*Securely Yours*	(80)
Hospital Pack	(36)	*Tape II**•	(8)
JC Penney		*Tranquility**	(85)
Kay Plus	(18)	*Unigard**	(87)

1.5 Absorbent Inserts—Contoured

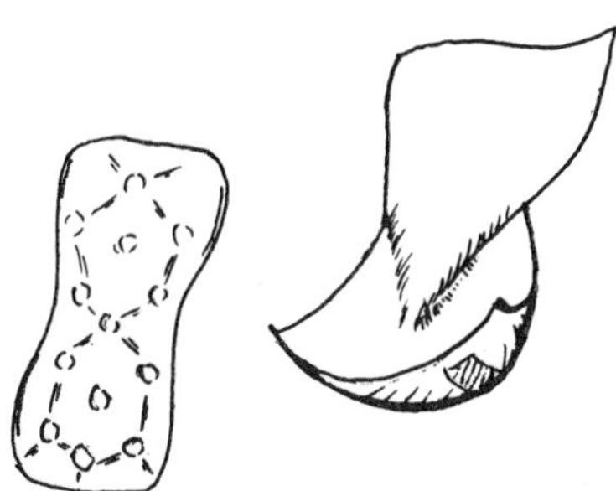

Insert liners shaped to improve comfort and fit. Held in place by incontinence pants or close-fitting underwear. Available with or without adhesive strips to hold pad in pant.

Brand Name:			
Attends	(86)	*Sears*	
Curity	(52)	*Serenity**	(82)
Depend	(53)	*Surety*	(46)
Full Life	(84)	*Promise*	(94)
Go-Ahead	(36)		

1.6 Undergarment

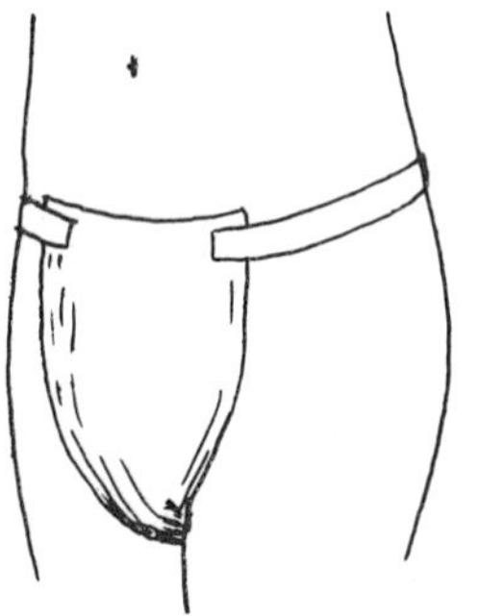

Held in place by their own straps. Can be worn without an incontinence pant. Waterproof cover.

Brand Name:	
Attends	(86)
*Depend**	(53)
Provide Trim	(27)
Surety	(46)

1.7 Underpads, Disposable

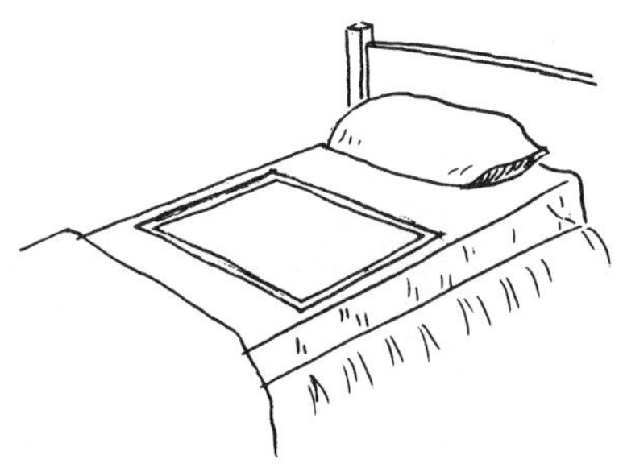

Flat pads with absorbent filler and waterproof backing. Designed to protect bedding. Available in various sizes and absorbencies.

Brand Name:

Attends	(86)	*Non-Skids*	(112)
Bio Clinic	(12)	*Paper-Pak*	(80)
Chux	(50)	*PolyCare**	(66)
Combosorb	(87)	*Polygard*	(87)
Curity	(51)	*Polygard II**	(87)
Curity	(52)	*Primapads*	(92)
Depend	(53)	*Revco*	
DisposEze•*	(112)	*Sabee*	
Dry Comfort	(42)	*Sani Pac**	(8)
Durasorb	(87)	*Sears*•*	
Excelgard		*Sorbeze*	
*Hosposable**	(44)	*Stanford*	(101)
JC Penney		*Tuckables*•*	(44)
Magnum	(44)	*Val-U-Sorb*	(87)
*Mark One**	(59)	*WingsPM**	(87)
*MaxiCare**	(66)		
Montgomery Ward			

1.8 Male Envelope-Style Dribble Collector

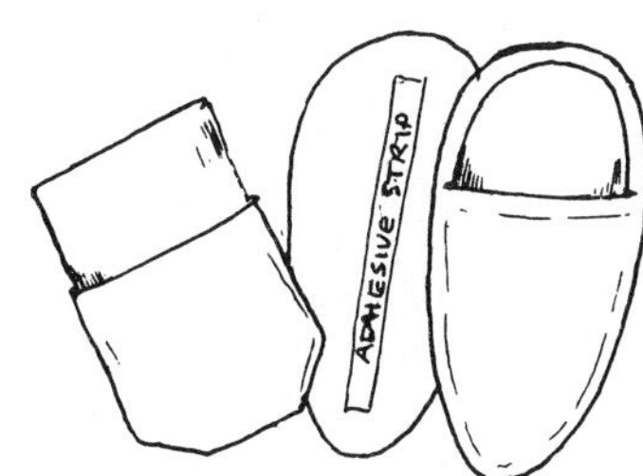

Shield slips over and around penis to absorb small amounts of urine. Waterproof backing. Designed for use with stretch mesh brief or close-fitting underwear.

Brand Name:

*Conveen**	(22)
Go-Ahead	(36)
Sears	
Tenasorb	(94)
Tranquility	(85)
Uri-Drain	(97)
*Uro-Tex**	(98)

REUSABLE PRODUCTS

2.1 Diaper—Flat

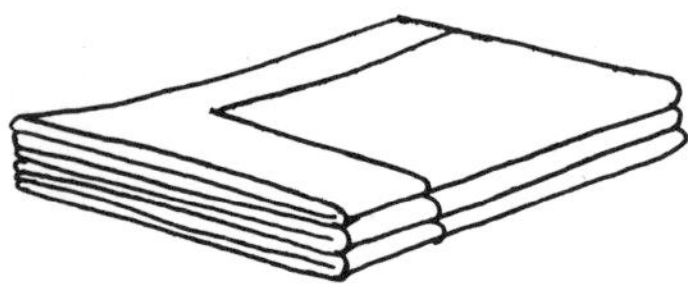

Washable, reusable adult cloth diaper. Some have plastic cover sewn into diaper. Needs to be pinned. Also available through a diaper or linen service.

Brand Name:

Absorb-Plus	(1)	*Geri-Care*	(37)
Allstate	(4)	*Mark-Clark*	(58)
Confidentially Yours	(31)	*Med-I-Pant*	(64)
Dundee Mills	(28)	*Sears*	

2.2 Diaper—Contoured

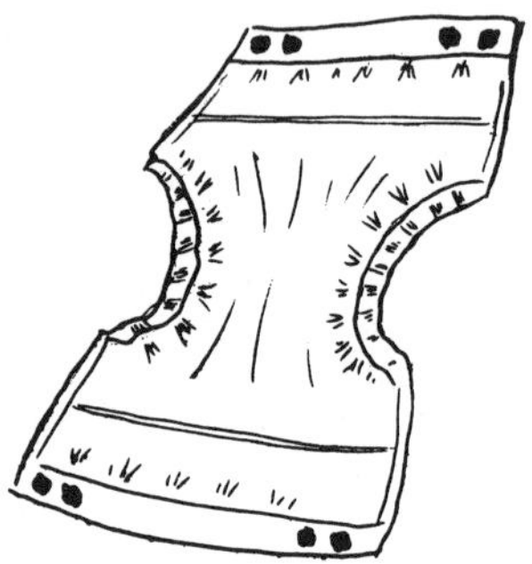

Washable reusable adult diaper made of cloth that is shaped. Some have elastic at legs and some have a plastic cover sewn into diaper. Held in place by elastic, snaps, or Velcro. Also available through diaper or linen service.

Brand Name:

Absorb-Plus	(1)	*Dydee*	
Allstate	(4)	*Geri-Care*	(37)
Confidentially Yours	(31)	*Med-I-Pant*	(64)
Dundee Mills	(28)	*Sears*	

2.3 Reusable Brief

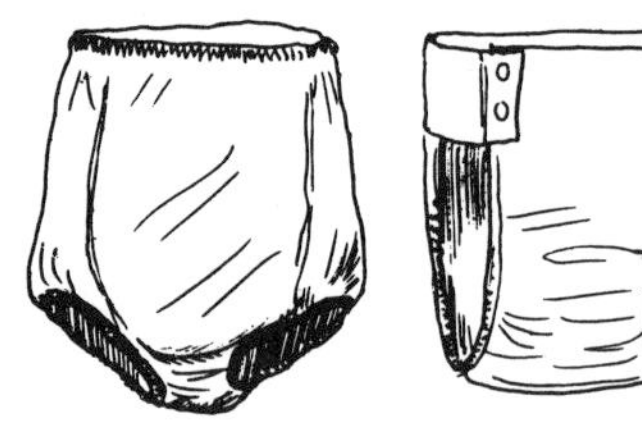

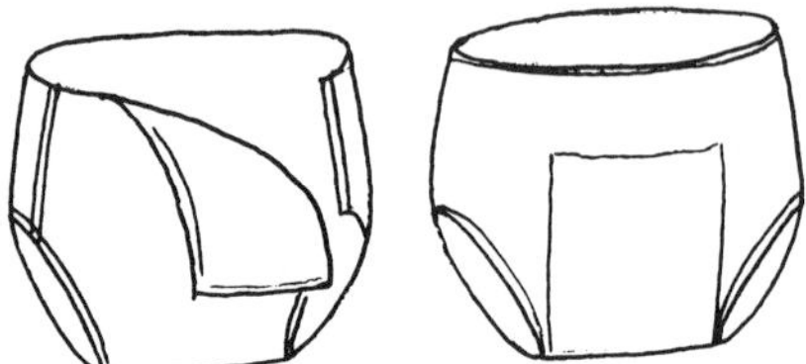

Pant of cotton, fabric blend, or waterproof material. Designed to hold reusable liners, pads, or diapers. Washable. Elastic legs for close fit. Held in place by elastic, snaps, or Velcro. Some have waterproof crotch panel. Liners and pads held in place with loops, snaps, pockets, Velcro shields, or self-adhesive strips.

Brand Name:

Absorb-Plus	(1)	*Lifespan*	(3)
Allstate	(4)	*Mark-Clark*	(58)
Bell-Horn	(10)	*Med-I-Pant*	(64)
Camp Int'l	(15)	*Montgomery Ward*	
Confidentially Yours	(31)	*Nikky*	(73)
Curity	(52)	*PCP-Champion*	(81)
Dignity	(45)	*PiPeer*	(72)
DRIpride	(27)	*Prefer*	(92)
Dundee Mills	(28)	*Rubber Duckies*	(89)
Geri-Care	(37)	*Safe and Dry*	(55)
Handicare	(66)	*Sani-Pant*	(92)
JC Penney		*Sears*	
		Tranquility	(85)

2.4 Mesh Stretch Brief

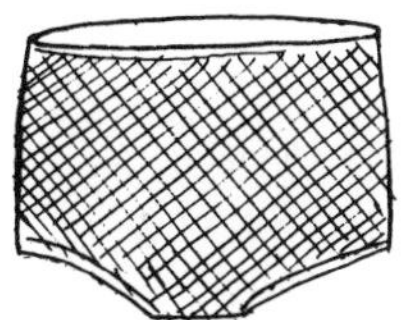

Highly elastic, soft, form-fitting, cool, discreet, comfortable mesh stretch pant to hold any size liner or pad that has plastic backing firmly but gently. Washable and reusable.

Brand Name:

Absorb-Plus	(1)	*K-Mart*	
Air-Flo	(66)	*MaxiShield*	(112)
Assurance	(33)	*Paper-Pak*	(80)
Cascade PSH	(18)	*Promise*	(94)
Conveen	(22)	*Revco*	
Curity	(51)	*Security*	(62)
Curity	(52)	*Sears*	
Depend	(53)	*X-Span*	(3)
DRIpride	(27)		
GEPCO	(35)		

2.5 Drawsheet

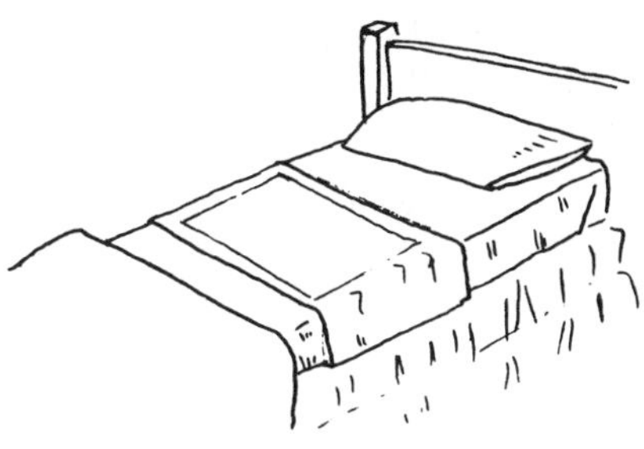

Plastic or cloth material that covers a portion of the bed. Can be waterproof or can encase a water-proof underpad. Drawsheet protects bed linen and mattress and assists in lifting and turning an immobile patient.

Brand Name:

Absorb-Plus	(1)	*Kylie*	(56)
Allstate	(4)	*Mark-Clark*	(58)
Curity	(52)	*Med-I-Pant*	(64)
Dundee Mills	(28)	*Promise*	(94)
GEPCO	(35)	*SuperCare*	(66)
Geri-Care	(37)	*Tendercare*	(100)
Intera	(47)		

2.6 Flat Reusable Liner

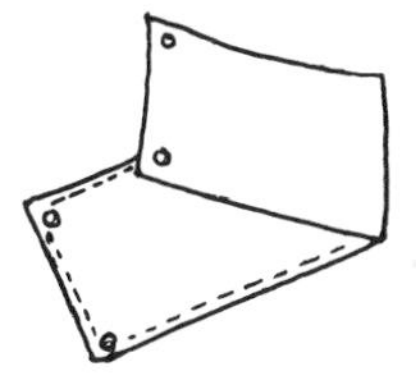

Rectangular absorbent washable cloth liner or pad. Held in place by waterproof pants. Some have waterproof backing.

Brand Name:

Absorb-Plus	(1)	*Mark-Clark*	(58)
Bell-Horn	(10)	*Med-I-Pant*	(64)
Curity	(52)	*Sears*	
Geri-Care	(37)		

2.7 Contoured Reusable Liner

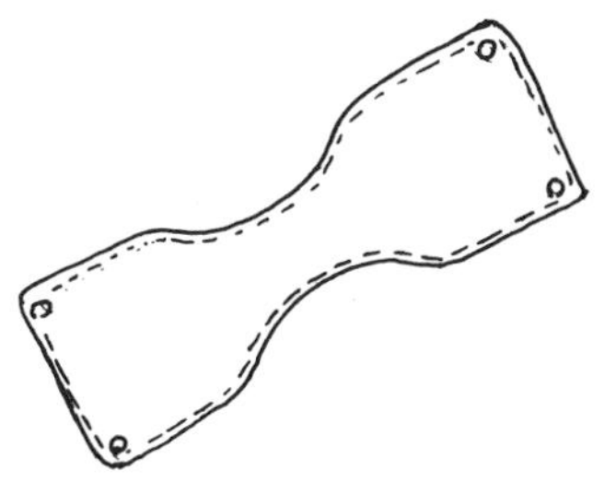

Shaped absorbent washable cloth liner or pad. Held in place by waterproof pants. Some have waterproof backing.

Brand Name:

Absorb-Plus	(1)
Geri-Care	(37)

2.8 Underpads, Reusable

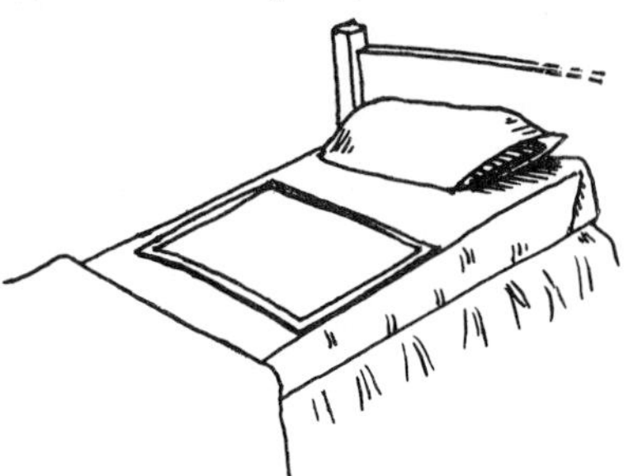

Absorbent cloth bed cover or linen protector with waterproof backing for use on beds or furniture or in wheelchairs. Also available through a diaper or linen service.

Brand Name:

Absorb-Plus	(1)	*Montgomery Ward*	
Alegra	(4)	*Sears*	
Dundee Mills	(28)	*Sure-Stay*	(4)
Med-I-Pad	(64)		

2.9 Men's Protective Support

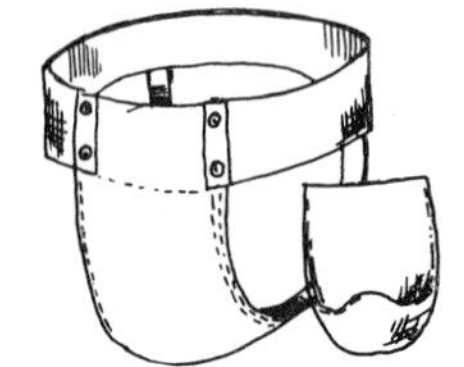

Resembles jockstrap (athletic supporter) with waterproof cup. Used with disposable or reusable cup inserts.

Brand Name:
PiPeer (72)
Salk Shells (92)
Sears

2.91 Men's Protective Brief

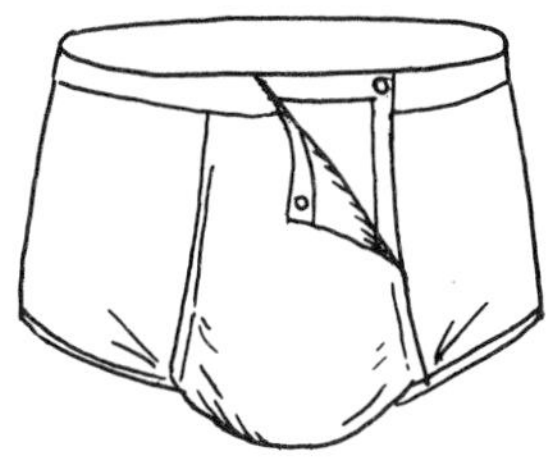

Tailored for men, with a fly. Some have zipper. Some have waterproof panel. Used with disposable and reusable pads or liners.

Brand Name:
Prefer (92)
Sears

2.92 Men's Collector

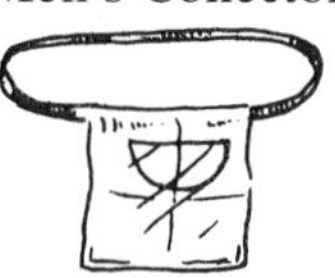

Cotton or vinyl pouch envelops the penis. Holds absorbent material.

Brand Name:
Male Bag (57)

2.93 Men's Protective Boxer-Style Short

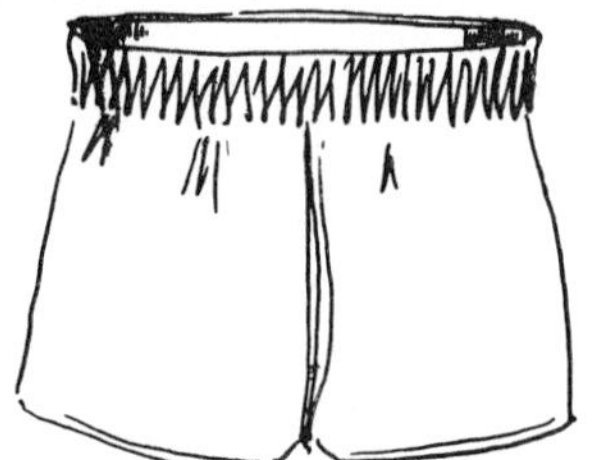

Boxer-style underwear with absorbent fabric in crotch.

Brand Name:
Security (62)

DEVICES

3.1 Condom Catheter for Men—Self-Adhesive

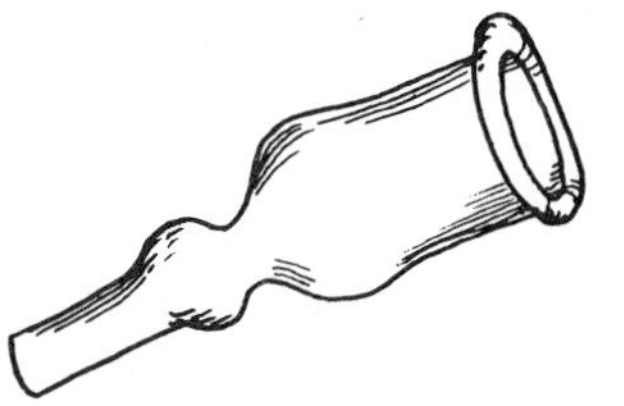

Soft latex sheath worn over the penis with attachment to leg bag or drain tube. No tapes, strips, straps, or pants necessary.

Brand Name:

Active-Cath	(69)	*Hollister*	(43)
Conveen Self-Sealing Urisheath	(22)	*Hollister-Removable Tip*	(43)
Freedom-Cath	(69)	*Weimer*	(99)

3.2 Condom Catheter for Men With Adhering Strips

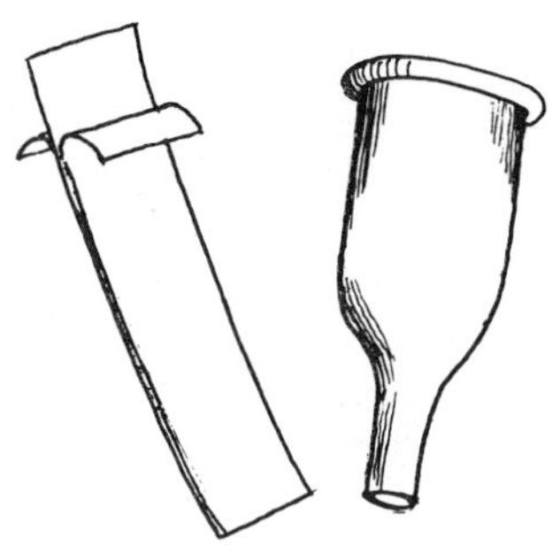

Soft latex sheath worn over penis. Attached to leg bag or drain tube. Requires adhering strips or encircling straps.

Brand Name:

Argyle	(97)	*MBS*	(70)
Baxter	(9)	*Sure Seal Golden Drain*	(67)
Comfort Mate	(98)	*TFX Medical*	(106)
Conveen—Uriliner	(22)	*Uri-Drain*	(97)
Conveen—Urisheath	(22)	*Urihesive*	(23)
Deluxe Golden Drain	(67)	*Uro-Cath*	(108)
Gizmo	(69)	*Uro-Con*	(108)
Golden Drain	(67)	*Uro-San Plus*	(69)
		Uro Sheath	(8)

3.21 Condom Catheter for Men With Inflatable Ring

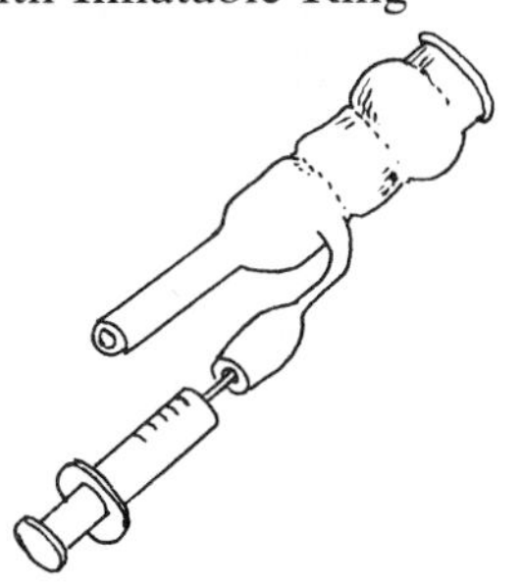

Reusable external catheter. Secured by filling an inflation ring with air. Syringe is furnished.

Brand Name:
Comfort-Seal (111)

3.3 Male Urinal With Supporter

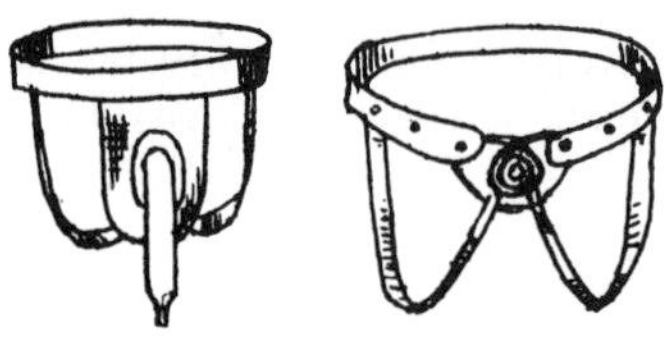

Latex sheath or vinyl collector worn over or around base of penis. Held in place by rubber or cloth supporter.

Brand Name:

McGuire	(98)	*Urocare*	(108)
Nu-Hope	(76)	*Weimer*	(99)
PiPeer	(72)	*Downs Pubic Pressure Urinal*	
Sears			

3.4 Female External Collecting Device

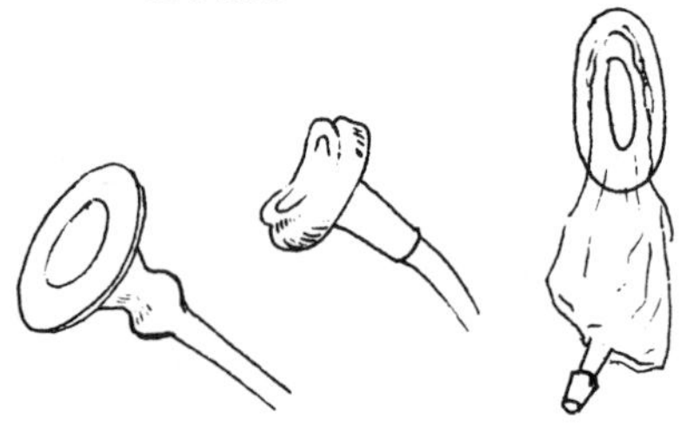

Special device or pouch held around the female urinary opening by glue, suction, or pressure. Leg bag is required.

Brand Name:

Freshette	(93)
Hollister	(43)
PiPeer	(72)
Uro-Cup	(108)

3.5 Leg Bag

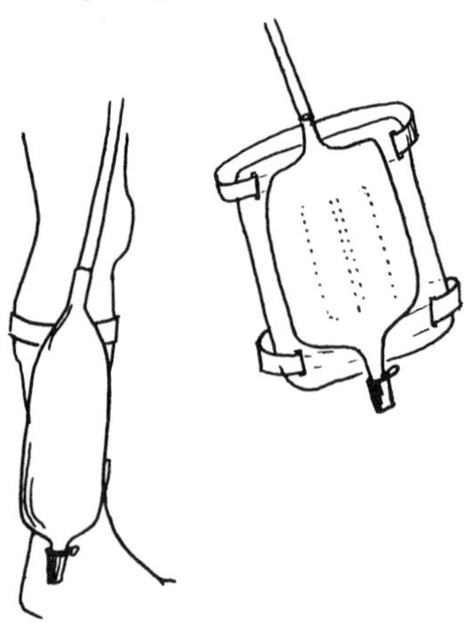

Bag worn with catheter to collect urine. Urine is drained from the bottom when bag fills. Many are called disposable, but can be washed and reused. Worn on leg with straps or carried in a holster-type holder.

Brand Name:

Argyle	(97)	*Mentor*	(69)
Baxter	(9)	*Nu-Hope*	(76)
MMG Button Bag	(67)	*Sears*	
Conveen	(22)	*Sierra*	(98)
Dis-Poz-A-Bag	(8)	*TFX Medical*	(106)
Freedom-Cath	(69)	*Teardrop*	(95)
Hollister	(43)	*Uri-Drain*	(97)
Mark-Clark	(58)	*Urocare*	(108)
Marlen	(60)	*Uro-Kit*	(108)
MDI Deluxe	(65)	*Uro-Safe*	(108)
MDI Rehab	(65)	*Weimer*	(99)

3.6 Leg Bag Straps or Holder

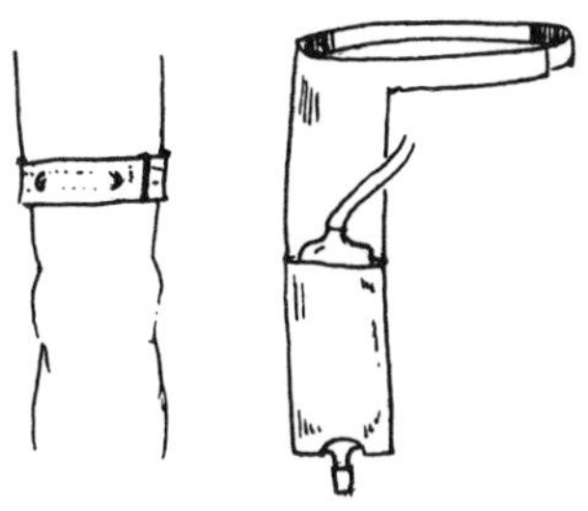

Replacing rubber straps, these straps are soft cloth. Close with Velcro or attach to the leg bag by buttons and buttonholes. Holder is a soft cloth leg bag holder, similar to a holster and suspended from a waistband.

Brand Name:

Argyle	(97)	*Hollister*	(43)
Bard	(8)	*Mark-Clark*	(58)
Comfort Straps	(67)	*Nu-Hope*	(76)
Conveen	(22)	*United*	(99)
Dale Medical	(26)	*Uri-Drain*	(97)
Fitz-All	(108)	*Urocare*	(108)
Freedom	(69)	*Velfoam*	(108)

3.61 Catheter Tube Holder

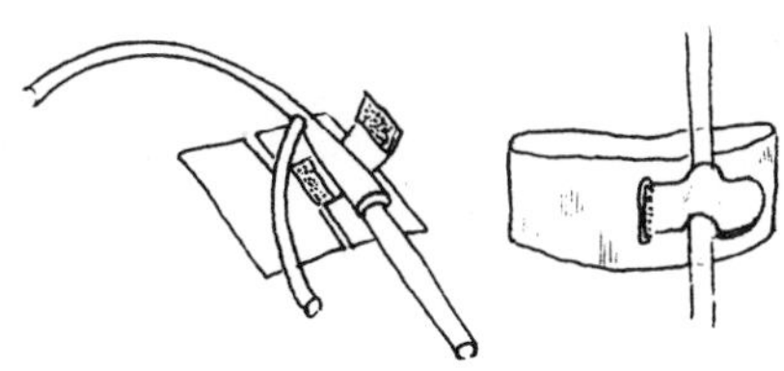

Catheter tube holders come in two styles: (1) adhesive, sticks to abdomen or to leg with Velcro loop to hold catheter in place; (2) soft leg band with Velcro loop to hold catheter in position.

Brand Name:

Cath-Secure-1	(63)
Conveen-2	(22)
Dale Medical-2	(26)
E-Z-Hold-1	(69)

3.7 Bedside Drainage Bag/Bottle and Cover for Leg Bag or Bedside Bag

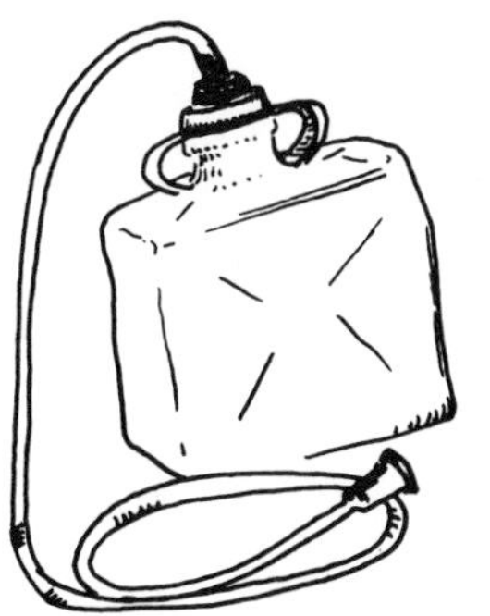

Urinary drainage bottle. Larger than a leg bag. Holds enough urine so user can sleep through the night. Covers (C) conceal drainage bag.

Brand Name:

Accuseal	(23)	*Mason*	(61)
Arnold/Dansac	(6)	*MDI*	(65)
Bard	(8)	*Mentor*	(69)
Baxter	(9)	*MMG*	(67)
Care-Bag (C)	(109)	*Permatype*	
Conveen	(22)	*Sur-Fit*	(23)
CPC (C)	(24)	*TFX Medical*	(106)
Curity	(51)	*Teardrop*	(95)
Dynacor		*United*	(99)
Lucky Leg (C)	(34)	*Urocare*	(108)
Marlen	(60)		

3.8 Penile Clamp or Compression Device

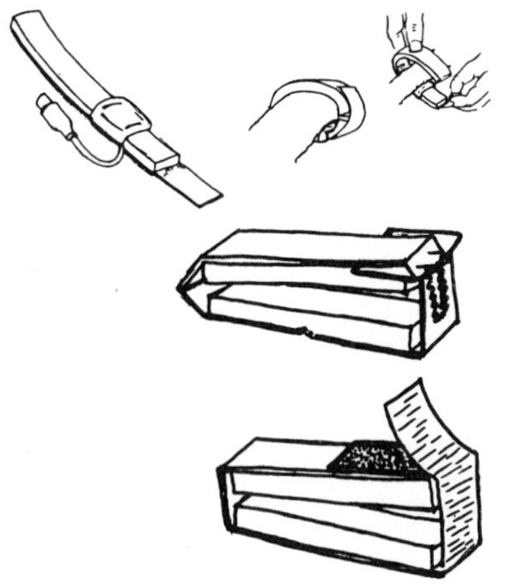

Clamps squeeze penis to stop urine flow. Metal or plastic frame with foam cushion. Adjustable size. Another type of compression device encircles the penis and stops urine flow when it is inflated with air. Adjustable size.

Brand Name:

Bard-Cunningham	(8)
Greenwald-Baumrucker	(38)
Greenwald-Cunningham	(38)
MMG-Cunningham	(67)
TFX-Cunningham	(106)
Cook Continence Cuff	(111)
Dacomed C^3	(25)

SKIN CARE PRODUCTS

4.1 Wet Wipes

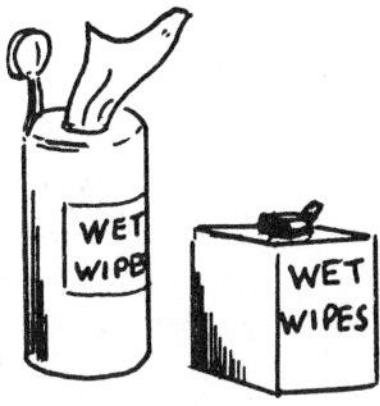

Nonirritating cleanser in handy, disposable wipe. Made to dissolve irritants gently.

Brand Name:

Arnold/Dansac	(6)
Clinipad	(21)
Depend	(53)
DRIpride	(27)
Kleen Ups	(44)
Wings	*(87)*

4.2 Cleanser

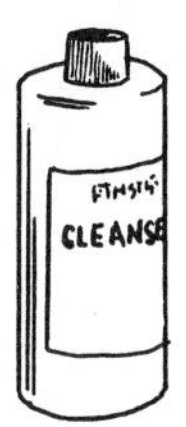

Soapless, nonirritating cleanser. Made to dissolve and remove feces and urine gently. Many contain deodorizers in their formula. Individuals with allergies to certain fragrances should read labels carefully.

Brand Name:

Adhese-Off	(69)	*Hygiene I*	(19)
Aloe Vesta	(14)	*Mark-Clark*	(58)
Arnold/Dansac	(6)	*Orchid Fresh*	(16)
Bard	(8)	*Osto-Zyme*	(96)
Baxter	(9)	*Pectin-Off*	(6)
Cara-Klenz	(17)	*Peri-Wash*	(105)
Care-Tech	(16)	*Peri-Wash II*	(105)
Confidant	(39)	*Promise*	(94)
Curity	(52)	*Soothe & Cool*	(68)
Davron—		*Triple Care*	(99)
Dailycare	(71)	*Ultra-Fresh*	(69)
Depend	(53)	*UniWash*	(99)
Hollister	(43)	*Uro-Wash*	(108)

4.3 Deodorizer

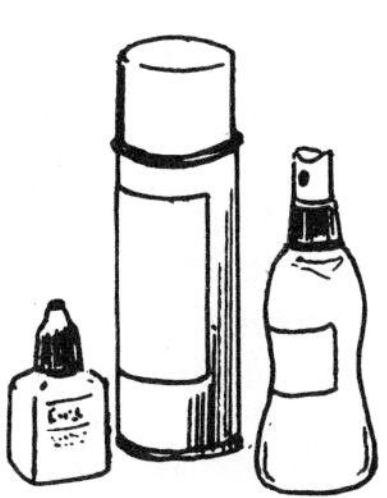

Spray or liquid drops neutralize or mask offensive odors. Not intended to be applied directly to skin or to products in contact with skin. Some liquids approved for use in leg bags and bedside drainage systems. Read directions carefully.

Brand Name:

AeroPURE	(41)	*Hollister*	(43)
Allstate	(4)	*Mason*	(61)
Arnold/Dansac	(6)	*Medi-Aire*	(19)
Banish II	(99)	*Nilodor*	(74)
Carrington	(17)	*Odour-Gard*	(60)
Confidant	(39)	*Odo-Way*	(99)
Dignity	(45)	*Tap-A-Drop*	(74)
Fresh Again	(107)	*Ultra-Fresh*	(69)
Fresh Choice	(11)	*Urolux*	(108)
Greer Guard	(69)	*Wick*	(74)
Hex-On	(105)		

4.4 Moisturizing Cream, Lotion, or Salve

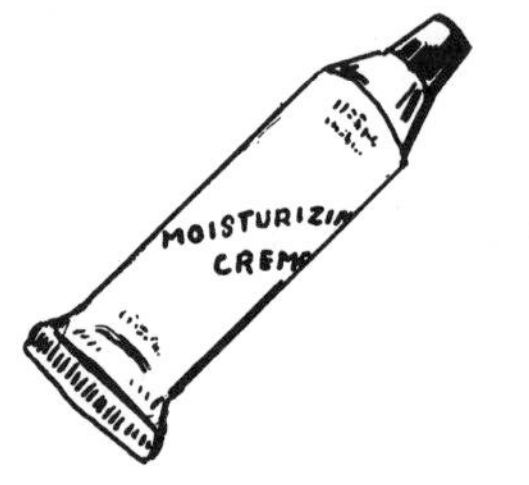

Protective moisturizer designed especially for incontinent people.

Brand Name:

Bard	(8)	*Nu-Hope*	(76)
Barri-Care	(16)	*Pharmaseal*	(9)
Carrington	(17)	*Skin Savvy*	(104)
Curity	(52)	*Soothe & Cool*	(68)
Davron—		*Special Care*	(19)
Dailycare	(71)	*Sween Cream*	(105)
Depend	(53)	*UniCare*	(99)
Hollister	(43)	*UniDerm*	(99)
Mark-Clark	(58)		

4.41 Antibacterial and Antifungal Cream

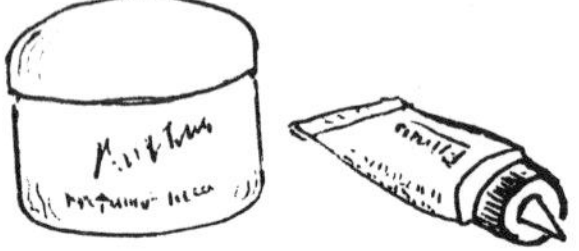

Cream or salve with nonprescription strength-ingredient to treat fungal skin infections.

Brand Name:

Aseptin	(19)
Micro-Guard	(105)
Prophyllin	(91)

4.5 Barrier Film, Cream, or Salve

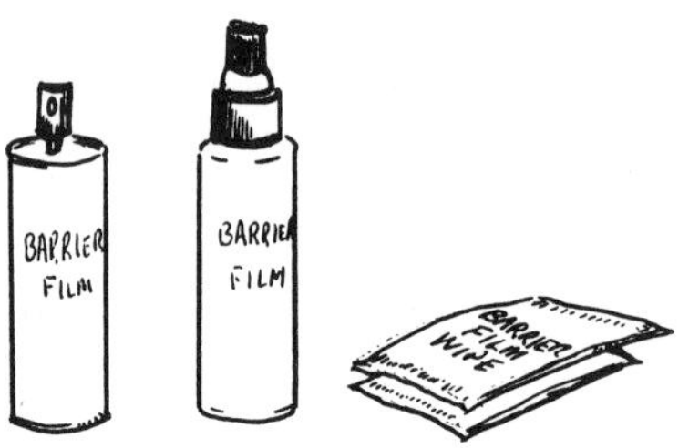

Barrier film is packaged in the form of wipes, aerosol spray, or pump spray. When film dries, skin is protected from irritation caused by stool and urine. Intended to prevent damage when used on broken skin, but stings somewhat because of alcohol content. Barrier creams are creams or salves designed for same purpose as films, but made from different ingredients. Can be used on broken skin.

Brand Name:

Aloe Vesta	(14)	*Peri-Care*	(105)
Bard	(8)	*Pharmaseal*	(9)
Carrington	(17)	*Skin-Prep*	(99)
Cliniguard	(21)	*Skin Savvy*	(104)
Curity	(52)	*Skincote*	(30)
Davron—		*Sooth & Cool*	(68)
Dailycare	(71)	*Special Care*	(19)
Depend	(53)	*Sween Prep*	(105)
Hollister	(43)	*UniDerm*	(99)
Mark-Clark	(58)	*UniSalve*	(99)
Mentor	(69)	*Wings*	(87)
Nu-Gard	(76)		

4.6 Body Powder

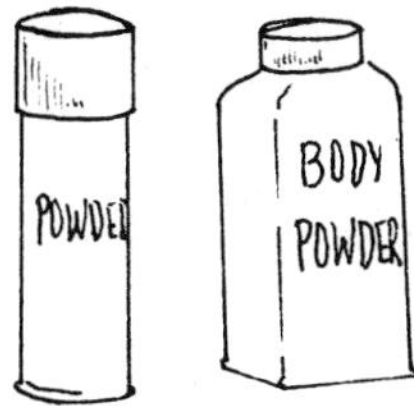

Special powders, usually with a cornstarch base. Help control dampness and perspiration. Some contain deodorizers as part of formula. Individuals with allergies to certain fragrances should read labels carefully.

Brand Name:
Davron—
Dailycare (71)
Soothe & Cool (68)
Fordustin (105)

MISCELLANEOUS

5.1 Catheters for Intermittent Catheterization

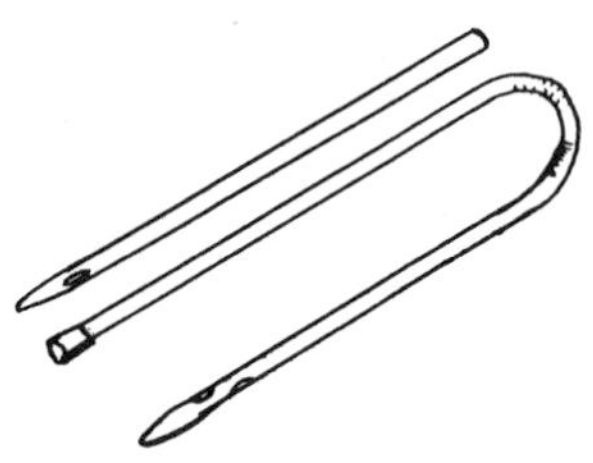

Variable-length catheters designed for repeated use in intermittent catheterization. Polished eyelets and round, smooth tips for easy insertion. Men should use water-soluble lubricant. Usually require a prescription.

Brand Name:

Argyle	(97)	*Rusch*	(90)
Clean-Cath	(8)	Seamless	(95)
Firlit-Sugar	(111)	*Self-Caths*	(69)
O'Neil	(67)	*Touchless*	(8)
Pharmaseal	(9)		

5.2 Enuresis Alarm

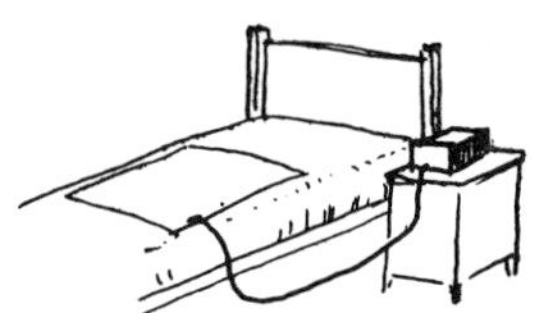

System consists of sensor for underpants or bed pad with built-in sensor. Connected to alarm that sounds when sensor gets wet.

Brand Name:

Eastleigh II System	(32)	*Nite Train-R*	(75)
Eastleigh System PEX2	(32)	*Nytone*	(77)
Eastleigh System PEX1	(32)	*Palco*	(78)
		Quietwake	(40)
		SleepDry	(103)

5.3 Fecal Incontinence Collection System

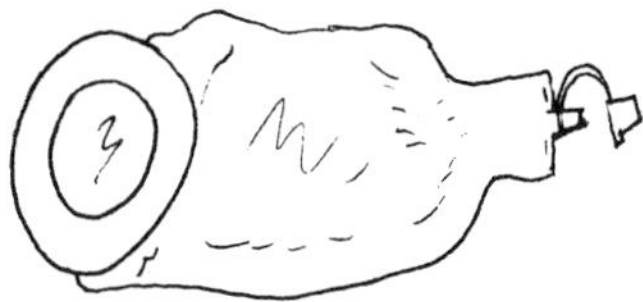

Bag with self-sticking surface for easy application around anus. Can be helpful for people with uncontrolled bowel movements.

Brand Name:

Avatar	(2)
Avatar 2000	(2)
Hollister	(43)
United	(99)

5.4 On-the-Go Urinals for Men and Women

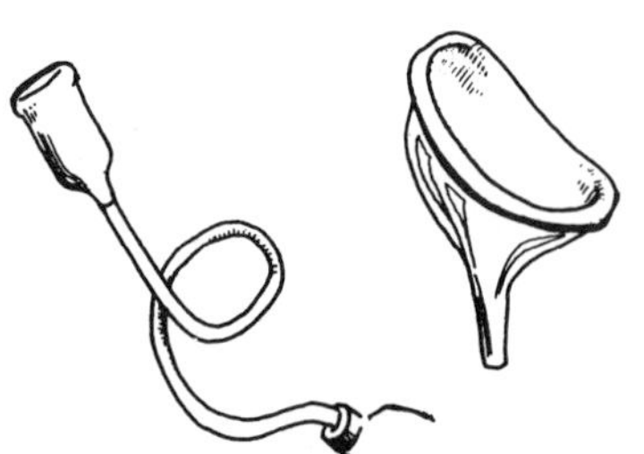

Urinals of various designs. Sold through supply houses and mail order companies.

Brand Name:

Auto-Go	(7)	*Millie*	(110)
Car John		*Restop*	(102)
Freshette	(93)	*Tinkle Tube*	
Mark Clark	(58)		

5.5 Oral Deodorant Tablets

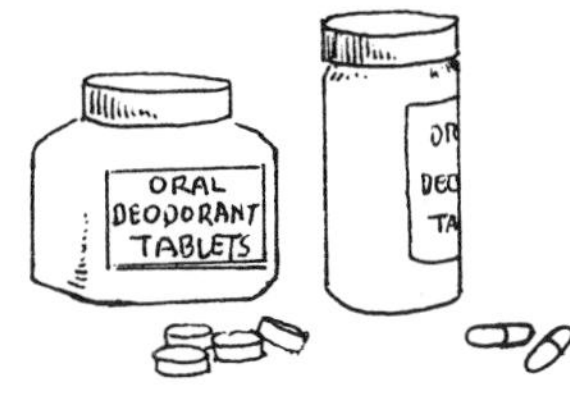

Tablets or capsules contain chlorophyllin copper complex. Helpful in controlling urine and bowel odors and other body odors.

Brand Name:	
Derifil	(91)
N'Odor	(83)
Nullo	(20)
Pals	(79)
Whoo-Noz	(54)

5.6 Perineometer and Pelvic Muscle Stimulator

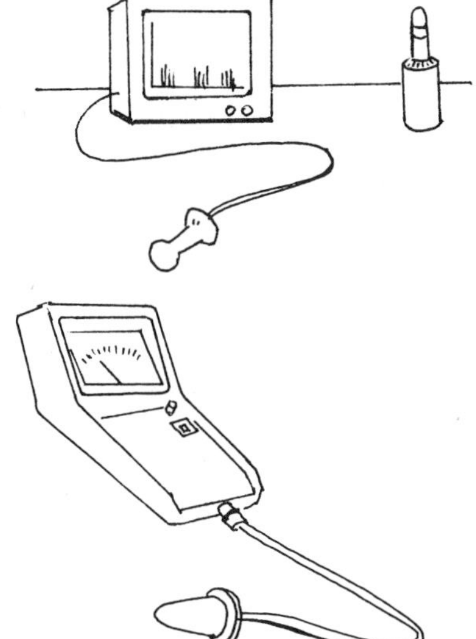

Perineometer is inserted into vagina of a female or anus of male to assist in teaching pelvic muscle exercises. Perineometer senses muscle activity and displays results on a computer screen or display gauge. Pelvic muscle stimulator is inserted into the vagina or anus and emits low-voltage electrical impuses that cause contractions of the pelvic floor muscles. Used under supervision of a physician or nurse.

Brand Name:	
Gynos	(48)
Perineometer	(13)
Restore	(48)
Conmax	

5.7 Specialty Leg Bag Emptiers, Valves, Drains, and Clamps

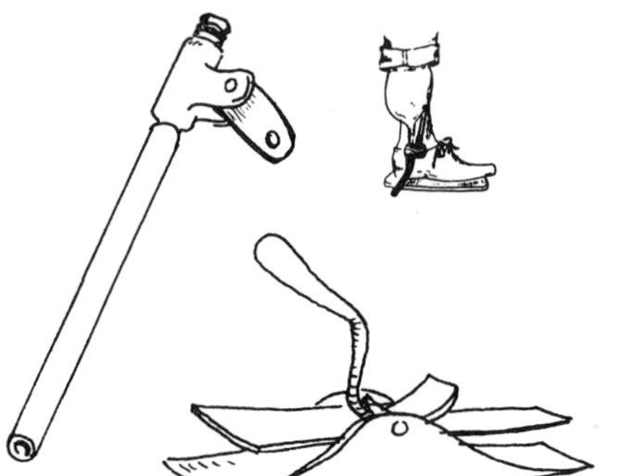

Accessories for leg bags. Help people with limited movement or use of hands.

Brand Name:	
JAECO	(49)
L.U.V.	(29)
MMG	(67)
R.D. Equipment	(88)
Urocare—Quick Drain	(108)

5.8 Artificial Urinary Sphincter

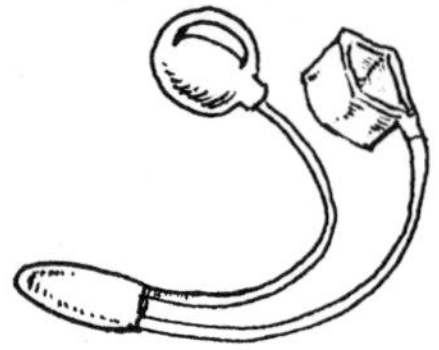

Mechanical device implanted in body by surgical procedure. Substitutes for a person's damaged sphincter.

Brand Name:
AMS (5)

MANUFACTURERS' INDEX

1. **Absorb-Plus Textiles, Inc.**
   1090, rue Dupuis
   Verdun, Quebec
   Canada H4G 2H7
   514-526-4444

   2.1 Flat diaper
   2.2 Contoured diaper
   2.3 Reusable brief
   2.4 Mesh brief
   2.5 Draw sheet
   2.6 Flat reusable liner
   2.7 Contoured liner
   2.8 Reusable underpad

2. **Aegis Medical, Inc.**
   370 17th Street, Suite 700
   P.O. Box 46506
   Denver, CO 80201-6506
   303-592-2050
   800-232-9919

   5.3 Avatar Personal Bowel Care System
   5.3 Avatar 2000 Bowel Evacuation System

3. **Alba Home Health Care Div. of Alba-Waldensian, Inc.**
   P.O. Box 100
   Valdese, NC 28690
   704-874-2191
   800-438-2167

   2.3 Lifespan incontinent pant
   2.4 X-Span perineum and rectal brief

4. **Allstate Medical Products, Inc.**
   3100 Ranchview Lane
   Minneapolis, MN 55447
   612-559-0030
   800-328-2915

   2.1 Flat diaper
   2.2 Contoured diaper
   2.3 Reusable brief
   2.5 Drawsheet
   2.8 Alegra underpad
   2.8 Sure-Stay underpad
   4.3 I-C incontinent spray

5. **American Medical Systems**
   11001 Bren Road East
   Minnetonka, MN 55343
   612-933-4666
   800-328-3881

   5.8 AMS artificial urinary sphincter

6. **Arnold/Dansac, Inc.**
   P.O. Box 471211
   Leesburg, FL 34749-471211
   904-326-5292
   800-451-8087

   3.7 Night drainage unit
   4.1 Skin Tissues
   4.2 Skin Lotion
   4.2 Pectin-Off
   4.3 Deodorizer

7. **Auto-Go**
   P.O. Box 303
   Plainfield, IN 46168

   5.4 Auto-Go Disposable Urinal

8. **Bard Home Health Division**
   111 Spring Street
   Murray Hill, NJ 07974
   201-277-8000
   800-526-4930

   1.1 Disposable brief with elastic legs
   1.2 Disposable brief
   1.4 Tape II liner
   1.7 Sani Pac underpad
   3.2 Uro Sheath disposable catheter
   3.2 Uro Sheath reusable catheter
   3.5 Dis-Poz-A-Bag leg bag
   3.6 Latex strap
   3.6 Soft fabric strap

3.7 Bedside drainage system
3.8 Cunningham penile clamp
4.2 Skin care cleanser with deodorizer
4.4 Skin care cream
4.5 Moisture barrier cream
4.5 Incontinence barrier film
5.1 Clean-Cath Intermittent Catheter
5.1 Touchless intermittent catheter

9. Baxter General Health Care
1 Parkway North
Suite 100, Box 851
Deerfield, IL 60015-0851
312-940-1990
800-423-2311

3.2 External catheter
3.5 Leg bag
3.7 Drainage bag
4.2 Incontinent wash
4.4 Pharmaseal skin cream
4.5 Pharmaseal barrier cream
5.1 Pharmaseal catheters for intermittent catheterization

10. Bell-Horn
(William H. Horn & Brothers, Inc.)
451 North Third Street
Philadelphia, PA 19123-4197
215-627-2773
800-366-4676

1.2 Disposable brief
1.3 Pad-and-pant starter kit
1.4 Replacement liner
2.3 Reusable brief
2.6 Flat liner

11. Bemis Company, Inc.
2705 University Avenue NE
Minneapolis, MN 55418
612-788-0100
800-231-6979

4.3 Fresh Choice Odor Eliminator

12. Bio Clinic Sunrise Medical
P.O. Box 1528
Rancho Cucamonga, CA 91730
714-989-2535
800-854-2369

1.7 Disposable underpad

13. Biotechnologies, Inc.
2 Bryn Mawr Avenue
Suite 107
Bryn Mawr, PA 19010
215-525-8778
800-537-3779

5.6 Perineometer

14. Calgon Vestal Laboratories
Subsidiary of Merck & Co., Inc.
5035 Manchester Avenue
St. Louis, MO 63110
314-535-1810
800-876-4357

4.2 Aloe Vesta perineal solution
4.5 Aloe Vesta protective ointment

15. Camp International, Inc.
P.O. Box 89
Jackson, MI 49204
517-787-1600

2.3 Reusable brief

16. Care-Tech Laboratories Div. of Consolidated Chemical
3224 South Kingshighway
St. Louis, MO 63139-1183
314-772-4610
800-325-9681

4.2 CC-500 skin cleanser
4.2 Orchid Fresh deodorizer
4.4 Barri-Care skin ointment

17. Carrington Laboratories, Inc.
1300 E. Rochelle Blvd.
Irving, TX 75062
214-541-2278
800-527-5216

4.2 Cara-Klenz cleanser
4.3 Odor eliminator
4.4 Aloe skin balm
4.5 Moisture barrier

18. Cascade PSH, Inc.
999 Farrel
Drummondville, Quebec
Canada J2C 5P6
819-477-5077

1.1 Kay Plus adult brief
1.4 Kay Plus insert
2.4 Mesh brief

19. Catalina Biomedical Corp.
1824 Flower Avenue
Duarte, CA 91010
818-357-0669
800-334-9966

4.2 Hygiene 1 cleanser
4.3 Medi-Aire deodorizer
4.4 Special Care cream
4.41 Aseptin antifungal cream
4.5 Special Care moisture barrier

20. Chattem, Inc.
1715 West 38th Street
Chattanooga, TN 37409
615-821-4578
800-366-6833

5.5 Nullo deodorant tablets

21. The Clinipad Corp.
P.O. Box 387
Guilford, CT 06437
203-453-6543
800-243-6548

4.1 Castile towelette
4.5 Cliniguard

22. Coloplast, Inc.
5610 W. Sligh Avenue
Tampa, FL 33634
813-886-5634
800-237-4555

1.8 Conveen drip collector
2.4 Conveen mesh brief
3.1 Conveen self-sealing Urisheath
3.2 Conveen Urisheath catheter
3.2 Conveen Uriliner catheter
3.5 Conveen leg bag
3.6 Conveen Velcro straps
3.61 Conveen leg bag hanger
3.7 Conveen night drainage bag

23. ConvaTec, A Squibb Company
200 Headquarters Park
Princeton, NJ 08543-5254
201-359-9200

3.2 Urihesive—male external system
3.7 Accuseal bedside drainage bag
3.7 Sur-Fit night drainage container

24. CPC (Creations for the Physically Challenged)
P.O. Box 27
Cedarlake, IN 46303
219-374-5154

3.7 Drainage bag cover

25. Dacomed Corp.
1701 E. 79th Street
Minneapolis, MN 55425
612-854-7522
800-328-1103

3.8 C³ Male Continence Device

26. Dale Medical Products, Inc.
7 Cross Street
P.O. Box 1556
Plainville, MA 02762
617-695-9316
800-343-3980

3.6 Waistband urinary leg bag support
3.61 Legband catheter tube holder

27. DRIpride, A Weyerhaeuser Company
5150 Nashville Road
Bowling Green, KY 42102
206-924-4092
800-253-3078

1.1 Provide adult brief
1.3 Pad-and-pant starter kit
1.4 Content I and II flat insert
1.4 Content I and II with adhesive strip
1.4 Regular Content insert
1.4 550- and 850-ml flat insert
1.6 Provide Trim Adult Brief
2.3 Pull-on pant
2.3 Cotton pant
2.4 Mesh brief
4.1 Washcloths

28. Dundee Mills, Inc.
111 West 40th Street
New York, NY 10018
212-840-7200

2.1 Adult flat diaper
2.2 Pin-free contoured diaper
2.3 Super fitted brief
2.5 Drawsheet
2.8 Underpad

29. Dynamic Mobility, Inc.
2068 Helena Street
Madison, WI 53704
608-249-1234

5.7 L.U.V. leg bag valve

30. Dynarex Corp.
1 International Blvd.
Brewster, NY 10509
914-279-9600
800-431-2786

4.5 Skincote protective dressing

31. Edley Enterprises, Inc.
P.O. Box 429
Old Stage Road
Sanbornville, NH 03872
603-473-2539

2.1 Confidentially Yours flat diaper
2.2 Confidentially Yours contoured diaper
2.3 Confidentially Yours vinyl brief

32. Electronic Monitors
P.O. Box 1087
101 East Fuller Drive
Euless, TX 76039
817-283-0859

5.2 Eastleigh II system
5.2 Eastleigh PEX1 extension alarm system
5.2 Eastleigh PEX2 audible or silent alarm system

33. Facelle Company, Ltd.
1551 Weston Road
Toronto
Canada M6M 4Y4
416-243-3011

1.1 Assurance adult brief
1.4 Assurance flat insert
2.4 Assurance mesh brief

34. Foxy Enterprises
P.O. Box 958
Brookhaven, PA 19015
215-566-8220

3.7 Lucky Leg bag holder

35. General Econopak, Inc. (GEPCO)
1725 North Sixth Street
Philadelphia, PA 19122
215-763-8200

2.4 GEPCO mesh brief
2.5 GEPCO incontinence sheets

36. George Disposables
P.O. Box 5887
Old Dunbar Road

West Columbia, SC 29171
803-796-9396

1.2 Go-Ahead disposable brief
1.2 Diaperbriefs
1.4 Hospital pack underpad
1.5 Go-Ahead stress pad
1.8 Go-Ahead drip shield

37. Geri-Care Products
252 Wagner Street
Middlesex, NJ 08846
201-469-7722

1.3 Pad-and-pant starter kit
2.1 Flat diaper
2.2 Contoured diaper
2.3 Reusable brief
2.3 Brief for partial incontinence
2.5 Reusable drawsheet
2.6 Reusable flat liner
2.7 Reusable contoured liner

38. Greenwald Surgical Company
2688 DeKalb Street
Lake Station, IN 46405
219-962-1604

3.8 Cunningham clamp
3.8 Baumrucker urinary incontinence clamp

39. Hallmark Industries
564 Kingshighway
West Springfield, MA 01089
413-739-9148

4.2 Confidant perineal cleanser
4.3 Confidant enzyme odor eliminator

40. Health & Comfort Products Corp.
2 Ridgedale Avenue
Suite 370
Cedar Knolls, NJ 07927
201-267-1871

5.2 Quietwake Enuresis Management Program

41. Health and Medical Techniques, Inc.
1175 Post Road East
P.O. Box 829
Westport, CT 06880/06881
203-222-0700
800-243-6375

4.3 AeroPURE lemon or mint air deodorizer

42. Health Tec, Inc.
First Street
Palmer, MA 01069-0720
413-289-1221
800-343-1205

1.1 Dry Comfort brief
1.4 Dry Comfort adult liners
1.7 Dry Comfort underpad

43. Hollister, Inc.
2000 Hollister Drive
Libertyville, IL 60048
312-680-1000
800-323-4060
800-942-1141 (in Illinois)

3.1 Self-Adhesive male external catheter
3.1 Self-Adhesive Male External Catheter with Removable Tip
3.4 Female urinary pouch
3.5 Leg bag
3.6 Leg bag straps/holder
4.2 Skin cleanser
4.3 Deodorizer and germicide
4.4 Skin conditioning cream
4.5 Barrier skin ointment
5.3 Fecal incontinence collector

44. Hosposable Products, Inc.
P.O Box 387
Bound Brook, NJ 08805
201-469-8700

1.7 Basic underpad
1.7 Magnum underpad
1.7 Tuckables underpad
4.1 Kleen Ups disposable washcloths

45. Humanicare International, Inc.
1200 Airport Road
P.O. Box 1939
North Brunswick, NJ 08902
201-214-0660
800-631-5270

1.3 Dignity pad and pant
1.4 Dignity pad
1.4 Free & Active pad
2.3 Dignity pant
4.3 Dignity odor eliminator

46. ICD Industries
630 Clark Avenue
King of Prussia, PA 19406
215-337-7200
800-262-0042

1.5 Surety pad
1.6 Surety undergarment

47. Intera Company, LTD.
P.O. Box 1166
222 Third Street, SE
Cleveland, TN 37311
615-476-3264

2.5 Reusable bed pad

48. Interactive Medical Technologies, Inc.
2646 Palma Drive, #290
Ventura, CA 93003
805-650-6235
800-752-8333

5.6 Gynos perineometer
5.6 Restore pelvic floor stimulator

49. JAECO
Orthopedic Specialties
P.O. Box 75
Hot Springs, AR 71901
501-623-5944

5.7 Leg bag clamp

50. Johnson & Johnson Products, Inc.
501 George Street
New Brunswick, NJ 08903
800-526-2459

1.7 Chux underpad

51. Kendall Canada
6 Curity Avenue
Toronto, Ontario
Canada M4B 1X2
416-750-4023

1.1 Curity shaped elastic leg diaper
1.4 Curity pad
1.7 Curity bed pad
2.4 Curity mesh brief
3.7 Curity bedside drainage system

52. Kendall-Futuro Company
5801 Mariemont Avenue
Cincinnati, OH 45227
513-271-3400
800-543-4452

1.1 Curity contoured brief
1.2 Curity adult brief
1.4 Curity liner
1.5 Curity shield
1.7 Curity underpad
2.3 Curity reusable brief
2.4 Curity mesh brief
2.5 Curity waterproof sheeting
2.6 Curity reusable liner
4.2 Curity skin cleanser
4.4 Curity moisturizing cream
4.5 Curity moisture barrier

53. Kimberly-Clark Corp.
401 North Lake Street
Neenah, WI 54956
414-721-2000
800-558-6423
800-242-6463 (in WI)

1.1 Depend fitted brief
1.5 Depend shield
1.6 Depend undergarment
1.7 Depend underpad

2.4 Depend mesh brief
4.1 Depend wet wipes
4.2 Depend perineal wash
4.4 Depend lotion
4.5 Depend barrier cream

54. King Ostomy & Healthcare Products
431 West 13th, #4
Eugene, OR 97401
503-345-0391

5.5 Whoo-Noz deodorant tablets

55. Kleinert's Inc.
120 W. Germantown Avenue
Suite 100
Plymouth Meeting, PA 19462
215-828-7261
800-633-7568

1.3 Safe and Dry Starter Kit
1.4 Safe and Dry Polymer Pad
2.3 Safe and Dry Cotton Snap Pant
2.3 Safe and Dry Pant and Shield

56. Kylie Healthcare Products
200 Berwyn Park
Berwyn, PA 19312
215-251-7815
800-426-8712

2.5 Incontinent draw sheet and chair pad

57. Longstreet Pharmacal Corp.
1218 50th Street
Brooklyn, NY 11219
718-436-9200
800-633-7878

2.92 Male bag
Replacement pouches
Embee absorbent tissue

58. Mark-Clark Products
3601 SW 29th, #250
Topeka, KS 66614
913-273-3990
800-255-3504

1.2 Adult disposable brief
1.3 Pad-and-pant starter kit
1.4 Flat insert
2.1 Flat diaper
2.3 Reusable brief
2.5 Drawsheet
2.6 Olefin liner
3.5 Urinary leg bag
3.6 Leg bag straps/holder
4.2 Cleanser
4.4 Moisturizing cream
4.5 Barrier film
5.4 On-the-Go urinal for men and women

59. Mark One Healthcare Products Div. of Struble & Moffitt
100 East 9th Avenue
Runnemede, NJ 08078
609-939-5400
800-631-3549

1.2 Passport adult brief
1.4 Flat insert
1.7 Underpad

60. Marlen Manufacturing & Development
5150 Richmond Road
Bedford, OH 44146
216-292-7060

3.5 Leg bag
3.7 Bedside drainage bag
4.3 Odour-Gard deodorizer

61. Mason Laboratories
119 Horsham Road
Horsham, PA 19044
215-675-6044
800-523-2302

3.7 Bedside drainage bag
4.3 M9 drop deodorant

62. MB Products, Ltd.
120 Swannanoa River Road
Asheville, NC 28805
704-253-8874

2.4 Security mesh brief

Easy mesh brief
Dispo mesh brief
Fancy Free V-brief
Sheer mesh brief
Security Plus mesh brief
2.93 Security boxer short

63. M.C. Johnson Co., Inc.
758 Main Street
Leominster, MA 01453
508-534-8483

3.61 Cath-Secure tube holder

64. Med-I-Pant, Inc.
P.O. Box 448
Champlain, NY 12919-0448
514-522-1224

2.1 Flat diaper
2.2 Contoured diaper
2.3 Reusable brief
2.5 Drawsheet
2.6 Reusable liner
2.8 Med-I-Pad reusable underpad

65. Medical Devices Intl. Corp.
3849 Swanson Court
Gurnee, IL 60031
312-336-6611
800-323-9035

3.5 MDI rehab leg bag
3.5 MDI deluxe leg bag
3.7 MDI urinary drainage bag

66. Medical Disposables Company
1165 Hayes Industrial Drive
Marietta, GA 30062
404-422-3036
800-241-8205

1.1 MaxiCare fitted brief
1.1 PrimeTime contoured brief
1.2 Ables regular brief
1.4 HandiCare flat insert
1.7 MaxiCare underpad
1.7 PolyCare underpad
2.3 HandiCare reusable brief
2.4 Air-Flo mesh brief
2.5 SuperCare underpad

67. Medical Marketing Group
P.O. Box 29187
Atlanta, GA 30359
404-981-2591

3.2 Deluxe Golden Drain
3.2 Golden Drain
3.2 Sure Seal Golden Drain
3.5 Button bag leg bag
3.6 Comfort straps
3.7 MMG urinary drainage bag
3.8 Cunningham clamp
5.1 O'Neil intermittent catheter
5.7 Bottom drain clamps

68. Medline Industries, Inc.
One Medline Place
Mundelein, IL 60060-4486
312-949-5500
800-323-5886

4.2 Soothe & Cool perineal wash
4.4 Soothe & Cool moisturizing cream
4.5 Soothe & Cool moisture barrier ointment
4.6 Soothe & Cool body powder

69. Mentor Corp.
2700 Freeway Blvd.
Minneapolis, MN 55430
612-560-3320
800-328-3863

3.1 Freedom-Cath condom catheter
3.1 Active-Cath condom catheter
3.2 Uro-San Plus catheter
3.2 Gizmo catheter
3.5 Freedom-Cath leg bag system
3.5 Leg bag
3.6 Freedom leg bag strap
3.61 E-Z-Hold catheter tube holder
3.7 Bedside drainage bag
4.2 Adhese-Off cleanser

4.2 Ultra-Fresh cleanser
4.3 Greer Guard deodorizer
4.3 Ultra-Fresh deodorizer
4.5 Shield skin cream
5.1 Self-Caths catheter

70. Minneapolis Society for the Blind (MSB)
1936 Lyndale Avenue South
Minneapolis, MN 55403
612-871-2222
800-843-0619

3.2 MBS external catheter

71. Minnetonka Medical
P.O. Box 1A
Minnetonka, MN 55343
612-448-4181
800-328-5928

4.2 Davron Dailycare cleanser
4.2 Davron Dailycare no-rinse
4.4 Davron Dailycare body cream
4.5 Davron Dailycare barrier cream
4.6 Davron Dailycare powder

72. Nelkin/Piper
811 Wyandotte Street
P.O. Box 807
Kansas City, MO 64141-0807
816-842-1711
800-821-5231

2.3 PiPeer Dri pant
2.9 PiPeer Dri (male)
3.3 PiPeer Easy Wear urinal
3.4 PiPeer Dri (female)

73. Nikky America
132 East 35th Street, 17E
New York, NY 10016
212-684-6625

2.3 Adult pull-on pants
2.3 Adult night pants
2.3 Adult Velcro diaper cover
2.3 Bedwetter pants

74. Nilodor, Inc.
7740 Freedom Avenue, NW
North Canton, OH 44720
216-499-4321
800-443-4321

4.3 Tap-a-Drop deodorizer
4.3 Wick deodorizer
4.3 Pump/aerosol deodorizer

75. Nite Train-r Enterprises, Inc.
9735 SW Sunshine Court
Suite 100
Beaverton, OR 97005
503-538-8717
800-544-4240

5.2 Enuresis alarm

76. Nu-Hope Laboratories, Inc.
2900 Rowena Avenue
Los Angeles, CA 90039
213-666-5248

3.3 Nu-Hope urinal
3.5 Leg bag with straps
3.6 Leg bag holder
4.4 Cream
4.5 Nu-Gard barrier film

77. Nytone Medical Products
2424 South 900 West
Salt Lake City, UT 84119
801-973-4090

5.2 Enuresis alarm

78. Palco Laboratories
1595 Soquel Drive
Santa Cruz, CA 95065
408-476-3151
800-346-4488

5.2 Alarm system

79. Palisades Pharmaceuticals, Inc.
219 County Road
Tenafly, NJ 07670
201-569-8502

5.5 Pals internal deodorant

80. Paper-Pak Products, Inc.
1941 White Avenue
LaVerne, CA 91750
714-392-1200

1.2 Disposable brief
1.4 Securely Yours flat insert
1.7 Underpad
2.4 Mesh brief

81. PCP-Champion
300 Congress Street
Ripley, OH 45167
513-392-4301
800-888-0867

2.3 Reusable brief

82. Personal Products Company
1 Van Liew Avenue
Milltown, NJ 08850
201-524-0400
800-338-2348

1.5 Serenity guards

83. Pharmacap, Inc.
P.O. Box 547
Elizabeth, NJ 07207
800-526-6993

5.5 N'Odor deodorant capsules

84. Pope & Talbot, Inc.
32 Dart Road
Shenandoah, GA 30265
404-253-2223

1.5 Full Life Inserts

85. Principle Business Enterprises, Inc.
Pine Lake Industrial Park
Dunbridge, OH 43414
419-352-1551

1.1 Tranquility SlimLine underpant
1.3 Tranquility pad and reusable brief
1.4 Tranquility flat shield
1.8 Tranquility male shield
2.3 Tranquility reusable brief

86. Procter & Gamble Company
6th and Sycamore Street
Cincinnati, OH 45201
513-983-5178
800-543-0400

1.1 Attends wrap-around pant
1.5 Attends pad
1.6 Attends undergarment
1.7 Attends underpad

87. Professional Medical Products
P.O. Box 3288
Greenwood, SC 29648
803-223-4281
800-845-4571

1.1 Wings fitted brief
1.1 Ultigard fitted brief
1.2 Unigard II disposable brief
1.4 Unigard flat insert
1.7 Polygard/Polygard II/Wings PM/Durasorb/Val-U-Sorb/Combosorb underpads
4.1 Wings cleansing wipes
4.5 Wings moisture barrier cream

88. R.D. Equipment, Inc.
12 Herring Run Road
Harwich, MA 02645
508-432-3948

5.7 Electric leg bag emptier

89. R. Duck Company
953 West Carillo Street
Santa Barbara, CA 93101
800-422-3825

2.3 Rubber Duckies pant

90. Rusch, Inc.
53 West 23rd Street
New York, NY 10010
212-675-5556

5.1 Intermittent catheter

91. Rystan Company, Inc.
47 Center Avenue
P.O. Box 214
Little Falls, NJ 07424-0214
201-256-3737

4.41 Prophyllin ointment
5.5 Derifil deodorant tablets

92. Salk Company, Inc.
P.O. Box 452
119 Braintree Street
Boston, MA 02134
617-782-4030
800-343-4497

1.1 PrimaCare II fitted brief
1.2 PrimaCare I brief
1.3 Salk-Knit system
1.4 Aquagel flat insert
1.4 Prefer flat insert
1.4 Salk-Knit flat insert
1.7 Primapads underpad
2.3 Prefer reusable brief
2.3 Sani-Pant reusable brief
2.9 Salk Shells protective supporter
2.91 Prefer brief for men

93. Sani-Fem Corp.
P.O. Box 4117
7415 Stewart and Gray Road
Downey, CA 90241
213-928-3435

3.4 Medical Freshette female collector
5.4 Freshette complete system on-the-go urinal

94. Scott Health Care Products
Scott Plaza One
Philadelphia, PA 19113
215-522-5000
800-992-9939

1.1 Skin-caring brief
1.4 Promise flat insert
1.5 Promise contoured insert
1.5 Promise overnight insert
1.8 Tenasorb pocket pad
2.4 Promise mesh brief
2.5 Promise drawsheet
4.2 Promise perineal cleanser

95. Seamless Hospital Products
P.O. Box 828
Wallingford, CT 06492
203-265-7671
800-243-3030

3.5 Teardrop leg bag
3.7 Teardrop urinary drainage bag
5.1 Intermittent catheter

96. Richard C. Shelton Company
P.O. Box 265
Wright Brothers Branch
Dayton, OH 45409
513-253-8662
800-223-5764

4.2 Osto-Zyme cleanser

97. Sherwood Medical
1831 Olive Street
St. Louis, MO 63103
314-241-5700
800-428-4400

1.8 Uri-Drain dribble collector
3.2 Argyle Flo-Rite condom catheter
3.2 Uri-Drain condom catheter
3.5 Argyle urinary leg bag
3.5 Uri-Drain leg bag
3.6 Argyle leg bag straps
3.6 Uri-Drain leg bag straps
5.1 Argyle catheter for intermittent catheterization

98. Sierra Laboratories, Inc.
P.O. Box 27005
Tucson, AZ 85726
602-624-0580

1.8 Uro-Tex male external collector
3.2 Comfort Mate male external catheter

3.3 McGuire urinal
3.5 Reusable latex leg bag

99. Smith & Nephew United, Inc.
11775 Starkey Road
P.O. Box 1970
Largo, FL 34649-1970
813-392-1261
800-553-7638

3.1 Weimer urinal sheath
3.3 Weimer male urinal
3.5 Weimer leg bag
3.6 Leg bag straps
3.7 Bedside drainage bag
4.2 UniWash cleanser with deodorizer
4.2 Triple Care incontinent cleanser
4.3 Odo-Way tablets
4.3 Banish II liquid ostomy deodorant
4.4 UniCare moisturizer
4.4 UniDerm protective moisturizer
4.5 Skin-Prep protective dressing wipe
4.5 Skin-Prep protective liquid barrier
4.5 UniDerm protective moisturizer
4.5 UniSalve protective ointment
5.3 Fecal incontinence bag

100. Spenco Medical Corp.
P.O. Box 2501
Waco, TX 76702
817-772-6000
800-433-3334

2.5 Tendercare drawsheet

101. Stanford Professional Products Corp.
1416 Union Avenue
Pennsauken, NJ 08110
609-665-4054
800-345-3929

1.7 Disposable underpad

102. Star Pioneer Products
2691 Dow Avenue, Suite D
Tustin, CA 92680
714-779-8833

5.4 Restop on-the-go urinal

103. StarChild/Labs.
P.O. Box 404
Aptos, CA 95001-0404
408-662-2659

5.2 SleepDry enuresis alarm

104. Strong Skin Savvy, Inc.
4 Lakeside Drive
New Providence, PA 17560
717-786-8947

4.4 Skin Savvy moisturizing cream
4.5 Skin Savvy barrier cream

105. Sween Corp.
101 Main Street
P.O. Box 980
Lake Crystal, MN 56055
507-726-6200
800-533-0464

4.2 Peri-Wash cleanser
4.2 Peri-Wash II cleanser
4.3 Hex-On deodorizer
4.4 Sween cream
4.41 Micro-Guard
4.5 Peri-Care
4.5 Sween prep barrier film
4.6 Fordustin powder

106. TFX Medical
100 Technology Drive
Alpharetta, GA 30201
404-442-0104
800-241-1926

3.2 Male external catheter
3.5 Leg bag
3.7 Bedside drainage
3.8 Cunningham penile clamp

107. Uncommon Conglomerates, Inc.
287 East 6th Street
St. Paul, MN 55101
612-227-7000
800-323-4545

4.3 Fresh Again deodorant spray

108. UROCARE Products, Inc.
2419 Merced Avenue
South El Monte, CA 91733
818-442-3477
800-423-4441

3.2 Uro-Con condom catheter
3.2 Uro-Cath condom catheter
3.3 Male urinal top
3.4 Uro-Cup female collector
3.5 Reusable latex leg bag
3.5 Uro-Safe vinyl leg bag
3.5 Uro-Kit latex leg bag
3.5 Disposable leg bag system
3.6 Fabric leg straps
3.6 Fitz-All fabric strap
3.6 Velfoam utility strap
3.7 Bedside drainage bag
3.7 Night drainage bottle
4.2 Uro-Wash medicated hygiene wash
4.3 Urolux cleaner and deodorant
5.7 Quick drain valve clamp

109. Van De Weghe Associates, Inc.
477 Colonial Road
Ridgewood, NJ 07450
201-652-7929

3.7 Care-Bag bedside drainage bag cover

110. Viscot Industries, Inc.
P.O. Box 351
32 West Street
East Hanover, NJ 07936
201-887-9273
800-221-0658

5.4 Millie female urinal

111. VPI
127 South Main Street
P.O. Box 266
Spencer, IN 47460
812-829-4891
800-843-4851

3.21 Comfort-Seal inflatable external catheter
3.8 Cook continence cuff
5.1 Firlit-Sugar intermittent catheter

112. Whitestone Products
40 Turner Place
Piscataway, NJ 08854
201-752-2700
800-526-3567

1.1 UltraShield fitted brief
1.2 Ambeze incontinent pant
1.4 MaxiShield flat insert
1.4 MiniGard flat insert
1.7 Non-Skids underpad
1.7 DisposEze underpad
2.4 Maxishield mesh brief

APPENDIX II

SELF-HELP GROUPS, AGENCIES, AND OTHER USEFUL ADDRESSES

American Society on Aging
833 Market Street, Suite 512
San Francisco, CA 94103
415-543-2617

American Uro-Gynecologic Society
c/o John DeLancey, MD
University of Michigan Medical Center
1500 Medical Center Drive
MPB D2230, Box 0718
Ann Arbor, MI 48109

Association of Continence Advisors
c/o Disabled Living Foundation
380-384 Harrow Road
London W9 2HU
England

Association of Rehabilitation Nurses
2506 Gross Point Road
Evanston, IL 60201
312-475-7300

Canadian Paraplegic Association
1500 Don Mills Road, Suite 201
Don Mills, Ontario M3B 3K4
Canada
416-391-0203

Canadian Urodynamic Professionals
Dr. Erik Schick
5415 boul. de l'Assomption
Montreal, Quebec H1T 2M4
Canada
514-376-7702

Canadian Urological Association
Dr. John P. Collins
1053 Carling Avenue, Suite B3
Ottawa, Ontario K1Y 4E9
Canada
613-725-4270

Continence Restored, Inc.
407 Strawberry Hill
Stamford, CT 06905
212-879-3131 (Daytime)
203-348-0601 (Evening)

Disabled Living Foundation
380-384 Harrow Road
London W9 2HU
England

HIP (Help For Incontinent People)
P.O. Box 544
Union, SC 29379
803-579-7900

International Association for Enterostomal Therapy
2081 Business Center Drive
Suite 290
Irvine, CA 92715
714-476-0268

International Continence Society
11 West Graham Street
Glasgow G4 9LF
Scotland
041-332-6061

KIT (Keeping In Touch)
National Kidney Foundation of Texas
13500 Midway Road
Suite 101
Dallas, TX 75244
214-750-1272

National Gerontological Nursing Association
1818 Newton Street, NW
Washington, DC 20010
202-667-6462

National Institute on Aging
National Institutes of Health
Federal Building, Room 6C12
Bethesda, MD 20892
301-496-1752

National Kidney Foundation, Inc.
Two Park Avenue
New York, NY 10016
212-889-2210

National Kidney and Urologic Diseases Information Clearinghouse
P.O. Box NKUDIC
Bethesda, MD 20892
301-468-6345

National Spinal Cord Injury Association
369 Elliot Street
Newton Upper Falls, MA 02164
617-964-0521

Simon Foundation
P.O. Box 815
Wilmette, IL 60091
800-23SIMON

Simon Foundation Canada
P.O. Box 3221
Tecumseh, Ontario N8N 2M4
Canada
800-265-9575

Spina Bifida Association of America
1700 Rockville Pike
Suite 540
Rockville, MD 20852
301-770-SBAA

Spina Bifida Association of Canada
633 Wellington Crescent
Winnipeg, Manitoba R3M OA8
Canada
204-452-7580

Self-Help Books

Burgio KL, Pearce KL, Lucco AJ: *Staying Dry.* Baltimore, MD: Johns Hopkins University Press, 1990.

Chalker R, Whitmore KE: *Overcoming Bladder Disorders.* New York: Harper & Row, in press.

Gartley CB: *Managing Incontinence: A Guide to Living with the Loss of Bladder Control.* Ottawa, IL: Jameson Books, Inc., 1985.

Millard RJ: *Overcoming Urinary Incontinence.* Northamptonshire, England: Thorsons Publishers Ltd., 1987.

Smith PS, Smith LJ: *Continence and Incontinence.* Beckenham, Kent, England: Croom Helm Ltd., 1987.

Appendix III

KIDNEY AND UROLOGIC DISEASE-RELATED ORGANIZATIONS

American Association of Genitourinary Surgeons
c/o Suite 1003
6560 Fannin
Houston, TX 77030
(713) 799-4001
C. Eugene Carlton, Jr., MD, Secretary/Treasurer
Professional society of urologists elected into membership because of their outstanding contributions to urology.

American Association of Kidney Patients (AAKP)
Suite LL1
1 Davis Boulevard
Tampa, FL 33606
(813) 251-0725
Richard B. Baumann, Executive Director
Mission: to serve the needs and interests of kidney patients and their families; founded by kidney patients to help others with kidney failure cope with its physical and emotional impact on their lives.
Publication: *Renalife* (quarterly journal).
Local Groups: 26

American Council on Transplantation (ACT)
Suite 505
700 North Fairfax Street
Alexandria, VA 22314
(703) 836-4301
Nancy Holland, Executive Director
Mission: To promote public awareness about the need for organ and tissue donation; to promote the successes of transplantation.
Publications: *Facts About Organ/Tissue Donation; From Here to Transplant; Exploratory Research Into Attitudes of Target Audiences About Organ and Tissue Donation; Report on Patient and Family Perspectives.*

American Diabetes Association (ADA)
1660 Duke Street
Alexandria, VA 22314
(703) 549-1500 or (800) ADA-DISC
Sheila Mylet, Coordinator, Patient Information
Mission: To improve the search for a prevention and cure for diabetes; to improve the well-being of all people with diabetes and their families.
Publications: *Diabetes; Diabetes Care; Diabetes Spectrum; Clinical Care; Diabetes Forecast.*
Local Groups: 58

From The National Kidney and Urologic Diseases Information Clearinghouse: Bethesda, MD, National Institutes of Health, Publ. No. 89-3052, January, 1989.

American Foundation for Urologic Diseases, Inc. (AFUD)
Suite 401
1120 North Charles Street
Baltimore, MD 21201
(301) 727-1100
David D. Shobe, Executive Director
Mission: To provide fund-raising, fund management, research grants, management, patient and public education, and Government relations.
Publications: Informational brochure of AFUD.

American Kidney Fund (AKF)
Suite 1010
6110 Executive Boulevard
Rockville, MD 20852
(301) 881-3052 or (800) 638-8299
M. Suzanne Popplewell, Information Specialist
Mission: To provide direct financial assistance, comprehensive educational programs, research grants, and community service projects for the benefit of kidney patients.
Publications: *AKF Nephrology Letter: AKF Torchbearer; AKF Newsletter* (for Health Professionals); patient and public education brochures.

American Nephrology Nurses' Association (ANNA)
Box 56
North Woodbury Road
Pitman, NJ 08071
(609) 589-2187
Ron Brady, Executive Director
Mission: To protect the future of quality care through continuing education, research, standards of clinical practice, quality assurance activities, certification, and interdisciplinary communication and cooperation.
Publications: *ANNA Journal; ANNA Update* (bimonthly newsletter); *Core Curriculum for Nephrology Nursing; Standards of Clinical Practice for Nephrology Nursing;* position statements and clinical monographs.
Local Groups: 4 regions, 62 chapters.

American Society of Artificial Internal Organs, Inc. (ASAIO)
National Office
P.O. Box C
Boca Raton, FL 33429
(407) 391-8589
Mrs. Karen K. Burke, Executive Director
Mission: To promote the increase of knowledge about artificial internal organs and of their utilization.
Publications: *ASAIO Transactions* (quarterly peer-reviewed journal); *ASAIO Abstracts* (for annual meeting).

American Society for Histocompatibility and Immunogenetics (ASHI)
Suite 301
211 East 43rd Street
New York, NY 10017
(212) 867-4193
Ellen Gordon
Mission: To provide investigators in the field with a mechanism for education and communication and to influence regulatory efforts; to provide a forum for the exchange of research and clinical data and offer technical workshops at an annual education meeting.
Publications: *Topics in Clinical Histocompatibility Testing, Volumes 1-3; Reports from the Educational Program for the 1978 & 1979 AACHT Meetings; Cellular Immunology, 1983; Paternity Testing, Data Analysis & Management in the Immunogenetics Lab; Third American Histocompatibility Workshop Report of HLA-A, B, C; Serology (Phases I and II) and B-Cell Serology (Phase II); Clinical Histocompatibility Testing, Laboratory Procedures Manual; Laboratory Directory; Human Immunology Journal;* membership directory.

American Society of Nephrology (ASN)
Suite 700
1101 Connecticut Avenue, NW
Washington, DC 20036
(202) 857-1190
Carolyn M. Del Polito, Ph.D.
Mission: To contribute to the education of member nephrologists and to improve the quality of patient care.
Publication: ASN abstract book.

American Society of Pediatric Nephrology (ASPN)
c/o University of Texas Health Science Center
5323 Harry Hines Boulevard
Dallas, TX 75234
(214) 688-3438
Billy S. Arant, Jr., M.D., Secretary/Treasurer
Mission: To promote public and professional educational programs in pediatric nephrology.

American Society of Transplant Physicians
c/o The Wright Organization
716 Lee Street
Des Plaines, IL 60016
(312) 824-5700
Mission: To promote and encourage education and research with respect to transplantation medicine and immunology; to provide a forum for exchange of scientific information; to provide an effective, unified voice in working with other organizations.

American Society of Transplant Surgeons
c/o Arnold Diethelm, M.D.
Department of Surgery
UAB Station
Birmingham, AL 35294
(205) 934-5200
Arnold Diethelm, M.D., President
Mission: To offer accreditation of training programs for transplant surgeons.

American Urological Association (AUA)
1120 North Charles Street
Baltimore, MD 21201
(301) 727-1100
Richard Hannigan, Executive Secretary
Mission: To encourage research, experiments, investigations, and analyses of conditions of the genitourinary tract and their treatments and corrections; to develop scientific methods for the diagnosis, prevention, and treatment of the genitourinary tract; to benefit the general public by encouraging the study of and maintaining the highest possible standards for urological education, practice, and research; to promote the publication of and encourage contributions to medical and scientific literature pertaining to urology.
Publication: *American Journal of Urology.*

American Urological Association Allied, Inc. (AUAA)
6845 Lake Shore Drive
Raytown, MO 64133
(816) 358-3317
Bruce R. Hagen, Executive Director
Mission: To unite urologic allied health professionals to promote the highest quality of urologic education and professional standards for the better and safer care of the urologic patient/client.
Publications: *Urogram Newsletter; Urologic Nursing* (official journal of AUAA); *Standards of Urologic Nursing Practice.*
Local Groups: 32

Continence Restored, Inc.
407 Strawberry Hill
Stamford, CT 06905
(212) 879-3131 (daytime)
(203) 348-0601 (evening)
Anne Smith-Young, President
Mission: To disseminate information on bladder control problems to all interested parties; to establish a network of Continence Restored Support Groups throughout the United States; to provide a resource for the public and professionals; to work with manufacturers who produce incontinence products.

Endourology Society
c/o Department of Urology
Long Island Jewish Medical Centre
New Hyde Park, NY 11024
(718) 470-7221
Arthur D. Smith, MD
Mission: To educate urologists about research and treatment in the management of endourological problems.
Publications: *Journal of Endourology.*

Help for Incontinent People, Inc. (HIP)
P.O. Box 544
Union, SC 29379
(803) 579-7900
Katherine F. Jeter, EdD, ET (Director)
Mission: To function as a clearinghouse of information about incontinence.
Publications: *The HIP Report* (quarterly newsletter); *Resource Guide of Continence Products and Services* (a complete listing of incontinence manufacturers and products).

Impotence Institute of America
119 South Ruth Street
Maryville, TN 37801
(615) 983-6064
Jane Rahe, Communications Director
Mission: To inform and educate the public about impotency and its causes and treatments; to maintain a referral list of urologists who work with impotence.
Publications: *It's Not All In Your Head* (book); *Impotence Worldwise* (newsletter); *Impotence: Help and Hope* (videotape).

International Pediatric Nephrology Association (IPNA)
Albert Einstein College of Medicine
1825 Eastchester Road
Bronx, NY 10461
(212) 904-2857
Ira Greifer, MD, Secretary General
Mission: To promote public and professional education and symposia.
Publication: *Pediatric Nephrology.*

International Society for Peritoneal Dialysis
3800 Reservoir Road, NW.
Washington, DC 20007
(202) 784-3662
James F. Winchester, MD, Secretary/ Treasurer
Mission: To advance knowledge of peritoneal dialysis.
Publication: *Peritoneal Dialysis International.*

Intersociety Council for Research of the Kidney and Urinary Tract
525 East 68th Street, Box 94
New York, NY 10021
(212) 879-7232
E. Darracott Vaughan, Jr., MD
Mission: To develop testimony about kidney and urologic diseases for Congress. Interested in the training of specialists in kidney and urologic diseases.

Interstitial Cystitis Association
East Coast
P.O. Box 1553
Madison Square Station
New York, NY 10159
(212) 983-7620
Debra Slade, East Coast Executive Director

West Coast
P.O. Box 151323
San Diego, CA 92115
(714) 495-6017
Sandi Bois, West Coast Executive Director
Mission: To assist the patients of IC; to educate the medical community about IC; to promote IC research.
Publications: ICA brochure; *ICA Update* (quarterly newsletter); and transcripts of annual meetings.

Interstitial Cystitis Foundation
Suite 210
120 South Spalding Drive
Beverly Hills, CA 90212
(213) 274-6307
Stephanie Rascoe
Mission: To provide education about interstitial cystitis, its management, and research.
Publication: *My Body, My Diet.*

Juvenile Diabetes Foundation International
432 Park Avenue South
New York, NY 10016
(212) 889-7575 or (800) JDF-CURE
Mary Kelly, Public Information Manager
Mission: To support and fund research to find the cause and cure of diabetes and its complications.
Publications: *Countdown* (magazine); patient education pamphlets.

National Association of Nephrology Technologists
c/o Plasma Office Center
234 Hudson Avenue
Albany, NY 12210
(518) 472-1772
Martin Hudson, President
(Dialysis technicians and technologists who emphasize and promote interaction between practitioners and industry).
Publication: Quarterly newsletter.

National Dialysis Association
Suite 840
1050 17th Street, NW
Washington, DC 20036
(202) 785-1197
Phillip Porte, Executive Director
Mission: To represent independent dialysis facilities to the public and the Federal Government.
Publications: *NDA Newsletter.*

National Kidney Foundation, Inc.
30 East 33rd Street
New York, NY 10016
(212) 889-2210 or (800) 622-9010
John Davis, Executive Director
Gigi Politoski, Communications Director
Mission: To seek the total answer to diseases of the kidney and urinary tract through prevention, treatment, and cure.
Publications: *The Kidney; American Journal of Kidney Diseases;* patient and public education materials; *CNSW* (newslettter); *CNSW Perspectives; CRN Quarterly; CNNT Action Update; Kidney '89.*
State Groups: 50
Other Services: Council of Nephrology Nurses and Technicians; Council of Nephrology Social Workers; Council on Clinical Nephrology; Dialysis and Transplantation; Council on Urology.

North American Transplant Coordinators Organization (NATCO)
P.O. Box 15384
Lenexa, KN 66215
(913) 268-9830
Dede Gish Panjada, Executive Director
Mission: To enhance the role of the transplant coordinator; to provide training courses for professionals.
Publications: *NATCO Newsletter.* Patient care brochures.

Peyronie's Society of America, Inc.
P.O. Box 3272
Wichita, KN, 67201
(800) 346-4875
Al Hybsha, Executive Director
Mission: To provide support to patients with Peyronie's disease; to increase patient and public knowledge of the condition; to provide a resource center of information about the disease.

Polycystic Kidney Research Foundation (PKRF)
922 Walnut Street
Kansas City, MO 64106
(816) 421-1869
Jean G. Bacon, Executive Director
Mission: To promote research into the cause and cure of polycystic kidney disease.
Publications: *Polycystic Kidney Disease?; Short History of the PKR Foundation; PKR Progress* (quarterly newsletter); *Your Diet and PKD; First International Workshop Book.*

Psychonephrology Foundation
c/o Westchester County Medical Center
Valhalla, NY 10595
Norman B. Levy, MD, President
Mission: To conduct conferences devoted to psychological issues surrounding patients with kidney failure.
Publications: *Psychonephrology I: Psychological Factors in Hemodialysis and Transplantation; Psychonephrology II: Psychological Problems in Kidney Failure and Their Treatment; Psychonephrology III and IV.*

Renal Physicians Association
Suite 500
1101 Vermont Avenue, NW.
Washington, DC 20005-3457
(202) 898-1562
M. Eileen Widmer, Executive Director
Mission: To ensure optimal care under the highest standards of medical practice for patients with renal disease and related disorders; to act as a national representative for physicians engaged in the study and management of patients with renal disease and related disorders; to serve as a major resource for the development of national health policy concerning renal disease.
Publications: Various publications available at no cost to members. A legal resource directory is presently being prepared, for which there will be a fee.

Simon Foundation
P.O. Box 815
Wilmette, IL 60091
(800) 23-SIMON
Cheryle B. Gartley, President
Canadian Office:
P.O. Box 3221
Tecumseh, Ontario N8N 2M4
Canada
(800) 265-9575
Mission: To remove the stigma from incontinence and provide help to sufferers, their families, and the professional care giver.
Publications: *Informer* (quarterly newsletter); *Managing Incontinence: A Guide to Living With the Loss of Bladder Control.*

Society of Government Service Urologists
720 Riverview Terrace
Annapolis, MD 21401
(301) 224-3610
Mr. H. G. Stevenson, Administrative Assistant
Professional membership organization of government service urologists.

Society for Pediatric Urology
c/o Dr. Richard M. Ehrlich
UCLA Medical Center
10833 Le Conte
Los Angeles, CA 90024
(213) 825-6865
Mission: To advance knowledge of pediatric urology; members have demonstrated interest and significant experience in pediatric urology.

Society of University Urologists
Division of Urology
Hershey Medical Center
Box 850
Hershey, PA 17033
Thomas J. Rohner, Jr., MD, Secretary/Treasurer
Mission: To provide educational and training programs for urologic residents and medical students; to represent organized academic urology.
Publications: Teaching objectives for urology residents

Society of Urologic Oncology
Urology Department
Brigham and Women's Hospital
45 Francis Street
Boston, MA 02115
(617) 732-6325
Jerome P. Richie, MD, Secretary
Mission: Professional society for people with primary interest in the field of urologic oncology.

Transplantation Society
c/o New England Deaconess Hospital
185 Pilgrim Road
Boston, MA 02215
(617) 732-8547
Mary L. Wood
Mission: To further knowledge in transplantation biology and medicine.
Publications: *Transplantation; Transplantation Proceedings.*

United Network for Organ Sharing (UNOS)
P.P. Box 28010
3001 Hungary Spring Road
Richmond, VA 23228
(804) 755-1600
Gene Pierce, Executive Director
Mission: To maintain the recipient registry for all patients in the United States who are waiting for donated organs; to maintain a followup database on transplants.
Publications: *UNOS Update; Transplant Perspective.*

Urodynamics Society
c/o Division of Urology
Hospital of the University of Pennsylvania
5 Silverstein
3400 Spruce Street
Philadelphia, PA 19104
(215) 662-2891
Alan J. Wein, MD
Mission: To act exclusively for charitable, scientific, and educational purposes, particularly in the advancement and dissemination of scientific knowledge in the fields of urology and the dynamics and bioengineering of the genitourinary system and of the application of such knowledge in the diagnosis and treatment of disease; to study all aspects of evaluation and management of voiding dysfunction, including incontinence, outlet obstruction, and other types of bladder and outlet-related abnormalities.
Publications: *Neurology and Urodynamics.*

Single copies of Appendix III may be obtained from the National Kidney and Urologic Diseases Information Clearinghouse, Box NKUDIC, Bethesda, MD 29892, (301) 468-6345.

Index

Note: Page numbers in *italics* refer to illustrations; page numbers followed by t refer to tables.